Critical Care: An Evidence-Based Approach

Critical Care: An Evidence-Based Approach

Editor: Eduardo Raymond

FOSTER ACADEMICS
www.fosteracademics.com

www.fosteracademics.com

FOSTER ACADEMICS

Cataloging-in-Publication Data

Critical care : an evidence-based approach / edited by Eduardo Raymond.
p. cm.
Includes bibliographical references and index.
ISBN 978-1-63242-636-9
1. Critical care medicine. 2. Emergency medicine. 3. Intensive care units.
I. Raymond, Eduardo.
RC86.7 .C75 2019
616.025--dc23

Foster Academics,
118-35 Queens Blvd., Suite 400,
Forest Hills, NY 11375, USA

ISBN 978-1-63242-636-9 (Hardback)

Printed and bound in China.

Contents

Preface

Care meant to support the life of extremely ill patients who are almost on the verge of death is known as critical care. An area in a hospital which is meant to provide intensive treatment medicine to critical patients is known as critical care unit. Trauma, acute respiratory distress syndrome (ARDS), multiple organ failure, and sepsis are some of the common conditions which are treated in a critical care unit. Some of the common equipment present in a critical care unit include equipment for performing hemofiltration, mechanical ventilation equipment, and nasogastric tubes. This book unfolds the innovative aspects of critical care which will be crucial for the progress of this field in the future. The topics included herein are of utmost significance and bound to provide incredible insights to readers. Doctors, experts, and students actively engaged in this field will find this book full of crucial and unexplored concepts.

All of the data presented henceforth, was collaborated in the wake of recent advancements in the field. The aim of this book is to present the diversified developments from across the globe in a comprehensible manner. The opinions expressed in each chapter belong solely to the contributing authors. Their interpretations of the topics are the integral part of this book, which I have carefully compiled for a better understanding of the readers.

At the end, I would like to thank all those who dedicated their time and efforts for the successful completion of this book. I also wish to convey my gratitude towards my friends and family who supported me at every step.

Editor

1

Complete Heart Block and Persistent Lactic Acidosis as an Initial Presentation of Non-Hodgkin Lymphoma in a Critically Ill Newly Diagnosed AIDS Patient

Mohsin Ijaz,[1] Hassan Tariq,[2] Masooma Niazi,[3] and Dmitry Lvovsky[1]

[1] *Division of Pulmonary and Critical Care Medicine, Department of Medicine, Bronx Lebanon Hospital Center, 1650 Selwyn Avenue, Suit No. 12 F, Bronx, NY 10457, USA*
[2] *Department of Medicine, Bronx Lebanon Hospital Center, 1650 Selwyn Avenue, Suit No. 10 C, Bronx, NY 10457, USA*
[3] *Department of Pathology, Bronx Lebanon Hospital Center, 1650 Selwyn Avenue, Suit No. 10 C, Bronx, NY 10457, USA*

Correspondence should be addressed to Mohsin Ijaz; doctor.mohsin@hotmail.com

Academic Editor: Claudius Diez

A 66-year-old male with newly diagnosed untreated acquired immunodeficiency syndrome (AIDS) presented with chronic nonspecific complaints of weakness, fatigue, myalgia, and weight loss. His initial EKG showed complete heart block necessitating temporary pacemaker placement. He had no previous history of cardiac disease. He was also found to have a persistent lactic acidosis and imaging studies showed abdominal lymphadenopathy. The patient underwent biopsy of these lymph nodes and was found to have diffuse large B-cell lymphoma. The hospital course was complicated by respiratory failure requiring mechanical ventilator support and cardiac arrest. Patient remained critically ill; he was not a candidate for chemotherapy and, after a month of hospitalization, he died. Lactic acidosis and heart block as an initial presentation of non-Hodgkin lymphoma in an AIDS patient are an unusual and unique presentation.

1. Introduction

Non-Hodgkin lymphoma (NHL) comprises a diverse group of hematological malignancies. The rate of NHL is estimated to be about 5–20% in human immunodeficiency virus (HIV) infected population, despite the availability of antiretroviral therapy (ART) [1–5]. The clinical presentation range greatly depends upon the subtype of lymphoma and body organ involved and can vary from indolent to very aggressive type. Cardiac infiltration of lymphoma is well recognized and remains asymptomatic in majority of the cases but there are some reports of lymphoma involving the heart presenting with third degree heart block [6–8]. Lactic acidosis is very frequently seen in intensive care unit (ICU) as a cause of anion gap metabolic acidosis and is a significant marker of mortality. Lactic acidosis is associated with a number of clinical entities; however, it is rarely associated with lymphoma, leukemia, and solid organ malignancies. In these conditions the pathogenesis of lactic acidosis remains poorly understood and the management is also a dilemma [9–11].

2. Case Presentation

A 66-year-old male was admitted to the ICU with complaints of chronic weakness, fatigue, myalgia, weight loss, and left flank pain. Comorbidities included hypertension, active smoking, and diabetes mellitus. Patient denied nausea, vomiting, diarrhea, hematemesis, melena, hematochezia, chest pain, or any shortness of breath. He had a recent admission due to community acquired pneumonia and was treated with antibiotics. He denied using any illicit drugs or alcohol abuse. He was retired truck driver by profession.

On examination, he was an elderly man with clinical signs of dehydration. Blood pressure was 155/56 mm Hg, heart rate was 67/min, respiratory rate was 16/min, was afebrile, and his oxygen saturation was 99% on room air. He had mild epigastric tenderness without guarding or rigidity. He had bilateral lower extremities chronic skin changes with scaling. The rest of the physical examination was normal.

Significant laboratory data revealed serum sodium 124 mEq/mL, potassium 5.1 mEq/mL, chloride 89 mEq/mL,

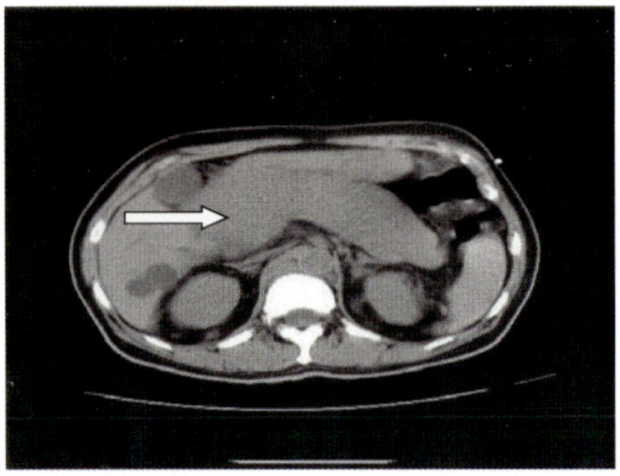

Figure 1: Diffuse enlargement of the pancreas with homogeneous attenuation and without significant peripancreatic inflammation.

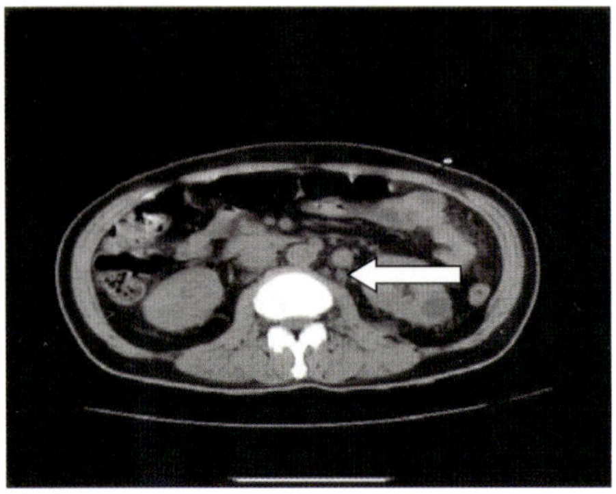

Figure 2: CT of abdomen without contrast showing lymphadenopathy.

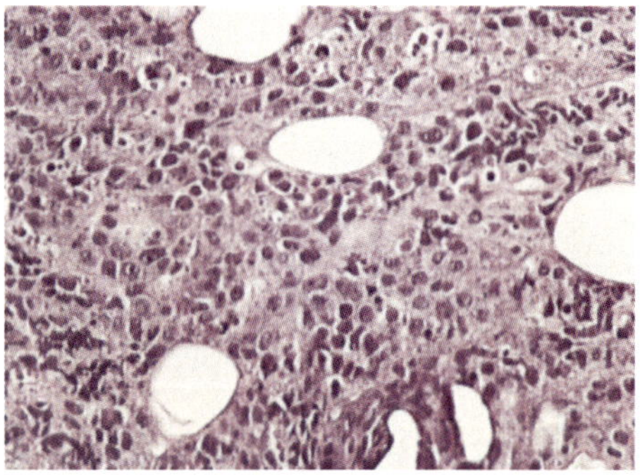

Figure 3: Diffuse large cell lymphoma with atypical lymphocytes, apoptosis, and mitotic figures.

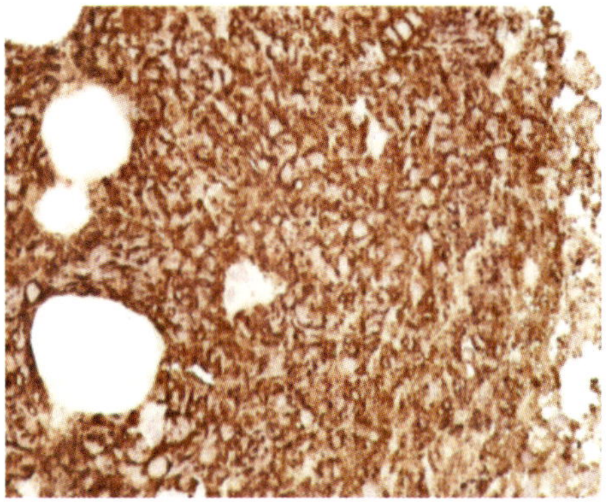

Figure 4: Lymphoma cells are strongly immunoreactive to CD 20.

bicarbonate 15 mEq/mL, blood urea nitrogen 44 mg/dL, creatinine 1.5 mg/dL, glucose 85 mg/dL, calcium 10.3 mg/dL, total protein 7.3 g/dL, and albumin 2.9 g/dL. The rest of the liver function tests were within normal limit. Anemia was with hemoglobin 9.4 g/dL, hematocrit 27%, platelets 558 k/μL, and white blood cells 10.4 k/μL. Arterial blood gas analysis showed pH of 7.36, pCO_2 of 25 mm Hg, pO_2 of 90.3 mm Hg, and oxygen saturation of 97% on room air. There was an anion gap of 20, lactic acid of 4.8 mmoles/L, serum lipase of 1540 U/L, amylase 406 unit/L, gamma GT 25 unit/L, INR 1.3, and lactate dehydrogenase (LDH) 950 unit/L; cancer antigen CA 19-9 was 49.9 μ/mL, TSH was 2.25 mIU/L, serum acetone was negative, and alcohol level was less than 10 mg/dL. His serial cardiac enzymes were negative and he was ruled out for an acute coronary event.

Chest X-ray (CXR) revealed bilateral patchy airspace disease. CT of abdomen and pelvis without contrast showed diffuse enlargement of the pancreas with homogeneous attenuation and without significant peripancreatic inflammation (Figure 1) with extensive retroperitoneal and pelvic adenopathy (Figure 2). A para-aortic lymph node measuring 2.1 cm and retrocaval lymph node measuring 1.6 cm were seen. A soft tissue density surrounding the right common iliac vessels likely representing confluent adenopathy was seen. His echocardiogram showed an ejection fraction of 67%; right ventricle systolic pressure was estimated to be 44 mm Hg. Pericardium was normal without any pericardial effusion. There was no significant valvular abnormality.

Initially, the patients EKG showed 2nd degree Mobitz type I block which later progressed to complete heart block. Patient was given atropine without improvement; hence, a temporary pacemaker was inserted. He was started on IV hydration and IV antibiotics and all his electrolyte abnormalities were corrected. His temporary pacemaker lead came out and it was removed. Subsequently he became unresponsive, was orally intubated, had four cardiac arrests, and was successfully resuscitated. Due to persistent pulmonary infiltrates he underwent fiberoptic bronchoscopy with bronchoalveolar lavage (BAL) and transbronchial biopsies which showed evidence of pneumocystis jiroveci pneumonia (PJP). He was started on Bactrim for the treatment of PJP. He tested positive for HIV and was found to have a CD 4 count of 12/uL.

A temporary pacemaker wire was again placed after ruling out the relevant reversible causes of third degree heart block. A repeat echocardiogram was unchanged from prior one. CT-guided biopsy of the para-aortic lymph nodes was consistent with diffuse large B-cell lymphoma with marked tumor necrosis (Figure 3). Immunoprofile showed that CD 20 (Figure 4), CD 79a, and CD 10 were positive. CD 43, CD 3, CD 7, and BcL were negative. Upper endoscopy for percutaneous endoscopic gastrostomy placement showed gastric polyps which revealed gastric lymphoma on biopsy.

Patient was not a candidate for chemotherapy or ART due to critical condition. Hospital course was complicated by acute respiratory distress syndrome, acute kidney injury, and eventual death a month into his hospital stay.

3. Discussion

NHL is the most common form of lymphoma in patients with HIV/AIDS and it is an AIDS defining condition as well. HIV viremia is thought to play a significant role in the pathogenesis of lymphoma [1]. The incidence of NHL has decreased after the advent of ART, however, it has been reported to be 4 to 23 times higher in HIV infected people as compared to those who are not HIV infected [2, 3]. In a large multicenter cohort study in the United States by Gopal et al., there was an increased risk of death among HIV-infected patients with high viral load and NHL, between six months and five years after diagnosis of lymphoma [4]. Advanced stage of extra nodal large B cell lymphoma can involve the heart as part of distant metastasis in 9–24% of cases in autopsy series [5].

Metastatic tumors of the heart are more common than primary cardiac tumors. Lung, breast, melanoma and lymphomas are the most common primary sites for heart metastasis. In an autopsy study, among various cardiac complications of lymphoma the incidence of atrioventricular (AV) block is reported to be about 12%, out of 33 patients with cardiac lymphoma one patient had first degree AV block, two patients had second degree AV block and one patient had third degree AV block [6]. In the same study, patients with lymphoma dying with cardiac involvement revealed that 16% of patients with Hodgkin's disease, 25% with non-Hodgkin's lymphoma, and 33% of cases of mycosis fungoides had cardiac involvement [6]. There have been about 20 reported cases of patients with lymphomas infiltrating the heart presenting with AV block [7], complete heart block was described in a very few cases [6–8]. Sudden appearance of heart block in a patient with lymphoma and no underlying cardiac disease should lead to a suspicion of cardiac involvement. In general, malignant lymphoma which is initially presenting with cardiac symptoms is rarely diagnosed premortally, and has a poor prognosis [8].

Lactic acidosis is a rare complication of lymphomas and its presence is considered an ominous sign [9]. Patients with lymphoma induced lactic acidosis are often critically ill and it is difficult to conclude whether the etiology of lactic acidosis is completely a result of malignancy and not other potential cause such as sepsis [10, 11]. Lactic acidosis secondary to lymphoma is considered a paraneoplastic syndrome [10]. Proposed mechanisms of pathogenesis include increased glycolytic activity causing an increase in lactic acid generation, overexpression of the glycolytic enzyme hexokinase II or increased IGF-binding protein (IGFBP) activity [9, 11]. In highly aggressive tumors, lactate production increases as the tumor outgrows its blood supply resulting in local hypoxia in the absence of any systemic hypoxia or hypoperfusion. The poor prognosis of lactic acidosis in malignancy can be judged from fact that among 29 published cases of lymphoma with lactic acidosis, 25 eventually died [11, 12].

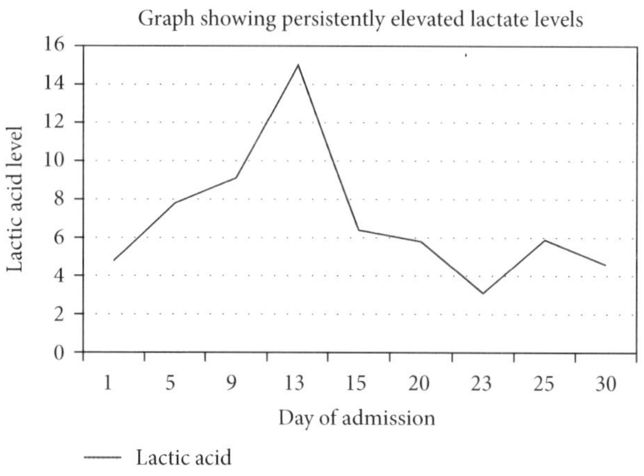

Figure 5: Graph showing persistently elevated lactic acid level.

Several imaging modalities, including echocardiography, cardiac CT, MRI and FDG PET may allow an early diagnosis and can suggest the tumor type. Cytology is diagnostic in two-thirds of cases [13]. If pericardial effusion is present, cytological analysis of pericardial fluid may demonstrate malignant lymphocytes [14]. The prognosis of cardiac involvement in lymphoma remains poor due to diagnostic delay and advanced stage of organ infiltration [13].

Systemic chemotherapy appears to be the only effective therapy for cardiac involvement by malignant lymphomas, and patients may require pacemaker for heart blocks [13]. The cyclophosphamide, adriamycin (doxorubicin), vincristine, prednisone (CHOP) regimen was among the first combinations to produce complete response rates and long-term survivors [13]. Complete AV block may be reversible in some patients with metastatic cardiac lymphoma treated by resection of the heart tumor and sequential combination chemotherapy [15, 16]. The addition of rituximab to the CHOP protocol (R-CHOP) increases the overall survival rate. Whenever a complete AV block caused by an infiltration of lymphoma cells occurs, chemotherapy is considered to be the treatment of choice, as well as the implantation of a pacemaker [13].

Considering no previous cardiac disease or invasive procedure, normal echocardiogram, no use of any nodal blocker medication and the presence of persistent lactic acidosis (Figure 5) our suspicion was that complete heart block was most likely from the lymphoma infiltrating the heart. Nevertheless, patients with advanced HIV disease can have various cardiovascular manifestations like cardiomyopathy, myocarditis, pericarditis, endocarditis, valvular disease, pericardial effusion and pulmonary hypertension [17, 18]. Our patient did not have any clinical or echocardiographic abnormality suggesting HIV related cardiac disease.

To the best of our knowledge this case represents the only case in English literature in which a patient with non-Hodgkin's lymphoma presented with both complete heart block and lactic acidosis which individually are rare presentations of NHL which makes this case very unusual and unique.

Authors' Contribution

All Authors have made contributions to the article and have reviewed it before submission.

References

[1] C. J. Achenbach, A. L. Buchanan, S. R. Cole et al., "HIV viremia and incidence of non-Hodgkin lymphoma in patients successfully treated with antiretroviral therapy," *Clinical Infectious Diseases*, vol. 58, no. 11, pp. 1599–1606, 2014.

[2] P. Patel, D. L. Hanson, P. S. Sullivan et al., "Incidence of types of cancer among HIV-infected persons compared with the general population in the United States, 1992–2003," *Annals of Internal Medicine*, vol. 148, no. 10, pp. 728–736, 2008.

[3] J. Polesel, G. M. Clifford, M. Rickenbach et al., "Non-Hodgkin lymphoma incidence in the Swiss HIV Cohort Study before and after highly active antiretroviral therapy," *AIDS*, vol. 22, no. 2, pp. 301–306, 2008.

[4] S. Gopal, M. R. Patel, E. L. Yanik et al., "Association of early HIV viremia with mortality after HIV-associated lymphoma," *AIDS*, vol. 27, no. 15, pp. 2365–2373, 2013.

[5] L. M. Bush, J. G. Urrutia, E. A. Rodriguez, and M. T. Perez, "AIDS-associated cardiac lymphoma—a review: apropos a case report," *Journal of the International Association of Providers of AIDS Care*, 2014.

[6] W. C. Roberts, D. L. Glancy, and V. T. Devita Jr., "Heart in malignant lymphoma (Hodgkin's disease, lymphosarcoma, reticulum cell sarcoma and mycosis fungoides). A study of 196 autopsy cases," *The American Journal of Cardiology*, vol. 22, no. 1, pp. 85–107, 1968.

[7] S. W. Cho, Y. J. Kang, T. H. Kim et al., "Primary cardiac lymphoma presenting with atrioventricular block," *Korean Circulation Journal*, vol. 40, no. 2, pp. 94–98, 2010.

[8] I. Aleksic, B. Herse, T. Busch, S. Lotfi, H. Sîrbu, and H. Dalichau, "Third degree atrio-ventricular-block caused by malignant non-Hodgkin's lymphoma: an unusual indication for epicardial pacing," *Cardiovascular Surgery*, vol. 7, no. 3, pp. 378–380, 1999.

[9] D. Hoogwerf, J. van Doorn, and E. Maartense, "The insulin-like growth factor-system in a patient with diffuse large B-cell non-Hodgkin's lymphoma and lactic acidosis," *Annals of Clinical Biochemistry*, vol. 50, no. 2, pp. 169–172, 2013.

[10] U. E. Martinez-Outschoorn, D. Whitaker-Menezes, M. Valsecchi et al., "Reverse warburg effect in a patient with aggressive B-cell lymphoma: is lactic acidosis a paraneoplastic syndrome?" *Seminars in Oncology*, vol. 40, no. 4, pp. 403–418, 2013.

[11] F. H. Chan, D. Carl, and L. J. Lyckholm, "Severe lactic acidosis in a patient with B-cell lymphoma: a case report and review of the literature," *Case Reports in Medicine*, vol. 2009, Article ID 534561, 6 pages, 2009.

[12] A. Kumar and V. Raina, " Non- hodgkins lymphoma with lactic acidosis at presentation: a case report of a rare oncologic emergency," *Indian Journal of Medical and Paediatric Oncology*, vol. 35, no. 1, pp. 83–85, 2014.

[13] V. C. Jorge, V. Bernardino, A. C. Araújo et al., "Complete heart block as a complicating feature of a mediastinal lymphoma," *BMJ Case Reports*, Article ID 22605004, 2012.

[14] J. G. Cho, Y. K. Ahn, S. H. Cho et al., "A case of secondary myocardial lymphoma presenting with ventricular tachycardia," *Journal of Korean Medical Science*, vol. 17, no. 4, pp. 549–551, 2002.

[15] T. Matsuo, R. Nishiura, Y. Tsumori et al., "Disappearance of complete atrioventricular block after chemotherapy for malignant lymphoma: a case report," *Journal of Cardiology*, vol. 34, no. 6, pp. 345–349, 1999.

[16] E. Takeuchi, H. Yanagawa, N. Nishikubo, F. Ogushi, and S. Sone, "Successful treatment of metastatic cardiac lymphoma with complete A-V block," *Anticancer Research*, vol. 18, no. 4B, pp. 2815–2817, 1998.

[17] G. Barbarini and G. Barbaro, "Incidence of the involvement of the cardiovascular system in HIV infection," *AIDS*, vol. 17, supplement 1, pp. S46–S50, 2003.

[18] P. Rerkpattanapipat, N. Wongpraparut, L. E. Jacobs, and M. N. Kotler, "Cardiac manifestations of acquired immunodeficiency syndrome," *Archives of Internal Medicine*, vol. 160, no. 5, pp. 602–608, 2000.

2

Dexmedetomidine as a Procedural Sedative for Percutaneous Tracheotomy

Jerrold L. Perrott,[1,2] Michelle T. Co,[3] Steven C. Reynolds,[4,5] and Derek J. R. Gunning[6]

[1] *Departments of Pharmacy and Critical Care, Royal Columbian Hospital, New Westminster, BC, Canada*
[2] *Faculty of Pharmaceutical Sciences, University of British Columbia, Vancouver, BC, Canada*
[3] *Department of Pharmacy, Ridge Meadows Hospital, Maple Ridge, BC, Canada*
[4] *Department of Critical Care, Royal Columbian Hospital, New Westminster, BC, Canada*
[5] *Department of Medicine, University of British Columbia, Vancouver, BC, Canada*
[6] *Departments of Cardiac Surgery and Critical Care, Royal Columbian Hospital, New Westminster, BC, Canada*

Correspondence should be addressed to Jerrold L. Perrott, jerrold.perrott@fraserhealth.ca

Academic Editors: M. Egi, W. J. Ko, and J. Starkopf

Purpose. To describe the successful use of dexmedetomidine as the primary procedural sedative for a percutaneous tracheotomy procedure and to systematically present the supporting literature. *Materials and Methods.* A Case report of our experience and systematic literature search. PubMed, Embase, and Google Scholar were searched without restriction using the key words *dexmedetomidine, percutaneous tracheotomy*, and *tracheotomy procedure.* All relevant published references were retrieved irrespective of their methodological quality. *Results.* In total, only 3 relevant references were found. These include one small placebo controlled randomized trial and 2 case reports. The randomized, placebo controlled trial enrolled patients already sedated on midazolam and included 64 total patients. The 2 other case reports both described the use of dexmedetomidine as the primary procedural sedative. All of the cases reported the successful completion of the percutaneous tracheotomy without any major complication, but none reported the subjective patient experience. *Conclusion.* Based on the available published literature and our experience, we suggest that dexmedetomidine be considered for use as the primary procedural sedative for percutaneous tracheotomy procedure. Dexmedetomidine's ability to provide adequate sedation and amnesia, without blunting the respiratory drive and protective reflexes of the patient, may make it an optimal agent in specific cases.

1. Introduction

Dexmedetomidine is a centrally acting alpha-2 agonist with licensed indications for an intensive care unit sedation and a conscious sedation for Monitored Anaesthesia Care and Awake Fiberoptic Intubation. Its pharmacology is such that it provides sedative, analgesic, and antishivering effects without attenuating respiratory drive and provides a state of "cooperative sedation" whereby the patient is sedated, but still able to interact with the healthcare team [1]. The primary adverse effects observed with the procedural use are bradycardia and hypotension [1]. Other agents for procedural sedation, such as benzodiazepines and propofol, can induce significant respiratory depression and loss of protective airway reflexes, making them suboptimal in certain clinical scenarios.

The properties of dexmedetomidine make it a viable option for procedural sedation when it is vital to maintain the respiratory drive of the patient. We present a case of a percutaneous tracheotomy performed under sedation with dexmedetomidine and fentanyl with lidocaine for local anaesthesia and a systematic literature review of the evidence supporting this indication.

2. Case Report

An 83-year-old male, who weighed 67 kg and was 170 cm tall, presented to our hospital in the spring of 2012 with a non-ST elevation myocardial infarction and congestive heart failure. He was referred for coronary artery bypass grafting (CABG) by the interventional cardiology after an angiogram demonstrated coronary disease not amenable to percutaneous intervention. Specifically, he had a significant triple-vessel disease which had progressed in the context of two previous angiograms with the placement of coronary stents in 1997 and 2000.

His past medical history included hypertension, dyslipidemia, a remote history of smoking, and of note, an episode of aspiration (of a carrot) at age 2 years that required a tracheostomy. Subsequent to his tracheostomy, multiple airway surgeries were completed over the following 8 years that resulted in significant supra and subglottic airway stenosis, as demonstrated on bronchoscopy approximately 10–15 years ago. As this stenosis did not impair his exercise tolerance, he elected to not pursue any corrective measures at that time.

Due to his airway concerns, anaesthesiology took special precautions in attempting to intubate the patient for his coronary artery bypass grafting. Despite multiple complex manoeuvres and the assistance of multiple airway experts, oral endotracheal intubation was unsuccessful and the process was abandoned. He was admitted to our intensive care unit awake and alert for observation on oxygen via nasal prongs at 3 L/min, with saturations of 99%.

After discussions between the cardiac surgery, interventional cardiology, anaesthesiology, and critical care teams and with consent from the patient, it was decided that an awake percutaneous tracheotomy would the best option to facilitate progression to CABG.

Owing to the complex airway issues, this was deemed a high risk procedure leading to the careful selection of the procedural sedation. Typical agents such as benzodiazepines and neuromuscular blocking agents were deemed unsuitable as they would impair the patient's respiratory drive and protective reflexes, especially in the event of an unsuccessful procedure. The pharmacological characteristics of dexmedetomidine were felt to provide the optimal effects to safely perform the percutaneous tracheotomy with the least risk. Specific aspects of dexmedetomidine that made it an excellent fit for this procedure were the sedative, amnestic, and opiate sparing effects, with the maintenance of respiratory drive and protective airway reflexes.

After confirming consent, the patient was prepared for tracheotomy. Preoxygenation was undertaken by administering 100% oxygen via face mask. Viscous lidocaine was applied topically to patient's tongue to reduce discomfort and gagging and upper airway topical anesthesia was obtained with atomized 2% lidocaine. A loading dose of dexmedetomidine 1 mcg/kg was infused intravenously (IV) over 20 minutes, followed by a maintenance infusion at a rate of 0.5 mcg/kg/hour. The prolonged loading time was used to reduce the likelihood of adverse cardiac effects developing. A bolus of 25 mcg of fentanyl IV was also administered. At this point, the patient was well sedated, but rousable to voice or physical stimulation, and was maintaining his airway and breathing spontaneously.

Upon the completion of the loading dose, the patient was put in the supine position with neck extension supported by a bolster under the upper torso. The larynx and previous tracheostomy sites were identified. A video bronchoscope was inserted into the airway and positioned immediately below the larynx. At this point, the patient was noted to be uncomfortable and coughing, so the maintenance infusion of dexmedetomidine was increased to 0.8 mcg/kg/hr, and an additional 25 mcg of IV fentanyl was administered.

The position of the bronchoscope was confirmed with the transillumination of the airway and with the manipulation of the trachea. The anterior neck was prepared with chlorhexidine/alcohol solution. A site was chosen in the midline in the previous tracheostomy scar well above the manubrium and 1-2 cm below the cricoid cartilage (approximating the 3rd tracheal ring which was not clearly identifiable). The Ciaglia Blue Rhino percutaneous tracheostomy set was used. This entailed airway access with a 16-gauge needle, introduction of a J tipped guide wire via the needle, serial dilation of the tract, and insertion of a no. 6 Shiley cuffed tracheostomy tube loaded on the tracheostomy loading catheter. Bronchoscopic guidance was maintained throughout each step. The bronchoscope was then inserted into the airway via the tracheostomy tube confirming its position. Following the insertion of the tracheostomy tube, the cuff was inflated, the inner cannula was inserted, and ventilation was initiated. Adequate oxygenation and carbon dioxide clearance were confirmed. The tube was secured in place with two 0 silk sutures and tracheostomy ties. Finally, the patient was allowed to emerge from sedation.

The patient's hemodynamic measurements were monitored continuously throughout the procedure and are presented in Table 1. As expected a small degree of hypotension and bradycardia evolved and were easily managed with an IV infusion of norepinephrine. There were no episodes of oxygen desaturation.

A few hours after the procedure, once he was fully recovered from the sedation, the patient reported that he did not recall the procedure, nor recall or feel any discomfort. He was very pleased with the whole procedure and was looking forward to having his coronary artery bypass grafting performed. When approached four days after his tracheotomy, he did not recall having had a conversation with the authors on the day of his procedure.

Two weeks following the insertion of the tracheostomy, when operating room time was next available, the patient underwent coronary artery bypass via lower hemisternotomy. This access was chosen to maintain the separation of the tracheostomy and sternotomy incisions. The perioperative course was uncomplicated. The patient was discharged home with plans for urgent otolaryngology followup for the management of his supraglottic stenosis.

3. Materials and Methods

The Fraser Health Authority Research and Ethics Board considers a case report to be a medical/educational activity and therefore, Fraser Health researchers are not required to obtain ethics approval for such publications as long as a written, informed consent is obtained from the patient, as was done in this case.

Table 1: Vital signs and infusions during tracheotomy procedure.

Time	HR	SBP	DBP	MAP	Dex. dose	NE dose	Comments
10:40	55	155	50	85	3	0	Dexmedetomidine load started
10:45	50	145	50	81	3	0	
10:50	55	115	45	68	3	2	
10:55	50	115	45	68	3	2	Dexmedetomidine load completed
11:00	50	135	50	78	0.5	2	Bronchoscope inserted
11:05	55	115	45	68	0.8	2	
11:10	50	130	55	80	0.8	0	
11:12	70	155	70	98	0	0	Procedure completed

DBP: diastolic blood pressure (mmHg); Dex. dose: dexmedetomidine infusion rate (mcg/kg/hr); HR: heart rate (beats per minute); MAP: mean arterial pressure (mmHg); NE dose: norepinephrine infusion rate (mcg/min); SBP: systolic blood pressure (mmHg).

For the literature search, PubMed, Embase, and Google Scholar were systematically searched up to May 1st, 2012 without restrictions using the terms *dexmedetomidine, percutaneous tracheotomy,* and *tracheotomy procedure*. Titles and abstracts were screened by 1 author (J. L. Perrott) and relevant full text articles were obtained. Only articles describing the use of dexmedetomidine as sedation for tracheotomy procedures, but not other airway surgical interventions or manoeuvres, were included.

4. Results

Three articles [2–4] were found to evaluate or describe the use of dexmedetomidine for a procedural sedation for a percutaneous tracheostomy.

Alhashemi et al. [2] reported in abstract only the results of a small randomized placebo controlled trial. They enrolled 64 intensive care unit patients already on the intermittent midazolam sedation to either a dexmedetomidine 1 mcg/kg or saline-placebo IV bolus over 10 minutes in addition to fentanyl 1 mcg/kg IV bolus just prior to skin incision. Their primary outcome was the amount of rescue propofol bolus needed during the procedure. They demonstrated no significant differences between the dexmedetomidine and placebo groups (median 40 mg versus 45 mg, $P = 0.7$). Their only positive secondary outcome was the median time to complete the tracheotomy procedure (dexmedetomidine 7 minutes versus placebo 10 minutes, $P = 0.04$). No details of the patients' experiences of the procedures were published.

David and de Marchi [3] reported a successful awake surgical tracheostomy procedure done in a 44-year-old woman with significant neck, upper airway, and facial swelling due to local after resection and chemoradiation therapy for a metastatic tonsillar squamous cell carcinoma. She received a loading dose of dexmedetomidine of 0.5 mcg/kg IV over 10 minutes followed by an IV infusion which was titrated from 0.2 mcg/kg/hour to 0.7 mcg/kg/hour for the procedure. They also administered a local anaesthetic with lidocaine 1% and a supplemental propofol 20 mg IV bolus for sedation during the initial airway instrumentation. Their patient had one episode of transient desaturation (down to an S_aO_2 of 86%), but no other complications were noted. They did not report any details of the patient's subjective experience.

Finally, Kunisawa et al. [4] reported a successful percutaneous tracheotomy procedure completed in a ninety-year-old 44 kg male who was one week after the evacuation of an intracranial hematoma. Clinically he had a persistently decreased level of consciousness and left hemiplegia. He was administered a dexmedetomidine 1 mcg/kg IV loading dose over 10 minutes, followed by an infusion of 0.7 mcg/kg/hour. Local anaesthesia with 1% lidocaine was also administered. They reported no complications during their procedure and did not report details of the patient's subjective experience.

5. Discussion

We present a case where dexmedetomidine was used successfully for a percutaneous tracheotomy in an 83-year-old male with a history of sub- and supraglottic airway stenosis. Adequate procedural sedation was maintained for completion of the procedure and for patient comfort and amnesia. The protracted period of amnesia after the full recovery of the level of consciousness was unexpected and should be examined in future studies to better characterize its total duration.

The literature reported on this topic is sparse and of overall low methodological quality [5]. The only randomized controlled trial was completed in patients already sedated with midazolam, whereas the case reports are more similar to the patient we present. Ideally, a controlled trial would be conducted to better define the place of dexmedetomidine for use as the primary procedural sedative for percutaneous tracheotomy procedures; however, this is unlikely to be completed. Future publication of further observational cases and data would, at the least, serve to better support this use for dexmedetomidine.

6. Conclusions

Dexmedetomidine in conjunction with small bolus dose narcotic provides adequate procedural sedation to complete percutaneous tracheotomy procedures without inhibiting the patient's protective airway reflexes or respiratory drive. The hemodynamic effects that can occur with dexmedetomidine can be easily managed with the judicious administration of vasopressors. Dexmedetomidine may induce an amnestic response, both during and for a number of hours after the infusion.

Based on our experience and the published literature of other similar cases, we recommend considering dexmedetomidine as the primary sedative for use during percutaneous tracheotomy procedures in patients for whom other agents are inappropriate or of a higher risk, though future research on this topic is necessary to fully characterize the efficacy and safety of dexmedetomidine for this use.

We suggest that dexmedetomidine be dosed following the manufacturers recommended administration for "Awake Fiberoptic Intubation" [6] with a loading dose of 0.5–1 mcg/kg IV over 10 minutes (with the lower dose used for elderly patients) followed by an infusion of 0.2–1 mcg/kg/hour IV, starting at 0.6 mcg/kg/hour. Careful monitoring of the vital signs and level of consciousness should be undertaken throughout the induction, maintenance, and recovery phase of the procedure.

Disclaimer

No funding was used for this paper. The authors report no relevant conflict of interests. None of this paper or any portion thereof has previously been presented or published.

References

[1] A. T. Gerlach and J. F. Dasta, "Dexmedetomidine: an updated review," *Annals of Pharmacotherapy*, vol. 41, no. 2, pp. 245–254, 2007.

[2] J. A. Alhashemi, Q. A. Alotaibi, G. M. Abdullah, H. M. Algethamy, and S. Shalaby, "Dexmedetomidine sedation for percutaneous tracheostomy in the intensive care unit: 536," *Critical Care Medicine*, vol. 34, supplement 12, p. A149, 2006.

[3] M. D. David and L. de Marchi, "Dexmedetomidine sedation for awake tracheotomy: case report and literature review," *Journal of Clinical Anesthesia*, vol. 22, no. 5, pp. 360–362, 2010.

[4] T. Kunisawa, S. Hanada, A. Kurosawa, and H. Iwasaki, "Tracheostomy in which dexmedetomidine alone was safely used in a high-risk elderly patient," *The Internet Journal of Anesthesiology*, vol. 29, no. 1, 2011.

[5] J. Howick, I. Chalmers, P. Glasziou et al., "The Oxford 2011 levels of evidence," Oxford Centre for Evidence-Based Medicine, 2012, http://www.cebm.net/index.aspx?o=5653 .

[6] *Product Monograph: Precedex—Dexmedetomidine Hydrochloride for Injection*, Hospira Healthcare Corporation, Quebec, Canada, 2009.

Boerhaave Syndrome, Pneumothorax, and Chylothorax in a Critically Ill Patient with Tuberous Sclerosis Complex

Mohsin Ijaz,[1] Arsalan Rafiq,[2] Sindhaghatta Venkatram,[3] and Gilda Diaz-Fuentes[3]

[1]*Division of Critical Care Medicine, Montefiore Medical Center, Albert Einstein College of Medicine, Bronx, NY 10467, USA*
[2]*Division of Cardiology, Mount Sinai St. Luke's Hospital, New York, NY 10025, USA*
[3]*Division of Pulmonary and Critical Care Medicine, Bronx-Lebanon Hospital Center, Bronx, NY 10457, USA*

Correspondence should be addressed to Mohsin Ijaz; doctor.mohsin@hotmail.com

Academic Editor: Nicolas Nin

Tuberous sclerosis complex (TSC) is an autosomal dominant, variably expressed multisystem disease. The predominant pulmonary features of TSC are identical to those of lymphangioleiomyomatosis (LAM). Pneumothorax, multifocal micronodular pneumocyte hyperplasia, and chylothorax are rare complications of TSC. We report a young male with pneumothorax, lung nodules, and chylous effusion who developed empyema thoracis after esophageal rupture. Hospital course was complicated by respiratory failure. Family opted to transfer to hospice care. Chylothorax is a rare complication of TSC with few scattered reports mostly in female patients. Patients with TSC are usually managed by multispecialists and it is important to be aware of the rare pulmonary manifestations of this disease. A male patient with TSC having lung nodules presenting with chylothorax and empyema thoracis from Boerhaave syndrome makes our case unique.

1. Introduction

Tuberous sclerosis complex (TSC) is a rare autosomal dominant, multisystem disorder that usually involves brain, heart, skin, eyes, lungs, liver, and kidneys [1]. Genes involved are TSC1 and TSC2 which encode hamartin and tuberin, respectively. Tuberous sclerosis complex was first described in 1862 by Von Recklinghausen [2]. This complex is involved in the inhibition of the mammalian-target-of-Rapamycin (mTOR) pathway which is involved in the control of cell proliferation and growth. Pulmonary manifestations of TSC include pulmonary cysts, multifocal micronodular pneumocytes (MMPH), and lymphangioleiomyomatosis (LAM) [3]. Chylothorax is the accumulation of chyle or lymph from the thoracic duct in the pleural space. This lymphocyte-predominant fluid can accumulate in the pleural space due to leakage from the thoracic duct [4]. Chylothorax can be seen in patients with pulmonary complications of tuberous sclerosis.

2. Case Discussion

A 21-year-old male patient was admitted to the intensive care unit with persistent vomiting of four days' duration, associated with progressive dyspnea, dry cough, and loss of appetite. As per the family, there was no history of fever, abdominal pain, dysuria, palpitations, chest pain, or any other associated complaints. There was no history of sick contacts or recent travel and he was up-to-date with immunizations. Medical history was significant for tuberous sclerosis with retinal hamartomas, renal mass, mental retardation, complex partial epilepsy, quadriparesis, severe kyphoscoliosis, iron deficiency anemia, reflux esophagitis with esophageal ulcers, chronic gastritis, and multiple pulmonary nodules.

His home medications included acetaminophen, carbamazepine, ferrous sulphate, folic acid, oral cyanocobalamin, ascorbic acid, multivitamins, omeprazole, and short acting bronchodilators. Patient was born in Dominican Republic and moved to USA at the age of 15; he has been wheelchair-bound since birth. He was born with normal spontaneous vaginal delivery but required oxygen supplementation for one week after birth. He had recurrent seizures since he was an infant. He had 3 siblings; elder brother also suffers from recurrent seizures.

On examination, the patient was hypoxic (oxygen saturation of 88% on ambient air which improved to 92% on 2

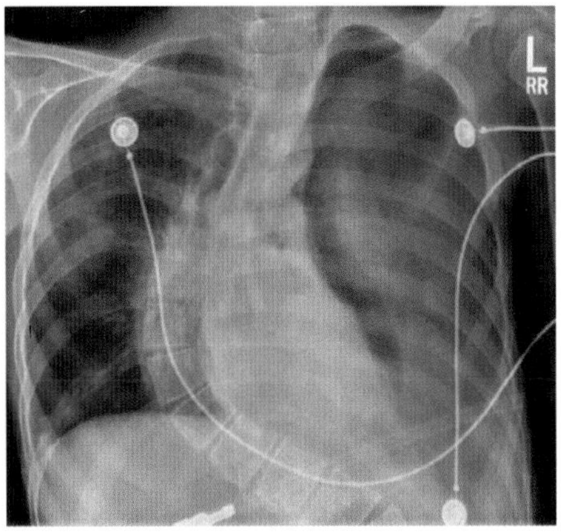

(a)

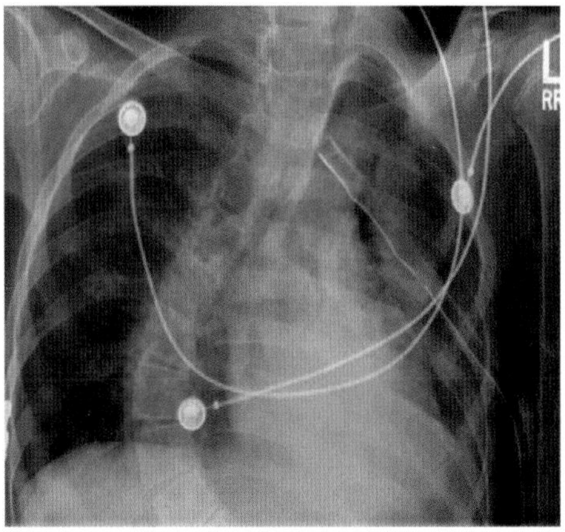

(b)

FIGURE 1: CXR showing (a) left side pneumothorax and pleural effusion. (b) Expansion of the left lung, chest tube, and left sided effusion.

liters oxygen), tachycardic (heart rate of 120/min), tachypneic (respiratory rate of 30/min), and hypotensive (blood pressure of 80/60 mmHg). Other findings on physical examination included decreased air entry on the left hemithorax, quadriparesis, and slow mentation. Chest X-ray (CXR) revealed large left hydropneumothorax (Figure 1(a)). A chest tube was inserted with 500 mL of purulent, brownish-green fluid drained; followup CXR showed expanded lung with residual pneumothorax (Figure 1(b)). Patient was treated for severe sepsis. Initial pleural fluid was exudative, neutrophilic with negative cytology for malignant cells (Table 1). A chest computerized tomography (CT) showed left pneumothorax with chest tube and multiple small nodules in right lung (Figure 2(a), lung window). There was no evidence of mediastinal air (Figure 2(b)). Subsequent pleural fluid drainage was noted to be milky and confirmed to be chylothorax with triglyceride level of 1041 mg/dL. Subcutaneous octreotide and medium chain triglycerides infusion were started and patient was started on orogastric tube feeding. Cultures from pleural fluid grew heavy growth of *Candida albicans* and Methicillin sensitive *Staphylococcus aureus* confirming the effusion to be empyema thoracis. Fluconazole and nafcillin were initiated and initial antibiotics (vancomycin and cefepime) were discontinued. Pleural fluid drainage remained elevated with daily output of 1.5–2 liters of chylous fluid/day despite octreotide.

A repeat chest CT scan with contrast 12 days later from the first CT scan revealed increasing left hydropneumothorax. Direct communication between the esophagus and left pleural space was seen, highly suggestive of esophageal tear (Figures 3 and 4). Repeat pleural fluid analysis showed amylase level of 12238 U/L also suggestive of esophageal tear.

Surgical intervention for management of the esophageal tear with possible repair of the thoracic duct was discussed with family who opted for conservative management and hospice care where he later died. We hypothesize that our patient initially presented with pneumothorax and empyema in the background of TSC related lung nodules. Chylothorax was probably related to a combination of lung disease and esophageal tear due to chronic esophagitis and esophageal ulcers.

TABLE 1: Description of pleural fluid analysis.

Pleural fluid	Day 1	Day 5	Day 20
pH	7.15		
Protein g/dL	3	2.1	
LDH U/L	5656	3628	
Glucose mg/dL	4	247	116
WBC	174000		
RBC	300		
Neutrophils %	96		
Lymphocytes %	4		
Cholesterol mL	—	15	
Triglycerides meq/L	—	1041	11
Amylase U/L	—		12238
Serum			
Protein g/dL	5.1	5.3	
LDH U/L	206		

3. Discussion

TSC is characterized by mental retardation, seizures, and cutaneous angiofibromas (Vogt's triad). Diagnosis is made when two major features, or one major and two minor features, are present [1]. Other manifestations include the most common renal angiomyolipomas (80% cases), isolated renal cysts, autosomal dominant polycystic kidney disease, and renal cell carcinoma. Retinal hamartomas and cardiac rhabdomyomas have been described in up to 50% of cases [1].

The pulmonary involvement in TSC is rare, seen in less than 1%, and is secondary to occlusion of the bronchus, vascular, and lymphatics by immature smooth muscle cells [5]. The three main pulmonary lesions found in TSC are

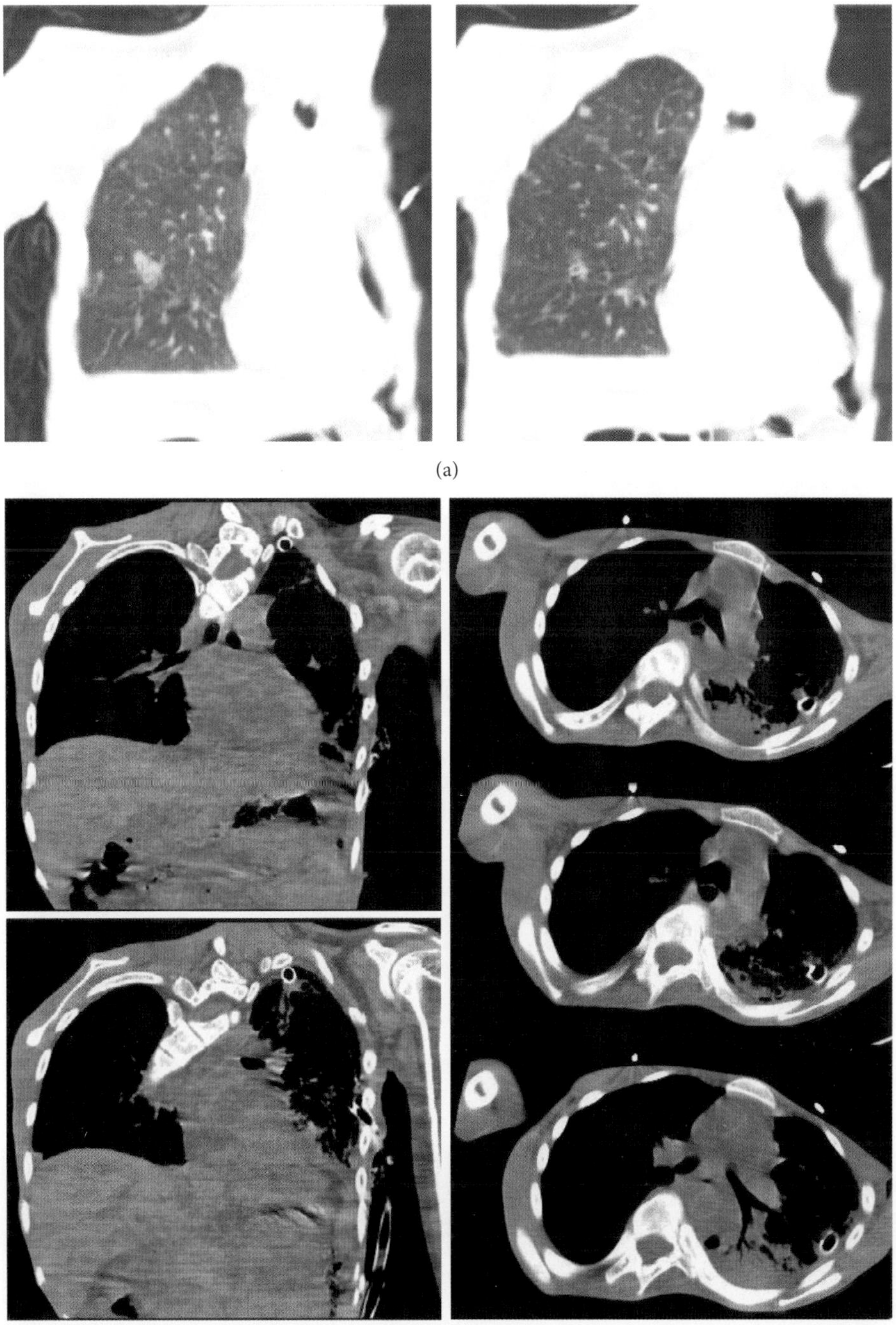

(a)

(b)

FIGURE 2: (a) Chest CT different cuts from lung showing right side multiple small nodules. (b) Mediastinal window showing no signs of air in the mediastinum.

LAM, MMPH, and clear cell tumor of the lung, with LAM being the most common. Average age of onset of pulmonary manifestation is 32 to 34 years of age and manifests mainly in women with TSC [6].

Dyspnea with mild exertion, spontaneous pneumothorax, or cough can be the first symptoms of lung involvement in patients with TSC. Progression to pulmonary failure usually does not occur until the third or fourth decade of life with some patients requiring lung transplantation. Clinical, radiological, and pathological manifestations of lung involvement in tuberous sclerosis and LAM are indistinguishable [7]. Radiological features include pneumothoraces, pleural effusion, ground glass opacification, and nodules [5].

Effort related esophageal perforation is usually called Boerhaave syndrome and is associated with high morbidity and mortality. In a study, spontaneous rupture of esophagus due to barotrauma resulting from increase in intraesophageal pressure due to vomiting represented 8 to 56% of all

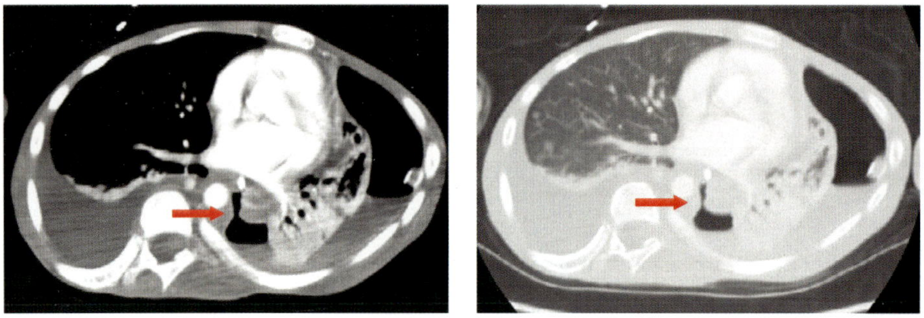

(a) (b)

Figure 3: Chest CT with wide window width: (a) mediastinal window, (b) lung window showing esophageal tear and communication with pleura (red arrow).

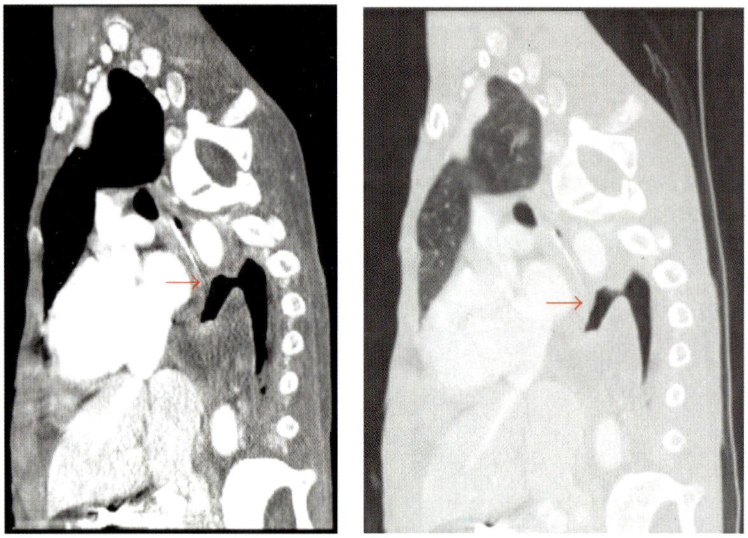

(a) (b)

Figure 4: Chest CT: (a) mediastinal window, (b) lung window. Sagittal view showing esophageal tear and communication with pleura (red arrow).

esophageal perforations [8]. The overall reported mortality of esophageal perforations is close to 20%. The intrathoracic rupture of esophagus can involve the overlying pleura due to inflammation and can cause a direct communication between the esophagus and the pleural cavity resulting in pleural effusions [8]. Management options include medical management and endoscopic or surgical repair.

The pleural fluid analysis in our patient also showed evidence of chylothorax, which is an uncommon condition resulting from either traumatic or nontraumatic damage of the thoracic duct. Trauma to the thoracic duct due to penetrating injuries, hyperextension of spine, and complications of surgeries involving the left side of neck, esophagus, and other cardiothoracic surgeries has been reported. These leaks usually heal spontaneously within 10–14 days [4, 9]. Nontraumatic chylothorax has been reported in association with malignancies, particularly lymphomas. Rare causes include subclavian vein thrombosis, filariasis, and thoracic duct tumors. The incidence of chylothorax in patients with LAM is as high as 75% [10]. The mechanism of formation of chylothorax in TSC is not well understood; proposed mechanisms include chyle leak, general oozing from pleural lymphatics or central vessels, and transdiaphragmatic flow of chylous ascites [11].

Pathological lung findings in patients with TSC are similar to LAM and include multiple air-filled small cysts comprised of bundles of smooth muscles with angiomatous new formation. Adenomatoid epithelial proliferation is a characteristic feature. Other findings include MMPH which is considered the second major form of pulmonary involvement in patients with TSC after LAM. MMPH represents benign overexpression of type II pneumocytes along with alveolar septa that reveal fibrous thickening, increase in elastic fibers, and aggregates of alveolar macrophages.

MMPH has an unclear prognosis and is very unlikely to have malignant progression, so management is conservative [12].

Management of pulmonary complications of TSC represents a challenge; due to the rarity of the condition, there are no established guidelines. Conservative management of chylothorax is indicated with avoidance of hypoproteinemia and electrolyte imbalance and monitoring for superimposed sepsis [13]. Success rate of conservative management is 16–75% [14]. Other modalities to reduce lymph flow include use of somatostatin or its analog octreotide. Response is assessed by a decrease in the output drain to around half within 48 hours as there are no prospective studies to guide evidence-based management [14]. Surgical interventions are indicated if other measures fail, and they include ligation of the thoracic duct, pleurectomy, pleurodesis, and pleuroperitoneal shunt [15]. Promising is the discovery of upregulation of the mTOR pathway in tumors associated with TSC and the use of mTOR inhibitors like sirolimus or analogs in the management of TSC [16].

Our patient developed sepsis secondary to empyema thoracis. The cause of empyema was initially unrecognized as the initial chest CT scan did not reveal evidence of esophageal rupture, which was found in the subsequent scan. We were not able to find any association between esophageal rupture and empyema thoracis in patients with tuberous sclerosis, as per our search of English literature. Our patient presented with persistent nausea and vomiting, likely leading to esophageal rupture and subsequent development of empyema thoracis causing patient's demise. Unfortunately, family opted for hospice care and no further evaluation or treatment was done.

4. Conclusions

Patients with TSC and pulmonary manifestations represent a diagnostic and management challenge with an overall poor prognosis. A male patient with TSC having lung nodules (likely MMPH) presenting with chylothorax and empyema thoracis from Boerhaave syndrome constitutes an extremely rare presentation and has not been reported before. ICU physicians caring for TSC patients should be aware of this presentation and consider a multidisciplinary approach towards early diagnosis and management in order to improve the overall grim prognosis.

Abbreviations

TSC: Tuberous sclerosis complex
mTOR: Mammalian-target-of-Rapamycin
LAM: Lymphangioleiomyomatosis
CT: Computerized tomography
MMPH: Multifocal micronodular pneumocyte hyperplasia.

Disclosure

None of the authors has a financial relationship with a commercial entity that has an interest in the subject of the paper. No financial support was used for this case report.

Authors' Contribution

Mohsin Ijaz treated the patient, searched the literature, and conceived and wrote the paper. Arsalan Rafiq searched the literature and wrote the paper. Gilda Diaz-Fuentes revised and edited the final paper for important intellectual content. Sindhaghatta Venkatram supervised the patient treatment and critically revised and edited the paper. All authors gave final approval of the paper to be published. All authors have made significant contributions to the paper and have reviewed it before submission. All authors have confirmed that the paper is not under consideration for review at any other journal. All authors have read and approved the final paper.

References

[1] P. B. Crino, K. L. Nathanson, and E. P. Henske, "The tuberous sclerosis complex," *The New England Journal of Medicine*, vol. 355, no. 13, pp. 1345–1356, 2006.

[2] H. Northrup and D. A. Krueger, "Tuberous sclerosis complex diagnostic criteria update: recommendations of the 2012 International Tuberous Sclerosis Complex Consensus Conference," *Pediatric Neurology*, vol. 49, no. 4, pp. 243–254, 2013.

[3] M. Castro, C. W. Shepherd, M. R. Gomez, J. T. Lie, and J. H. Ryu, "Pulmonary tuberous sclerosis," *Chest*, vol. 107, no. 1, pp. 189–195, 1995.

[4] V. Agrawal, P. Doelken, and S. A. Sahn, "Pleural fluid analysis in chylous pleural effusion," *Chest*, vol. 133, no. 6, pp. 1436–1441, 2008.

[5] M. E. A. P. M. Adriaensen, C. M. Schaefer-Prokop, D. A. C. Duyndam, B. A. Zonnenberg, and M. Prokop, "Radiological evidence of lymphangioleiomyomatosis in female and male patients with tuberous sclerosis complex," *Clinical Radiology*, vol. 66, no. 7, pp. 625–628, 2011.

[6] L. C. Costello, T. E. Hartman, and J. H. Ryu, "High frequency of pulmonary lymphangioleiomyomatosis in women with tuberous sclerosis complex," *Mayo Clinic Proceedings*, vol. 75, no. 6, pp. 591–594, 2000.

[7] V. Foresti, O. Casati, R. Zubani, and A. Villa, "Chylous pleural effusion in tuberous sclerosis," *Respiration*, vol. 57, no. 6, pp. 398–401, 1990.

[8] M. Chirica, A. Champault, X. Dray et al., "Esophageal perforations," *Journal of Visceral Surgery*, vol. 147, no. 3, pp. e117–e128, 2010.

[9] C. H. Doerr, D. L. Miller, and J. H. Ryu, "Chylothorax," *Seminars in Respiratory and Critical Care Medicine*, vol. 22, no. 6, pp. 617–626, 2001.

[10] A. J. Fairfax, W. R. McNabb, and S. G. Spiro, "Chylothorax: a review of 18 cases," *Thorax*, vol. 41, no. 11, pp. 880–885, 1986.

[11] J. H. Ryu, C. H. Doerr, S. D. Fisher, E. J. Olson, and S. A. Sahn, "Chylothorax in lymphangioleiomyomatosis," *Chest*, vol. 123, no. 2, pp. 623–627, 2003.

[12] H. Kamiya, K. Shinoda, N. Kobayashi et al., "Tuberous sclerosis complex complicated by pulmonary multinodular shadows," *Internal Medicine*, vol. 45, no. 5, pp. 275–278, 2006.

[13] J. R. Breaux and C. Marks, "Chylothorax causing reversible T-cell depletion," *Journal of Trauma*, vol. 28, no. 5, pp. 705–707, 1988.

[14] H. H. Schild, C. P. Strassburg, A. Welz, and J. Kalff, "Treatment options in patients with chylothorax," *Deutsches Ärzteblatt International*, vol. 110, no. 48, pp. 819–826, 2013.

[15] M. Liu, B. Wu, Y. Cui, D. Chang, S. Zhang, and M. Gong, "Surgical treatment of chylothorax caused by lymphangioleiomyomatosis," *Journal of Thoracic Disease*, vol. 6, no. 2, pp. E11–E14, 2014.

[16] P. Curatolo and R. Moavero, "mTOR inhibitors in tuberous sclerosis complex," *Current Neuropharmacology*, vol. 10, no. 4, pp. 404–415, 2012.

4

Fluctuation of Spuriously Elevated Troponin I

Sam Ghali, Keith Lewis, Viviane Kazan, Neezam Altorok, Jamil Taji, Mohammad Taleb, Kiranmayee Lanka, and Ragheb Assaly

The University of Toledo Medical Center, Toledo, OH 43614, USA

Correspondence should be addressed to Sam Ghali, sam_ghali@yahoo.com

Academic Editors: M. Egi, P. Kopterides, C. Lazzeri, Z. Molnar, and C. D. Roosens

Serum troponin is a useful laboratory study for the diagnosis of acute myocardial infarction. However, elevations can also be seen in a variety of other diseases processes. Falsely positive troponin values caused by interference with current troponin assays have been reported. We report a unique case that demonstrates the fluctuation of falsely elevated troponin correlating with hemoglobin, serving as a marker of heterophile antibody levels. A 74-year-old gentleman presented to our Emergency Department with a several-day history of increasing shortness of breath associated with a new-onset chest pain and a troponin I level of 77.28 ng/mL. Throughout his stay, fluctuations in measured troponin levels correlated strongly with fluctuations in hemoglobin levels. Several investigations confirmed false elevated troponin levels secondary to heterophile antibody interference. We conclude that hemoglobin trending in our patient represented a surrogate measure of his heterophile antibody titers with time and that fluctuations in these levels correlated with respective fluctuations in the falsely elevated troponin levels.

1. Introduction

Cardiac troponins T (cTnT) and I (cTnI) are regulatory proteins that control the calcium-mediated interaction between actin and myosin [1]. The skeletal and cardiac isoforms of cTnT and cTnI are distinct, and skeletal isoforms are not detected by the monoclonal antibody-based assays currently in use [2]. This specificity for cardiac isoforms is the basis for the clinical utility of cTnT and cTnI assays.

Relying on history, physical examination, and ECG abnormalities to diagnose acute myocardial infarction may often lead the clinician astray. Thus, the diagnosis of an acute myocardial infarction has become increasingly dependent upon the evaluation of cardiac enzymes, particularly cardiac troponins [2, 3].

In addition to acute myocardial infarction, elevated serum troponins can also be seen in a variety of other diseases including sepsis or critical illness, tachycardia, LVH, heart failure, pulmonary embolism, myocarditis, myocardial trauma, and renal failure [4, 5]. Although irreversible myocyte damage is the usual presumed mechanism responsible for troponin elevation, several additional mechanisms are believed to be responsible for elevated serum troponins in the aforementioned pathological states, including endothelial dysfunction, loss of membrane integrity with leakage of the free cytosolic troponin pool, stretch-mediated troponin release, and impaired renal excretion [6].

Falsely elevated troponin values caused by interference with current troponin assays have been reported. We report a unique case that demonstrates the fluctuation of falsely elevated troponin correlating with hemoglobin, serving as a marker of heterophile antibody levels [7–17].

2. Case Presentation

A 74-year-old man, a retired railroad conductor, with a history of hypertension, hyperlipidemia, and noninsulin-dependent diabetes mellitus presented to our Emergency Department with a several-day history of increasing shortness of breath associated with a new-onset chest pain. ECG performed in the Emergency Department showed a right bundle branch block, left ventricular hypertrophy, and left atrial enlargement. Troponin I was elevated at 77.28 ng/mL. (Beckman-Coulter's Access AccuTnl Assay; reference range 0.00–0.04) The remainder of the cardiac enzymes were essentially normal: myoglobin (50 ng/mL), CK-MB (5.2 ng/mL), and creatine kinase (74 IU/L). D-Dimer was normal at 0.33 mcg/mL. BUN was 13 mg/dL and creatinine was normal at 0.65 mg/dL (reference range 0.64–1.27). Standard Acute Coronary Syndrome protocol was initiated, and the patient was admitted to the hospital. Transthoracic echocardiography showed left ventricular hypertrophy, mild diastolic dysfunction, and a normal ejection fraction with no evidence of wall motion abnormality. Troponin levels remained elevated throughout the entire hospitalization, in continued disproportion to the other cardiac enzymes, (Myoglobin, CK-MB, and CK) which remained either normal or very mildly elevated throughout.

His hospital course was complicated by bibasilar pneumonia and atelectasis requiring multiple bronchoscopies, intubation with ventilatory support, and ultimately a tracheostomy; bilateral lower extremity deep venous thromboses, for which he underwent successful inferior vena cava filter placement; a progressive thrombocytopenia which proved to be Heparin-Induced Thrombocytopenia-antibody positive; and finally, a life-threatening bleeding duodenal ulcer.

A complete blood count trend analysis revealed a significant two-week down-trending of the patient's hemoglobin and hematocrit values; retrospectively a result of the slowly bleeding ulcer. Troponin levels was obtained serially throughout. Figure 1 is a graph showing all the patient's troponin I levels recorded at our hospital, with a juxtaposed graphing of his hemoglobin levels.

As the duodenal ulcer proved to be incendiary, and refractory to temporizing measures, the patient ultimately developed hemorrhagic shock and was taken emergently to the operating room where he underwent an exploratory laparotomy with pyloroplasty and successful suture ligation of the ulcer.

In addition to extensive resuscitation with normal saline, the patient had required a total of 18 units of PRBC. 12 of these units were given within 24 hrs. Intraoperatively, the patient received 5 units of PRBC, 10 units of FFP, and 5 units of platelets.

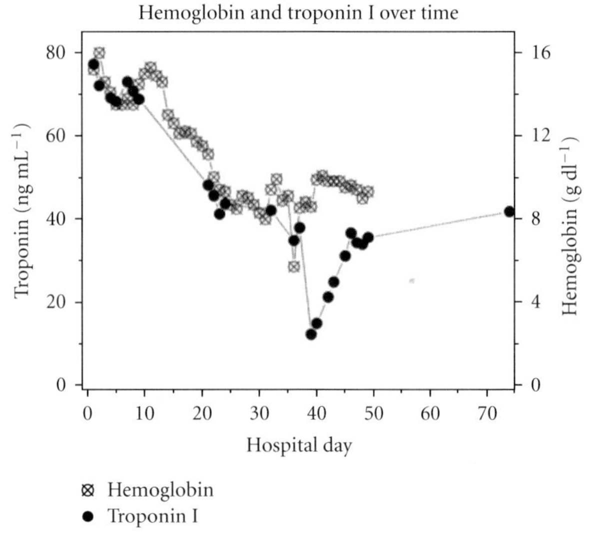

Figure 1

3. Investigations

A patient's blood sample was sent out for a troponin I level on two separate occasions to a near-by hospital laboratory that used the Siemens ADVIA Centaur Immunoassay as opposed to the Beckman-Coulter Access AccuTnl Assay used by our hospital. Both times the result returned at <0.01 ng/mL. Additionally, a random troponin T level measured by Associated Regional and University Pathologists Laboratories using the Electrochemiluminescent Immunoassay was only 0.13 ng/mL.

A heterophile antibody by latex agglutination was also sent out to ARUP Laboratories and returned negative. However, since this screen only tests for those heterophile antibodies known to develop in response to infection with Epstein-Barr Virus, this test was of limited value. Rheumatoid factor, which also may induce heterophilic antibodies [18], was also negative in our patient.

We contacted Beckman-Coulter and request a formal investigation for Heterophile antibodies for our patient. The following blocking reagents, produced by Scantibodies Laboratory, were introduced into the patient's serum and again run through the immunoassay: Goat IgG, Mouse IgG, Rabbit IgG, Bovine IgG, Poly Mak 33, Scavenger ALP, AP Mutein, HBR-1, HBR-Non Murine, and TRU Block [19].

A blocking reagent is a preparation which, when added to immunoassay reagents, has the ability to block the binding of heterophile antibodies, effectively preventing heterophilic interference with another measured value. This is manifested by normalization or near-normalization of the measured value (in this case troponin I) after introduction of the blocking reagent. A blocking reagent can be either a specific blocking reagent, meaning that it has the ability to block only one specific heterophile antibody, or a nonspecific blocking reagent, meaning that it is capable of block heterophile antibodies in general, "nonspecifically" [19].

The first 7 reagents listed previously are specific heterophile antibody blocking reagents. The last 3 are nonspecific heterophile antibody blocking reagents. 9 out of the 10 blockers had no effect on the resulting troponin I level. However, the addition of HBR-1, a nonspecific blocking reagent, reduced the troponin result by greater than 90% of the original value, indicating successful blockage of our patient's heterophile antibodies, drastically diminishing the spurious elevation, with near-normalization of the level.

4. Discussion

We suspected heterophile antibody interference in our patient for several reasons. The troponin elevation could not be explained by acute myocardial damage. There was no evidence of wall motion abnormalities, there was no clinical suggestion of myocarditis, the degree of LVH was moderate at best, and the degree of troponin elevation was inappropriate and inconsistent with what would be expected for any of these pathologies. Also, the troponin elevations were in extreme disproportion to the remainder of the cardiac enzymes, and the typical pattern of decay known of the troponin was not demonstrated. Finally, the presence of immune interference was suspected due to the dramatic fluctuations in troponin levels correlating with blood loss, blood transfusions (replacements), and overall volume status.

The term "heterophile antibodies" has historically been used in reference to specific heterophile antibodies, produced by the human immune system in response to Epstein-Barr virus infection. These specific heterophile antibodies react to antigens from phylogenetically unrelated species. They agglutinate sheep erythrocytes, used in the classic Paul-Bunnell test, horse erythrocytes, used in the "Monospot" test, as well as ox and goat erythrocytes [20].

Probably a better term, antianimal antibodies, encompasses the many different human heterophile antibodies that have the ability to bind to immunoglobulins of many different animal species. It is estimated that 10–40% of humans possess antianimal antibodies. "Anti-animal antibodies (IgG, IgA, IgM, IgE class, anti-isotype, and anti-idiotype specificity) arise as a result of iatrogenic and noniatrogenic causes and include human anti-mouse, -rabbit, -goat, -sheep, -cow, -pig, -rat, and -horse antibodies and antibodies with mixed specificity. Circulating antibodies can reach gram per liter concentrations and may persist for years" [20].

Reagents used in contemporary troponin immunoassays are derived from immunoglobulins of other species. These antianimal antibodies, or "heterophile antibodies", have the capability to interfere with the assays by simply binding these immunoglobulins, resulting in spurious troponin elevations. Even the newer ultrasensitive three-site sandwich troponin I immunoassays have been found to produce similar false positive results [21].

Figure 1 demonstrates two key drops in the measured troponin values. The first drop was from 68.83 ng/mL to 47.11 ng/mL (a net of –21.72 ng/mL) and occurred over a period of 13 days. The patient was transfused 6 units of PRBC's during this time period. No additional troponins were drawn during this 13-day period. The hemoglobin levels essentially mirrored the steady drop in troponin. The continued loss and dilution of the patient's blood steadily overcame the rate of heterophile antibody production, effectively mitigating the interference with the troponin assay. This manifested as a consistent, gradual decline in measured troponin levels observed on the graph.

The second troponin drop produced a glaring, abrupt dip on the troponin curve, as this drop was from 35.23 ng/mL to 11.20 ng/mL (a net of –24.03 ng/mL) over a period of only less than 32 hours. This highly precipitous decrease in troponin was the result of the patient's extensive upper gastrointestinal bleeding, copious fluid resuscitation, and massive blood transfusions described previously, which served to purge and dilute his heterophile antibodies, again mitigating interference with the troponin assay. Furthermore, according to our theory it follows that his troponin levels should gradually but steadily climb back up, once given an opportunity for his antibody levels to build back up to his baseline. Looking at the graph we can see that this trend too was demonstrated.

Since the in vitro addition of HBR-1 to the patient's serum reduced the troponin result by greater than 90% of the original value, we know that the patient does indeed posses heterophile antibodies that interfere with the Beckman-Coulter Access AccuTnI Assay. Since HBR-1 is a nonspecific heterophile antibody blocker, it remains unknown what the specific heterophile antibody(ies) are.

Several sources have been implicated as possible causes for inducing heterophile antibodies in humans, including exposure to animals, special diets, deliberate immunization, rheumatoid factors, blood transfusions, autoimmune diseases, dialysis, certain medications, and cardiac myopathy [19]. The elicitation of heterophile antibodies in our patient may have been the result of one or several of these causative factors.

We conclude that hemoglobin trending in our patient represented a surrogate measure of his heterophile antibody titers with time and that fluctuations in these levels correlated very strongly with respective fluctuations in the falsely elevated troponin levels.

References

[1] A. M. Katz, *Physiology of the Heart*, Raven Press, New York, NY, USA, 2nd edition, 1992.

[2] D. A. Morrow, C. P. Cannon, R. L. Jesse et al., "National Academy of Clinical Biochemistry Laboratory Medicine Practice Guidelines: clinical characteristics and utilization of biochemical markers in acute coronary syndromes," *Circulation*, vol. 115, no. 13, pp. e356–e375, 2007.

[3] K. Thygesen, J. S. Alpert, and H. D. White, "Universal definition of myocardial infarction," *Circulation*, vol. 116, no. 22, pp. 2634–2653, 2007.

[4] T. K. Bakshi, M. K. F. Choo, C. C. Edwards, A. G. Scott, H. H. Hart, and G. P. Armstrong, "Causes of elevated troponin I with a normal coronary angiogram," *Internal Medicine Journal*, vol. 32, no. 11, pp. 520–525, 2002.

[5] S. M. Hamwi, A. K. Sharma, N. J. Weissman et al., "Troponin-I elevation in patients with increased left ventricular mass," *American Journal of Cardiology*, vol. 92, no. 1, pp. 88–90, 2003.

[6] H. D. White, "Pathobiology of troponin elevations: do elevations occur with myocardial ischemia as well as necrosis?" *Journal of the American College of Cardiology*, vol. 57, no. 24, pp. 2406–2408, 2011.

[7] M. Cassin, P. Cappelletti, D. Rubin, M. Zaninotto, F. Macor, and G. Luigi Nicolosi, "Two cases of false-positive troponin I in patients with heterophilic antibodies," *Italian Heart Journal Supplement*, vol. 3, no. 2, pp. 235–238, 2002.

[8] R. J. Knoblock, C. M. Lehman, R. A. Smith, F. S. Apple, and W. L. Roberts, "False-positive AxSYM cardiac troponin I results in a 53-year-old woman," *Archives of Pathology and Laboratory Medicine*, vol. 126, no. 5, pp. 606–609, 2002.

[9] S. M. Fleming, L. O'Byrne, J. Finn, H. Grimes, and K. M. Daly, "False-positive cardiac troponin I in a routine clinical population," *American Journal of Cardiology*, vol. 89, no. 10, pp. 1212–1215, 2002.

[10] A. O. K. Chan, J. P. S. Chan, K. L. Choi, and C. C. Shek, "A patient with an increased troponin level without evidence of

ischaemic cardiac injury," *Hong Kong Medical Journal*, vol. 10, no. 4, pp. 277–279, 2004.

[11] M. L. Garciá-Mancebo, M. T. Aguiló-Otuno, J. R. Gimeno, M. D. Navarro-Martinez, J. Ruiz-Gomez, and J. A. Noguera-Velasco, "Heterophile antibodies produce spuriously elevated concentrations of cardiac troponin I in patients with Legionella pneumophilia," *Clinical Biochemistry*, vol. 38, no. 6, pp. 584–587, 2005.

[12] C. Bionda, D. Collin-Chavagnac, K. Chikh, A. Charrié, M. Manchon, and R. Rousson, "Unnecessary coronary angiography due to false positive troponin I results in a 51-year-old man," *Clinica Chimica Acta*, vol. 378, no. 1-2, pp. 225–226, 2007.

[13] A. N. Makaryus, M. N. Makaryus, and B. Hassid, "Falsely elevated cardiac troponin I levels," *Clinical Cardiology*, vol. 30, no. 2, pp. 92–94, 2007.

[14] A. K. Salah, S. M. Gharad, K. Bodiwala, and D. C. Booth, "You can assay that again!," *American Journal of Medicine*, vol. 120, no. 8, pp. 671–672, 2007.

[15] P. Pernet, B. Bénéteau-Burnat, C. Hermand, and M. Vaubourdolle, "Point-of-care testing: false elevation of cardiac troponin I assayed in the emergency department," *American Journal of Emergency Medicine*, vol. 26, no. 8, pp. 969.e1–969.e2, 2008.

[16] M. A. R. Ginés, J. M. R. Martín, J. A. R. Ginés, and M. Y. R. Martín, "Heterophil antibodies and false positive troponin I results in the diagnosis of myocardial ischemia," *Medicina Clinica*, vol. 130, no. 3, pp. 117–118, 2008.

[17] N. Shayanfar, L. Bestmann, G. Schulthess, and M. Hersberger, "False-positive cardiac troponin T due to assay interference with heterophilic antibodies," *Swiss Medical Weekly*, vol. 138, no. 31-32, article 470, 2008.

[18] G. H. White, P. A. Tideman, D. Mangold, and R. Zerback, "Heterophilic antibody interference with CARDIAC T quantitative rapid assay," *Clinical Chemistry*, vol. 48, no. 1, pp. 201–203, 2002.

[19] B. Seitanidis, "A comparison of the Monospot with the Paul-Bunnell test in infectious mononucleosis and other diseases," *Journal of Clinical Pathology*, vol. 22, no. 3, pp. 321–323, 1969.

[20] L. J. Kricka, "Human anti-animal antibody interferences in immunological assays," *Clinical Chemistry*, vol. 45, no. 7, pp. 942–956, 1999.

[21] Y. Zhu, M. M. Jenkins, D. A. Brass et al., "Heterophilic antibody interference in an ultra-sensitive 3-site sandwich troponin I immunoassay," *Clinica Chimica Acta*, vol. 395, no. 1-2, pp. 181–182, 2008.

Gas-Forming Pyogenic Liver Abscess with Septic Shock

Muhammad S. Khan,[1] Muhammad K. Ishaq,[2] and Kellie R. Jones[2]

[1]*Department of Medicine, University of Oklahoma Health Sciences Center, Williams Pavilion 1130, P.O. Box 26901, Oklahoma City, OK 73190, USA*
[2]*Department of Pulmonary & Critical Care Medicine, University of Oklahoma Health Sciences Center, Williams Pavilion 1130, P.O. Box 26901, Oklahoma City, OK 73190, USA*

Correspondence should be addressed to Muhammad S. Khan; muhammad-khan@ouhsc.edu

Academic Editor: Mehmet Doganay

The pyogenic liver abscess caused by *Clostridium perfringens* (*C. perfringens*) is a rare but rapidly fatal infection. The main virulence factor of this pathogen is its α-toxin (lecithinase), which decomposes the phospholipid in cell membranes leading to cell lysis. Once the bacteria are in blood stream, massive intravascular hemolysis occurs. This can present as anemia on admission with evidence of hemolysis as indicated by low serum haptoglobin, high serum lactate dehydrogenase (LDH), elevated indirect bilirubin, and spherocytosis. The clinical course of *C. perfringens* septicemia is marked by rapidly deteriorating course with a mortality rate ranging from 70 to 100%. The very rapid clinical course makes it difficult to diagnose on time, and most cases are diagnosed at autopsy. Therefore it is important to consider *C. perfringens* infection in any severely ill patient with fever and evidence of hemolysis. We present a case of seventy-seven-year-old male with septic shock secondary to pyogenic liver abscess with a brief review of existing literature on *C. perfringens*.

1. Introduction

Pyogenic liver abscess caused by *Clostridium perfringens* is a rare disease and progression to septicemia has been associated with adverse outcomes. Early recognition and intervention are cornerstone of management due to aggressive course of the disease. This paper discusses an interesting case of elderly gentleman presenting with septic shock secondary to gaseous pyogenic liver abscess and also provides a brief review of the current literature on the topic.

2. Case

A seventy-seven-year-old native American male with past medical history of hypertension and diabetes mellitus presented at an outside hospital with two-day history of fever, generalized fatigue, nausea, vomiting, and abdominal pain. The patient was in usual state of health prior to presentation and was attending a church camp at a lake. He began to have nonbloody vomiting, nausea, and abdominal pain. He was checked by the camp nurse and was found to have a temperature of 101.7 degrees Fahrenheit. He was taken to the emergency room at a nearby hospital where he was found to be hypotensive with systolic blood pressure in 80s and subsequently transferred to the University of Oklahoma Medical Center for higher level of care. On arrival, the patient was confused. His temperature was 95 degrees Fahrenheit, blood pressure was 85/40 mmHg, pulse was 120/min, respiratory rate was 30/min, and oxygen saturation was 90% on room air. On examination, the patient was markedly confused and had cold and clammy extremities, pallor, and severe right upper quadrant pain on deep palpation coupled with abdominal distension. Significant labs on admission consisted of white blood cell count (WBC) of 33 K/cc^3 (normal range 4–11 K/cc^3), hemoglobin of 6 g/dL (normal range Hb 13–18 g/dL), platelet count of 278 k/cc^3 (normal range 140–440 k/cc^3), creatinine of 2.9 mg/dL (normal range 0.8–1.1 mf/dL), total bilirubin of 9.5 mg/dL (normal range 0.3–1.2 mg/dL), aspartate aminotransferase (AST) of 1179 IU/L (normal range 8–41 IU/L), alanine aminotransferase (ALT) of 370 IU/L (normal range 12–48 IU/L), alkaline phosphatase

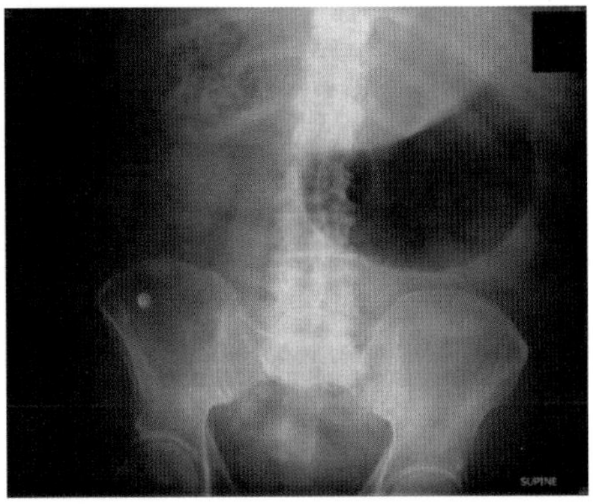

FIGURE 1: Abdominal radiograph showing right upper quadrant gas bubbles.

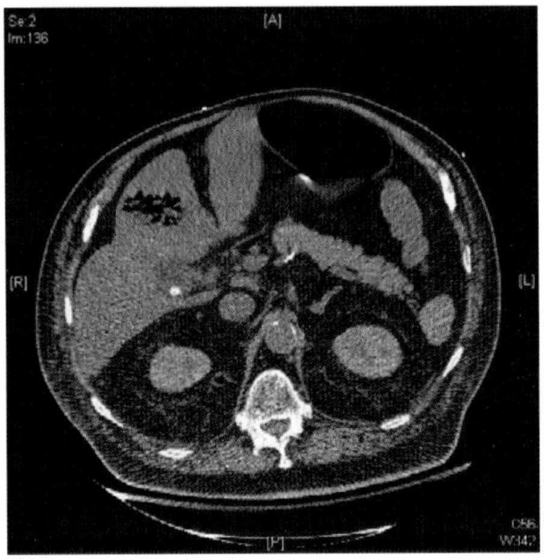

FIGURE 2: CT abdomen showing gas in left liver lobe.

(AlkP) of 238 IU/L (normal range 70–178 IU/L), and lactic acid of 3.1 mmol/L (normal range 0.5–2.0 mmol/L). The patient was intubated on arrival due to inability to protect his airway. A central line was placed and normal saline (NS) fluid bolus was started. After three liters of NS was infused, the patient remained hypotensive and was started on norepinephrine infusion. Blood cultures, urine analysis, and urine cultures were obtained and the patient was initiated on broad spectrum antibiotics with intravenous (IV) vancomycin, piperacillin/tazobactam, and ciprofloxacin. Given marked abdominal tenderness and distension, an abdominal X-ray was obtained which showed radiographic findings concerning intra-abdominal abscess (Figure 1).

Due to concern for liver abscess, a computed tomography scan (CT scan) of abdomen was done which revealed an ovoid air and debris containing structure in the left hepatic lobe concerning for hepatic abscess (Figure 2).

IV metronidazole was then initiated and surgery was consulted emergently. The patient required transfusion of packed red blood cells on arrival and his hemoglobin increased to 10 g/dL after transfusion but 3 hours later dropped to 6.4 g/dL. Lactate dehydrogenase (LDH) and haptoglobin were checked for concerns of hemolysis and were found to be 3442 U/L (normal range 112–236) and 90 mg/dL (normal range 38–195 mg/dL), respectively. A disseminated intravascular coagulation panel (DIC panel) was normal. Seven hours after admission the patient became bradycardiac with heart rate of 30 beats/min and quickly went into asystole. Cardiopulmonary resuscitation (CPR) was initiated and patient received multiple rounds of epinephrine during CPR. He developed ventricular tachycardia (VT) twice during CPR and was shocked without return of circulation. The resuscitation efforts were continued for 45 minutes and at that time the family indicated that they wanted no further resuscitative efforts. The family requested an autopsy limited to the abdominal cavity, which revealed a necrotic and hemorrhagic hepatic abscess with a myriad of Gram positive anaerobic rods in the liver parenchyma (Figure 3). The gallbladder had chronic cholecystitis and a black, friable calculus. The common bile duct was dilated without any evidence of ascending cholangitis. The blood cultures obtained on admission remained negative; therefore the cause of septic shock is unknown but we believe it was linked to gas-forming hepatic infection. The differential diagnosis of gas-forming anaerobic rods includes *Clostridium perfringens* and *Clostridium septicum*. Other common Gram negative gas-forming organisms include *Klebsiella pneumoiae* and *Escherichia coli*. However, due to anaerobic Gram negative rods on liver biopsy we believe that the most likely pathogen was *Clostridium* species.

3. Discussion

Gas-forming pyogenic liver abscess accounts for 7% to 24% of cases of pyogenic liver abscess cases [1]. The most common organism implicated is *Klebsiella pneumonia* which is a Gram negative rod and has a high fatality rate [1]. In patients with diabetes, the high levels of glucose may provide gas-forming microorganisms with a more favorable environment for forming gas via acid fermentation of glucose. In our case, even though the blood cultures remained negative, the morphology of organism on autopsy was most compatible with Gram positive anaerobic bacteria, raising the concern that this might represent *Clostridium* pyogenic liver abscess. Furthermore, the presence of gaseous pyogenic liver abscess and otherwise unexplained massive intravascular hemolysis with increased numbers of spherocytes and multiorgan failure supports the diagnosis of *Clostridium* septic shock. Our discussion in this paper will focus on *Clostridium perfringens* pyogenic liver abscess and septic shock.

C. perfringens is a Gram positive, anaerobic spore-forming bacterium which is responsible for a broad spectrum of human diseases resulting in considerable morbidity and mortality [2]. It is part of commensal flora of human digestive tract and female genital tract and is found in soil and fresh water sediments [3]. In cases of severe life threatening infections, *C. perfringens* can cause septicemia following food borne infection, wound associated soft tissue infection, and liver abscess, as well as lung abscess [4–7]. Risk factors include advanced age, diabetes mellitus, malignancy, liver cirrhosis, and immunocompromised states [8]. In some reports, *C. perfringens* infection has followed invasive procedure in

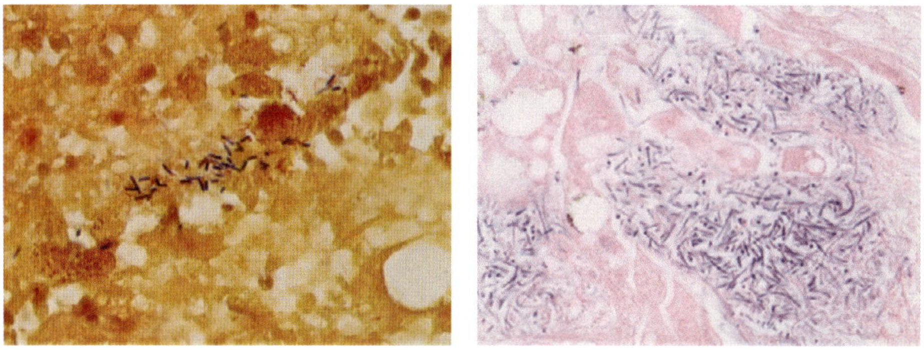

(a) (b)

FIGURE 3: Pathology slides showing Gram positive rods in the liver parenchyma.

the hepatobiliary and gastrointestinal tract, after central venous line insertion and routine gynecological procedures [9–11]. The septicemia may also occur without any underlying risk factors via bacterial translocation.

The mechanism of action is via secretions of toxins causing hemolysis and cell damage. Of these toxins, alpha-toxin is a major cause of hemolysis [12]. The alpha-toxin of *C. perfringens* has two domains with a loop in between. The N-terminal domain has phospholipase activity while C-terminal domain is hydrophobic in nature and enters into cell membrane [12]. The loop between C- and N-terminal contains GM1 ganglioside-binding motifs and specifically binds to GM1a. The phospholipase part disrupts the cell membrane phospholipids, while the alpha-toxin binding to GM1a triggers specific signaling events which leads to activation of tyrosine kinase A (TsKA) and the subsequent signaling cascade results in the release of tumor necrosis factor-alpha (TNF-A) which causes catastrophic hemolysis and inflammation [13]. Other virulence factors work primarily on vascular endothelium, causing capillary leakage. Like other clostridia, *C. perfringens* grows rapidly with the doubling time of about 7 minutes [14].

The incidence of pyogenic liver abscess and septicemia from *C. perfringens* is rare. Kasai et al. reported 119 cases of gas-forming abscess in diabetic patients of which only 8 cases were positive for *Clostridium* [15]. Another study from Japan reported that, among 5011 blood samples that were positive for any bacteria, only 41 were positive for *Clostridium*. Of the 41 samples, 16 were confirmed as septicemia, and 9 of the 16 were positive for *C. perfringens* [16]. The incidence of *C. perfringens* septicemia was reported to be 0.7 in 100000 per year in Canada [17]. Similarly, in a large hospital based study of 7989 positive blood cultures, only 7 cases of *C. perfringens* infection were reported [18].

The clinical course of *C. perfringens* septicemia and liver abscess is usually aggressive with high mortality ranging up to 70% to 100% [19]. The initial presentation can be variable, but fever and abdominal pain are common symptoms [16]. The abdominal pain has been strongly associated with a ruptured liver abscess. Once the bacteria are in blood stream, massive intravascular hemolysis occurs [20–22]. This can present as anemia on admission with evidence of hemolysis as indicated by low haptoglobin, high LDH, elevated indirect bilirubin, and spherocytosis [23]. Therefore, it is important to consider *Clostridium perfringens* infection in severely ill patient with fever and evidence of hemolysis.

Overall, the infection carries significant morbidity and mortality and early intervention has been shown to decrease mortality. Once the infection is suspected based on clinical picture, aggressive management with timely debridement of the focus, early initiation of antibiotics, and a multidisciplinary team approach is necessary [16]. Recently, van Bunderen et al. reported 40 cases of *C. perfringens* septicemia and hemolysis between 1990 and 2010 and the mortality rate was found to be 80% [24]. Law and Lee reported a review of 20 cases of which only 6 patients survived [23]. Among the patients who survived in both reports, an early attempt to remove the focus of infection was strongly associated with favorable outcomes [23, 24]. Similarly, Kurasawa et al. reported a review of 30 cases of *C. perfringens* liver abscess in which only 3 patients survived after receiving early surgical intervention via laparotomy and drainage [16]. The median time between admission and death varied between 6 and 11 hours signifying the aggressive course of disease [16, 23, 24].

There are no clear guidelines regarding any specific antibiotic use against *C. perfringens* infection. The antibiotics classified as appropriate for *Clostridium* are penicillin G, clindamycin, cefoxitin, metronidazole, ampicillin/sulbactam, piperacillin/tazobactam, and imipenem/cilastatin [25]. Patients who are treated with inappropriate antibiotics have significantly higher mortality rate of 75%, compared to patients treated with adequate antibiotic coverage [25]. Clindamycin, metronidazole, and rifampicin have been shown to be effective in reducing alpha-toxin release [26]. Additionally, the use of erythromycin pretreatment is thought to reduce TNF-alpha release from activated neutrophils, thus reducing hemolysis [27].

In summary, *C. perfringens* liver abscess and septicemia are a rare but lethal entity. Given the high mortality, index of suspicion should be very high in at-risk patients presenting with fever, unexplained hemolysis, and blood cultures positive for Gram positive rods. Early surgical intervention has been shown to be the most effective mode of treatment. In our patient the clinical course was very aggressive and, despite initiating appropriate antibiotics, the patient was never hemodynamically stable enough to permit surgery.

References

[1] H.-L. Lee, H.-C. Lee, H.-R. Guo, W.-C. Ko, and K.-W. Chen, "Clinical significance and mechanism of gas formation of pyogenic liver abscess due to *Klebsiella pneumoniae*," *Journal of Clinical Microbiology*, vol. 42, no. 6, pp. 2783–2785, 2004.

[2] G. S. A. Myers, D. A. Rasko, J. K. Cheung et al., "Skewed genomic variability in strains of the toxigenic bacterial pathogen, Clostridium perfringens," *Genome Research*, vol. 16, no. 8, pp. 1031–1040, 2006.

[3] J. I. Rood and S. T. Cole, "Molecular genetics and pathogenesis of *Clostridium perfringens*," *Microbiological Reviews*, vol. 55, no. 4, pp. 621–648, 1991.

[4] K. Mcilwaine and M. T. J. Leach, "*Clostridium perfringens* septicaemia," *British Journal of Haematology*, vol. 163, no. 5, p. 549, 2013.

[5] D. Kitterer, N. Braun, M. C. Jehs, B. Schulte, M. Dominik Alscher, and J. Latus, "Gas gangrene caused by *Clostridium perfringens* involving the liver, spleen, and heart in a man 20 years after an orthotopic liver transplant: a case report," *Experimental and Clinical Transplantation*, vol. 12, no. 2, pp. 165–168, 2014.

[6] E. Okon, E. Bishburg, S. Ugras, T. Chan, and H. Wang, "*Clostridium perfringens* meningitis, plesiomonas shigelloides sepsis: a lethal combination," *The American Journal of Case Reports*, vol. 14, pp. 70–72, 2013.

[7] G. Rajendran, P. Bothma, and A. Brodbeck, "Intravascular haemolysis and septicaemia due to *Clostridium perfringens* liver abscess," *Anaesthesia and Intensive Care*, vol. 38, no. 5, pp. 942–945, 2010.

[8] E. Schröpfer, S. Rauthe, and T. Meyer, "Diagnosis and misdiagnosis of necrotizing soft tissue infections: three case reports," *Cases Journal*, vol. 1, article 252, 2008.

[9] H. Nakanishi, Y. Chuganji, K. Uraushihara et al., "An autopsy case of the hepatocellular carcinoma associated with multiple myeloma which developed fatal massive hemolysis due to the *C. perfringens* septicemia following TAE," *Nihon Shokakibyo Gakkai Zasshi*, vol. 100, pp. 1395–1399, 2003.

[10] N. W. Hendrix, A. D. Mackeen, and S. Weiner, "*Clostridium perfringens* sepsis and fetal demise after genetic amniocentesis," *American Journal of Perinatology Reports*, vol. 1, no. 1, pp. 25–28, 2011.

[11] C. Determann and C. A. Walker, "*Clostridium perfringens* gas gangrene at a wrist intravenous line insertion," *BMJ Case Reports*, vol. 2013, 2013.

[12] J. Sakurai, M. Nagahama, and M. Oda, "*Clostridium perfringens* alpha-toxin: characterization and mode of action," *The Journal of Biochemistry*, vol. 136, no. 5, pp. 569–574, 2004.

[13] M. Oda, M. Kabura, T. Takagishi et al., "*Clostridium perfringens* alpha-toxin recognizes the GM1a-TrKA complex," *The Journal of Biological Chemistry*, vol. 287, no. 39, pp. 33070–33079, 2012.

[14] S. Ohtani, N. Watanabe, M. Kawata, K. Harada, M. Himei, and K. Murakami, "Massive intravascular hemolysis in a patient infected by Clostridium perfringens," *Acta Medica Okayama*, vol. 60, no. 6, pp. 357–360, 2006.

[15] K. Kasai, N. Manabe, K. Tateishi, N. Ichihara, Y. Ohta, and C. Fujimoto, "Severe infections in diabetic patients of reported 568 cases in Japan," in *Proceedings of the Kagawa Prefectural College Health Sciences*, vol. 1, pp. 1–10, 1999.

[16] M. Kurasawa, T. Nishikido, J. Koike, S. Tominaga, and H. Tamemoto, "Gas-forming liver abscess associated with rapid hemolysis in a diabetic patient," *World Journal of Diabetes*, vol. 5, no. 2, pp. 224–229, 2014.

[17] J. T. Ngo, M. D. Parkins, D. B. Gregson et al., "Population-based assessment of the incidence, risk factors, and outcomes of anaerobic bloodstream infections," *Infection*, vol. 41, no. 1, pp. 41–48, 2013.

[18] J.-R. Zahar, H. Farhat, E. Chachaty, P. Meshaka, S. Antoun, and G. Nitenberg, "Incidence and clinical significance of anaerobic bacteraemia in cancer patients: a 6-year retrospective study," *Clinical Microbiology and Infection*, vol. 11, no. 9, pp. 724–729, 2005.

[19] H. Ng, S. M. Lam, H. P. Shum, and W. W. Yan, "*Clostridium perfringens* liver abscess with massive haemolysis," *Hong Kong Medical Journal*, vol. 16, no. 4, pp. 310–312, 2010.

[20] B. Pastene, E. Gregoire, V. Blasco, and J. Albanese, "Alpha and theta toxin *C. perfringens* infection complicated by septic shock and hemolysis," *Annales Françaises d'Anesthésie et de Réanimation*, vol. 33, no. 9-10, pp. 552–553, 2014.

[21] T. G. Simon, J. Bradley, A. Jones, and G. Carino, "Massive intravascular hemolysis from *Clostridium perfringens* septicemia: a review," *Journal of Intensive Care Medicine*, vol. 29, no. 6, pp. 327–333, 2014.

[22] B. Juntermanns, S. Radunz, M. Heuer et al., "Fulminant septic shock due to *Clostridium perfringens* skin and soft tissue infection eight years after liver transplantation," *Annals of Transplantation*, vol. 16, no. 3, pp. 143–146, 2011.

[23] S.-T. Law and M. K. Lee, "A middle-aged lady with a pyogenic liver abscess caused by *Clostridium perfringens*," *World Journal of Hepatology*, vol. 4, no. 8, pp. 252–255, 2012.

[24] C. C. van Bunderen, M. K. Bomers, E. Wesdorp, P. Peerbooms, and J. Veenstra, "*Clostridium perfringens* septicaemia with massive intravascular haemolysis: a case report and review of the literature," *Netherlands Journal of Medicine*, vol. 68, no. 9, pp. 343–346, 2010.

[25] M. Shah, E. Bishburg, D. A. Baran, and T. Chan, "Epidemiology and outcomes of clostridial bacteremia at a tertiary-care institution," *TheScientificWorldJournal*, vol. 9, pp. 144–148, 2009.

[26] D. L. Stevens, K. A. Maier, and J. E. Mitten, "Effect of antibiotics on toxin production and viability of *Clostridium perfringens*," *Antimicrobial Agents and Chemotherapy*, vol. 31, no. 2, pp. 213–218, 1987.

[27] M. Oda, A. Kihara, H. Yoshioka et al., "Effect of erythromycin on biological activities induced by *Clostridium perfringens* α-toxin," *The Journal of Pharmacology & Experimental Therapeutics*, vol. 327, no. 3, pp. 934–940, 2008.

6

Recurrent Febrile Neutropenia and Thrombocytopenia in a Chronic Cocaine User: A Case of Levamisole Induced Complications

Eduardo Martinez,[1,2] Raza Alvi,[3,2] Sindhaghatta Venkatram,[1,2] and Gilda Diaz-Fuentes[1,2]

[1] *Division of Pulmonary and Critical Care Medicine, Bronx Lebanon Hospital Center, Bronx, NY 10457, USA*
[2] *Albert Einstein College of Medicine, Bronx, NY 10461, USA*
[3] *Department of Internal Medicine, Bronx Lebanon Hospital Center, Bronx, NY 10457, USA*

Correspondence should be addressed to Eduardo Martinez; eduardo.martinez1@gmail.com

Academic Editor: Ricardo J. Dinis-Oliveira

Cocaine is used by approximately 1.5 million Americans each month and up to 69% of the cocaine seized contains levamisole. The real incidence of cocaine-levamisole induced neutropenia is unclear but probably underestimated. Associated complications include fever, thrombocytopenia, skin-vasculitis disorders, and rarely kidney injury. We present a young male, with chronic active cocaine use presenting with recurrent episodes of febrile neutropenia and thrombocytopenia. He underwent extensive work-up and was treated with many antibiotics and we suspect that his neutropenia and thrombocytopenia were caused by recurrent cocaine-levamisole use.

1. Introduction

The etiology for neutropenia is extensive and includes medications, sepsis, and hematological or oncological conditions. Neutropenia has been well described as one of the common side effects of levamisole, an imidazothiazole previously used as an anthelminthic and adjuvant to 5-fluorouracil (5-FU) in the treatment of colon cancer [1]. Due to its serious adverse effects, it was discontinued in the year 2000 [2]. In the past decade there has been resurgence in the use of levamisole, not as a prescribed medication but as an adulterant of up to 69% of the cocaine found in the United States [3]. Analysis of street samples of cocaine has shown an average purity rate of 50%. Average purities fell substantially from 2004 to 2010, decreasing from 69.1% to 50.5% for crack cocaine and from 65.2% to 37.0% for powder cocaine [4]. Therefore, adulterants represent more than half of the composition of all cocaine sold. Adulterants are added to cocaine to promote the perceived potency of the drug or to increase the volume of the drug [5]. Drug dealers may respond to changing drug market and law enforcement pressure by manipulating cocaine quality using adulterants rather than adjusting prices. Adulterants are pharmacologically active substances that are intentionally added to cocaine in order to potentiate its effect. Levamisole, along with its metabolite aminorex, has been proven to enhance noradrenergic neurotransmission by inhibiting reuptake, by acting on ganglionic nicotinic receptors, and by increasing the concentration of endogenous opiate compounds [6, 7]. Levamisole also shares very similar chemical properties with cocaine, such as color and melting point, which makes it almost imposible to distinguish between the two [8]. The fact that patients not only deny the use of cocaine but also are unaware of this combination of drugs makes the diagnosis of cocaine-levamisole associated neutropenia very difficult.

This is relevant to physicians in New York where in 2011, in a yearly survey distributed by the Substance Abuse and Mental Health Services Administration, 2.24% of persons aged 18 years or older stated that they had used cocaine within the past year (3rd behind Rhode Island and Colorado) [9].

Cocaine-levamisole associated neutropenia is frequently self-limited and usually resolves after withdrawing the use of the contaminated cocaine but tends to recur with reexposure [1, 2]. Another adverse effect with similar presentation is thrombocytopenia. This associated thrombocytopenia and the recurrent episodes are seldom reported in the literature.

We present a patient with recurrent episodes of febrile neutropenia and thrombocytopenia which improved after discontinuing the use of cocaine.

2. Case Report

A 36-year-old man was admitted to the intensive care unit with fever and right gluteal pain and swelling of three-day duration. He denied trauma, rash, flu-like symptoms, or sick contacts. Medical history included continuous cocaine abuse (sniffing), paroxysmal atrial fibrillation, and two episodes of febrile neutropenia in the past.

On examination, the patient was awake, alert, comfortable, febrile 103.1 F, and tachycardic (120 bpm) nontoxic looking. An abscess was found on the gluteal area. The rest of the skin was intact and the rest of the exam was unremarkable. Laboratory findings showed severe leucopenia with neutropenia and thrombocytopenia. Urine toxicology by immunoassay was reported to be positive for cocaine and cannabinoids.

He was managed for severe sepsis and febrile neutropenia with drainage of his gluteal abscess, fluids, broad spectrum antibiotics, including caspofungin, and granulocyte colony-stimulating factor (G-CSF). Serum and urine levamisole levels performed by high performance liquid chromatography/tandem mass spectrometry (LC-MS/MS) five days after admission were negative. Flow cytometry, cultures, serology, HIV, and vasculitis work-up were done and ruled out other common causes of neutropenia and thrombocytopenia (Table 1). Despite high fevers, the patient remained stable and asymptomatic. Clinical course was complicated by acute kidney injury on day 5 of admission. Urine analysis revealed no eosinophils and benign sediment.

On review of medical records, the patient had been admitted to our institution twice during the last 12 months for febrile neutropenia. Table 1 shows summary of presentations during all admissions including the current one.

Patient became afebrile on day 7 of admission with resolution of thrombocytopenia and some improvement of WBC. He was discharged home in stable condition and he was lost to follow-up.

3. Discussion

Approximately 1.5 million Americans use cocaine each month and, according to a report from the Drug Enforcement Administration (DEA) in July 2009, 69% of the cocaine seized coming into the United States contained levamisole [10]. Levamisole, neutropenia, thrombocytopenia, and other serious side effects associated with levamisole use were first reported in the 1970s when it was used for inflammatory conditions and as an adjuvant treatment of colon and breast cancer [11, 12]. Neutropenia has been reported in 60–69% of cases of cocaine-levamisole induced complications [1, 13].

The pathophysiology of this syndrome is not completely understood, but drugs with reactive thiol groups, such as levamisole, behave as haptens and trigger immune or cytotoxic response, causing opsonization and destruction of white blood cells leading to agranulocytosis [14]. Autoantibody formation and human leukocyte antigen B27 (HLA B27) status have also been proposed [15, 16]. Pure cocaine has recognizable cardiovascular and neurological toxic effects, but there is no evidence that it can cause neutropenia and thrombocytopenia [5, 17].

The most common reported complications are skin involvement with a retiform purpura with or without bullae on the helix of the ears or extremities and a self-limited neutropenia. These can occur as isolated manifestations or simultaneously. Although thrombocytopenia has been reported as an adverse effect of levamisole when used for medical purposes, a literature review of 203 cases by Larocque et al. revealed only 4 (2%) cases with thrombocytopenia. Other less common complications are fever, arthralgias, hyponatremia, and kidney injury. Although recurrence is seen with reexposure to the contaminated cocaine, it is not commonly reported [1, 18]. Our patient presented with febrile neutropenia and thrombocytopenia and developed acute kidney injury (AKI). Lee et al. reported 30 cases of anti-neutrophil cytoplasmic antibodies (ANCA) positivity associated with cocaine ingestion; they all had anti-myeloperoxidase antibodies (MPO) and 50% also had anti-proteinase 3 antibodies. Two of the thirty cases (6.6%) had AKI [18]. It is unclear whether our patient developed AKI due to levamisole or neprotoxicity due to medications and contrast.

On review of all the admissions for our patient, it is interesting to note that the nadir for the thrombocitopenia occured between day 5 and 8 and, similarly, the fever curve improved between days 5 and 8 of presentation with marginal improvement in WBC count (Figure 1).

The diagnosis of cocaine-levamisole complications is a diagnosis of exclusion. It is difficult to distinguish this condition from other forms of vasculitis. A high-titer c-ANCA, p-ANCA, human neutrophil elastase ANCA (HNE-ANCA), with concomitant antinuclear, anti-phospholipid antibodies and 11 isolated skin vasculitis suggests of cocaine-levamisole as etiological agent [11]. The detection of levamisole in the serum or urine assists in the diagnosis, but the absence does not rule out levamisole as the etiology since its half-life is only approximately 5.6 hours [2, 19]. In our patient the vasculitis work-up and the levamisole levels were negative.

Management of the condition is conservative with discontinuation of the levamisole contaminated cocaine and treatment of complications. This usually leads to a rapid clinical improvement in 2-3 weeks. Other modalities such as systemic steroids and G-CSF are also recommended without consensus about their benefits [10, 14]. Use of G-CSG is supportive and suggested for patients with very severe febrile neutropenia with absolute neutrophil count (ANC) less than 0.1×10^9/L. Our patient was initially treated with G-CSF in two of the admissions with no improvement in WBC count.

TABLE 1: Comparison of characteristics during the three admissions.

	Admission number 1	Admission number 2	Current admission
Presentation	Fever and sore throat	Fever, neck stiffness, cough, macular rash with whitish central papules on chest and extremities	Fever, gluteal abscess
WBC (ANC)	2.8 k/uL (600 cells/uL)	1.9 k/uL (100 cells/uL)	1.3 k/uL (100 cells/uL)
Platelets lowest	176 k/uL	53 k/uL	33 k/uL
Urine toxicology	Cocaine and cannabinoids	Cocaine	Cocaine and cannabinoids
Imaging	Chest X-ray-negative Chest CT negative Abdomen/pelvis CT-possible colitis	Chest X-ray-negative CT head-negative CT facial bones negative Echocardiogram-normal	Chest X-ray-negative Abdomen/pelvis CT-perianal abscess Echocardiogram-normal
Serology-negative	HIV-negative Thyroid panel-normal Cardiac markers-negative	HIV, HTLV, BCR-abl, malaria smear, dengue titer, hepatitis panel serum cryptococcal antigen, collagen vascular disease work-up negative, RPR	ANCA, ANA, MPO, antiphospholipid antibodies, anti-cardiolipin, complement, HLA B27, malaria, hepatitis, HIV, HTLV-all negative
Other tests		Flow cytometry neg.	Flow cytometry neg.
Urine and serum for levamisole	Not done	Not done	Sent at day 5 of admission-negative
Cultures-blood, urine, stools	Negative	Negative	Negative
Procedures	None	Spinal tap normal Bone marrow biopsy ×2 (hypercellular marrow with myeloid predominance and trilineage maturation)	Perianal abscess drainage at the bed side
Antibiotics	Ciprofloxacin Metronidazole Moxifloxacin	Vancomycin, meropenem, acyclovir, fluconazole, doxycycline, daptomycin, metronidazole, cefepime, clindamycin	Vancomycin, cefepime, Zosyn, caspofungin, amikacin, and meropenem
G-CSF (duration-days)	Not given	5 days of administration	8 days of administration
Others			Platelets transfusion
Hospital complications	None	None	Acute renal failure. Serum Creatinine 1.4 → 2.9 → 4.4 Gastrointestinal bleeding
Fever resolution-time days	2 days	8 days	7 days
Outcome	Discharged after 4 days-symptoms improved	Discharged after 23 days-symptoms improved	Discharged after 16 days-symptoms improved, abscess healing

ANA = antinuclear antibodies; ANCA = antineutrophil cytoplasmic antibodies; HIV = human immunodeficiency virus; HTLV = human T-lymphotropic virus; MPO = anti-myeloperoxidase; human leukocyte antigen B27.

4. Conclusion

Cocaine-levamisole induced febrile neutropenia should be highly suspected in patients presenting with a positive cocaine test and neutropenia, vasculitis, thrombocytopenia, and positive ANCA. A careful review of prior admissions is warranted and we speculate that there is a relationship between improvement in platelets count and fever resolution in those patients.

Awareness of this entity will allow clinicians to early identify serum and urine levamisole levels and, if no readily identifiable source of fever, take these into consideration to avoid extensive and potentially costly and dangerous procedures and medications.

Patients should be advised of possible recurrence as long as they continue using these substances.

Disclosure

None of the authors has a financial relationship with any commercial entity that has interest in the subject of the paper.

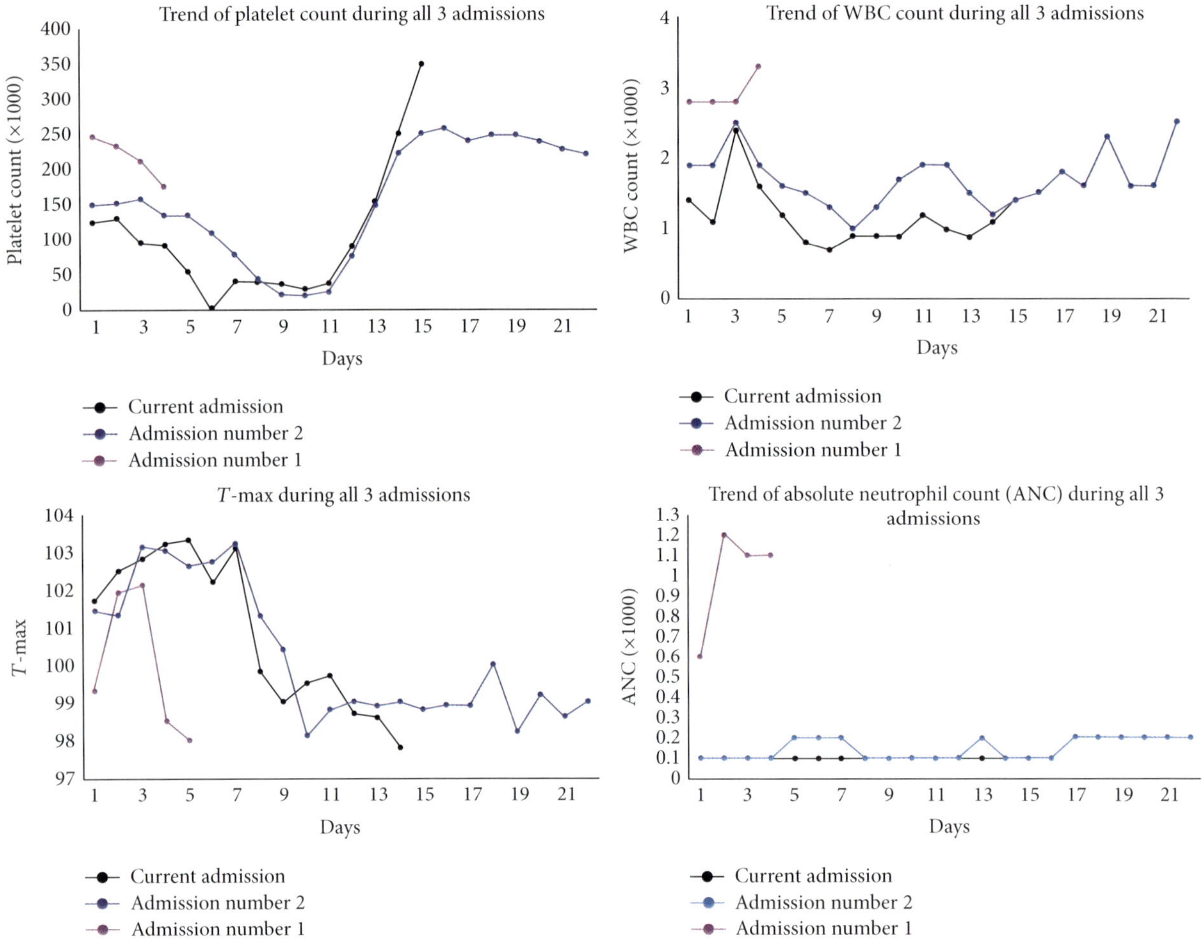

Figure 1: Graph of trend for platelets, temperature, and WBC and ANC count.

References

[1] A. Larocque and R. S. Hoffman, "Levamisole in cocaine: unexpected news from an old acquaintance," *Clinical Toxicology*, vol. 50, no. 4, pp. 231–241, 2012.

[2] A. Goyal, "A self destructing reaction to a self destructive habit: levamisole tainted cocaine causing autoimmune vasculitis," *New York Medical Journal*, vol. 8, no. 1, p. 1, 2014.

[3] Centers for Disease Control and Prevention (CDC), "Agranulocytosis associated with cocaine use—four states," *Morbidity and Mortality Weekly Report*, vol. 58, no. 49, pp. 1381–1385, 2009.

[4] H. Zhu, "Correlation between cocaine prices and purity with trends in emergency department visits in a major metropolitan area," *Journal of Urban Health*, vol. 91, no. 5, pp. 1009–1018, 2014.

[5] R. A. Goldstein, C. DesLauriers, A. Burda, and K. Johnson-Arbor, "Cocaine: history, social implications, and toxicity: a review," *Seminars in Diagnostic Pathology*, vol. 26, no. 1, pp. 10–17, 2009.

[6] T. Hofmaier, A. Luf, A. Seddik et al., "Aminorex, a metabolite of the cocaine adulterant levamisole, exerts amphetamine like actions at monoamine transporters," *Neurochemistry International*, vol. 73, pp. 32–41, 2014.

[7] C. Hess, N. Ritke, S. Broecker, B. Madea, and F. Musshoff, "Metabolism of levamisole and kinetics of levamisole and aminorex in urine by means of LC-QTOF-HRMS and LC-QqQ-MS," *Analytical and Bioanalytical Chemistry*, vol. 405, no. 12, pp. 4077–4088, 2013.

[8] A. Chang, J. Osterloh, and J. Thomas, "Levamisole: a dangerous new cocaine adulterant," *Clinical Pharmacology & Therapeutics*, vol. 88, no. 3, pp. 408–411, 2010.

[9] Substance Abuse and Mental Health Services Administration and Center for Behavioral Health Statistics and Quality, *The DAWN Report: Highlights of the 2011 Drug Abuse Warning Network (DAWN) Findings on Drug-Related Emergency Department Visits*, Substance Abuse and Mental Health Services Administration, Center for Behavioral Health Statistics and Quality, Rockville, Md, USA, 2013.

[10] Substance Abuse and Mental Health Services Administration (SAMHSA), *Results from the 2013 National Survey on Drug Use and Health: Summary of National Findings*, U.S. Department of Health and Human Services, Rockville, Md, USA, 2014.

[11] D. R. Parkinson, P. O. Cano, L. M. Jerry et al., "Complications of cancer immunotherapy with levamisole," *The Lancet*, vol. 309, no. 8022, pp. 1129–1132, 1977.

[12] L. Teerenhovi, E. Heinonen, P. Gröhn, P. Klefström, M. Mehtonen, and A. Tiilikainen, "High frequency of agranulocytosis in breast-cancer patients treated with levamisole," *The Lancet*, vol. 2, no. 8081, pp. 151–152, 1978.

[13] T. Pearson, M. Bremmer, J. Cohen, and M. Driscoll, "Vasculopathy related to cocaine adulterated with levamisole: a review of the literature," *Dermatology Online Journal*, vol. 18, no. 7, p. 1, 2012.

[14] I. A. Dy and P. H. Wiernik, "Cocaine-levamisole thrombotic vasculopathy," *Seminars in Thrombosis and Hemostasis*, vol. 38, no. 8, pp. 780–782, 2012.

[15] S. I. Drew, B. M. Carter, D. S. Nathanson, and P. I. Terasaki, "Levamisole-associated neutropenia and autoimmune granulocytotoxins," *Annals of the Rheumatic Diseases*, vol. 39, no. 1, pp. 59–63, 1980.

[16] E. M. Veys, H. Mielants, and G. Verbruggen, "Levamisole-induced adverse reactions in HLA B27-positive rheumatoid arthritis," *The Lancet*, vol. 311, no. 8056, p. 148, 1978.

[17] M. B. Ellis, "Treating vasculitis arising from levamisole-contaminated cocaine," *Podiatry Today*, vol. 27, no. 8, 2014.

[18] K. C. Lee, B. Ladizinski, and D. G. Federman, "Complications associated with use of levamisole-contaminated cocaine: an emerging public health challenge," *Mayo Clinic Proceedings*, vol. 87, no. 6, pp. 581–586, 2012.

[19] E. Kouassi, G. Caille, L. Lery, L. Larivière, and M. Vézina, "Novel assay and pharmacokinetics of levamisole and p-hydroxylevamisole in human plasma and urine," *Biopharmaceutics and Drug Disposition*, vol. 7, no. 1, pp. 71–89, 1986.

7

An Elusive Bullet in the Gastrointestinal Tract: A Rare Case of Bullet Embolism in the Gastrointestinal Tract and a Review of Relevant Literature

Saptarshi Biswas, Catherine Price, and Sunil Abrol

Brookdale University Hospital and Medical Center, 1 Brookdale Plaza, Brooklyn, NY 11212, USA

Correspondence should be addressed to Saptarshi Biswas; saptarshibiswas@comcast.net

Academic Editors: C. Lazzeri and G. Pichler

Bullet embolism within the gastrointestinal system is extremely rare. Such bullet injuries are infrequently covered in the general literature, but the surgeon should be aware of the phenomenon. Smaller caliber bullets are more common in civilian gunshot wound (GSW) events. These bullets are able to tumble through the gastrointestinal tract and cause perforation of the intestinal lumen which is small enough to be easily missed. Bullets retained in the abdominal cavity should not be dismissed as fixed and should be carefully monitored to ensure that they do not embolize within the bowel and cause occult lesions during their migration. We present a unique case wherein a bullet caused a minute perforation in the small bowel, before migrating to the distal colon, which resulted in late presentation of sepsis secondary to peritonitis.

1. Introduction

Bullet emboli are rare complications of gunshot injuries [1]. The relative rarity of the condition, along with potential lack of early symptoms, often leads to significant delay in diagnosis and treatment of the problem. Consequences of such a missed injury can be devastating and prove fatal as shown in our case. The easy availability of guns in the United States, complimented by the upsurge of gun violence in a civilian urban setting, has increased the possibility of encountering bullet embolism [2].

The majority of such emboli are notoriously asymptomatic and thus can be missed on initial evaluation. Whenever initial workup fails to visualize the bullet or the entry and exit wounds do not match up, a need for detailed interrogation should be triggered in the mind of the clinician. Unexplained trajectories of bullets should raise the suspicion of bullet embolism.

In this paper, we describe a rare case of gastrointestinal bullet embolism where a small-caliber bullet perforated the small bowel, migrated distally, and eventually lodged in the distal colon, which resulted in a missed injury, leading to sepsis and the demise of the patient.

2. Case Report

An 18-year-old male was brought into an urban, level-one trauma center by emergency medical service after reportedly being shot in the buttocks. On arrival, the patient was awake, alert, and oriented to person, place, and time. Airway and breathing were determined to be patent and adequate. The patient's initial vitals were T97.5°F, BP109/75, HR103, and RR20. Venous access was secured via placement of two large-bore intravenous catheters and insertion of a femoral vein triple lumen catheter. Patient was moving all four extremities upon arrival.

All clothes were removed and, while stabilizing the cervical spine, the patient was rolled and evaluated for injuries on all surfaces. Noted GSWs included one near the coccyx, two in the left lateral gluteal region, one in the right lateral gluteal region, and one in the left upper medial thigh. A secondary

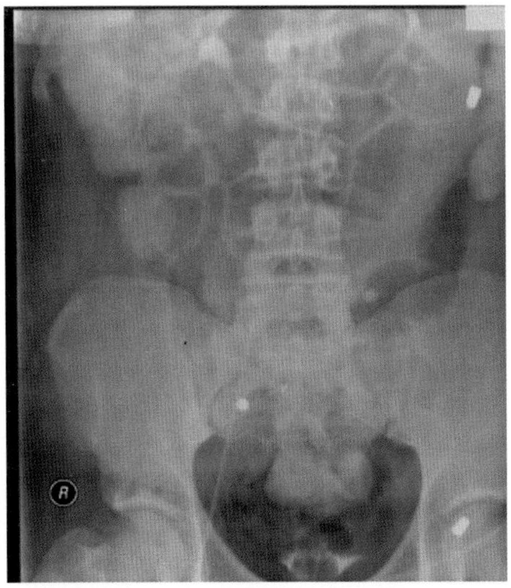

FIGURE 1: Note the bullet in the left upper quadrant of the abdomen.

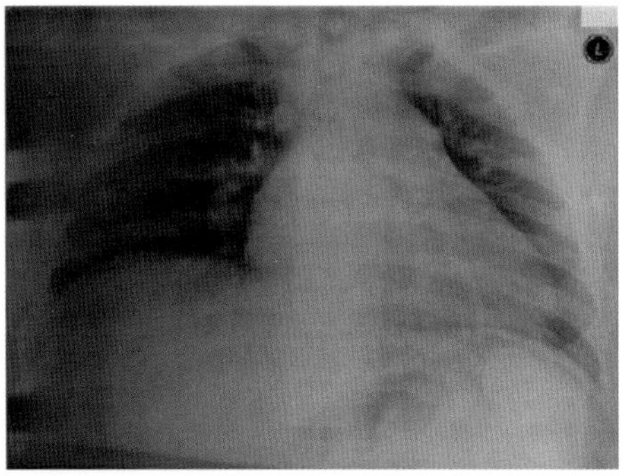

FIGURE 2: The initial chest X-ray on presentation to the emergency department shows no pathology.

survey revealed a soft, nondistended abdomen with active bowel sounds and a rectum with good tone and no bleeding on the examining finger. Patient's initial laboratory values were WBC 9.9, hemoglobin 14, hematocrit 41.7, platelets 241, sodium 141, potassium 4.3, chloride 101, bicarbonate 28, BUN 14, creatinine 0.9, and glucose 127. X-rays of the chest, abdomen, and pelvis were taken (Figures 1 and 2).

A CT scan with triple contrast enhancement of the chest, abdomen, and pelvis was obtained. The CT revealed a bullet in the left upper quadrant of the abdomen, a bullet in the right hemisacrum, and a bullet lodged in the posterior column of the left acetabulum. There were air bubbles in the peritoneum, which could be secondary to entrance of the bullet into the peritoneal cavity or secondary to intestinal injury. There was a minute amount of free fluid in the pelvis. There was no evidence of colonic or vascular contrast extravasation (Figure 3).

The patient was taken to the operating room for an exploratory laparotomy to rule out intra-abdominal hollow viscus or intraperitoneal injury. The small bowel, from the ligament of Treitz to the ileocecal valve, was evaluated independently by two surgeons. The large colon was mobilized starting with the left colon down to the sigmoid colon, then the transverse colon, and finally the right colon. Intraoperatively, neither gross bowel nor intraperitoneal injuries were noted. The patient was transferred to the postanesthesia care unit in stable condition.

The patient's postoperative course was uneventful with the exception of vomiting and an associated WBC count rise from 7.9 to 11.3, on post operative day 3. An abdominal X-ray was performed to determine small bowel ileus versus obstruction. A small, rounded metallic density was again noted overlying the right sacrum. The bullet previously seen overlying the left upper quadrant was no longer visualized at that site. There was a similar-appearing bullet seen in the right abdomen at the level of L4, possibly just inferior to the right colon. It is possible this bullet was within the small bowel. If it were, this would explain its transit. If it was in the bowel, it may have been lodged at the ileocecal valve. There was also associated small bowel dilatation with air-fluid levels seen. Small bowel obstruction could not be excluded and, theoretically, might be attributed to the bullet. It was also possible the bullet may have moved due to the exploratory laparotomy. There was retained contrast material noted in the colon and rectum, which were not significantly dilated. If there was a small bowel obstruction it was either incomplete or early (Figure 4).

On POD 4, the patient's WBC count increased to 19 and he spiked a fever of 38.4°C. Cultures of blood, urine, and sputum were obtained. No bacterial growth was ever realized from these cultures. A chest X-ray was obtained and deemed to be unremarkable. On POD 5, the patient was afebrile for a period greater than 24 hours, ambulating, and tolerating diet. He had stable vitals, a normal WBC count, and normal bowel function; therefore a decision was made to discharge the patient to his home.

The patient presented to the emergency room on POD 8 with hypotension and abdominal pain since that morning, which was accompanied by coffee ground emesis. Physical examination revealed a jaundiced male who was awake, alert, and oriented to person, place, and time but in obvious discomfort. His abdomen was distended with positive signs for peritonitis. Labs obtained at this time were WBC 24.2, hemoglobin 12.4, hematocrit 37, platelets 496, sodium 131, potassium 6.1, chloride 94, bicarbonate 15, BUN 30, creatinine 3.4, glucose 124, ALT 150, AST 200, total bilirubin 2.2, creatine kinase 203, lactate 7.18, ammonia 180, INR 1.3, PT 14.7, and PTT 23.7. Arterial blood gas measurements (pH 7.27/pCO_2 33.7/pO_2 96.1/HCO_3 15/O_2 sat 96%/base deficit −10.9) showed significant metabolic acidosis. Volume resuscitation was started, and an NGT and Foley catheter were placed.

A CT of the chest, abdomen, and pelvis showed pneumatosis intestinalis (Figure 5) of the small bowel. Dilated loops of the small bowel in the right mid-abdomen had peripheral curvilinear air, which was consistent with air in the bowel wall and was due to pneumatosis, probably due to ischemia. In addition, there were tiny bubbles of air between the dilated small bowel loops which was most likely air in the blood vessels or extraluminal air. Jejunal loops were markedly distended and contained air and fluid without wall

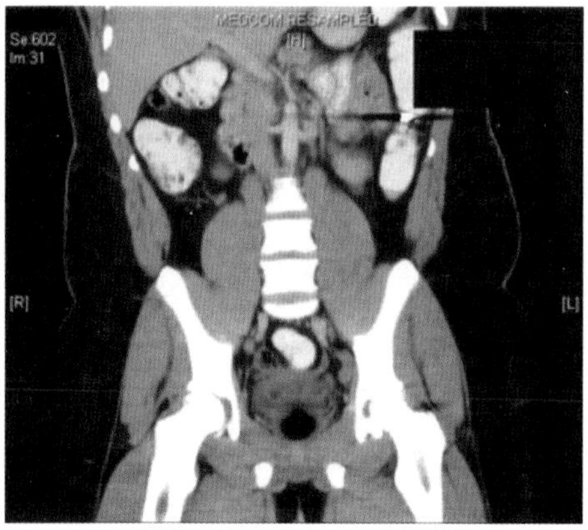

Figure 3: A CT reveals a bullet in the lumen of the small intestine in the right upper quadrant.

thickening. These changes are more consistent with proximal small bowel obstruction than with ileus. The cecum and proximal ascending colon contained air and fluid and were normal sized. The hepatic flexure, transverse colon, and splenic flexure were moderately dilated and contained air. The descending colon was totally collapsed. The sigmoid colon was collapsed and contained minimal air. There was a large amount of pelvic and right upper quadrant ascites, which was increased in size in comparison to the last CT. There was a bullet located in the right lower quadrant, perhaps in the small bowel loops, which was previously in the left upper quadrant. A metallic bullet fragment was on the right side of the sacrum and posterior column of the left acetabulum (Figures 5 and 6). There was a moderate amount of fluid in the lower abdomen and right upper quadrant, which was partly loculated and could represent infected fluid.

After CT, the patient started having bilious vomiting, and his blood pressure plummeted to 99/66. A right internal jugular triple lumen catheter was placed and normal saline boluses were begun. The patient was intubated and received IV cefoxitin and piperacillin/tazobactam for empiric polymicrobial coverage.

The patient was taken to the operating room. Coffee ground-appearing emesis was now present in the suction canister of the NGT. Urine output was scant. Intraoperatively, ischemic bowel was noted. The small bowel was resected from an area distal to the ligament of Treitz to the distal ileum, and the remaining portion was anastomosed. A portion of the large bowel proximal to the splenic flexure was resected with the proximal portion brought to the skin to form a colostomy.

Intraoperatively, the patient received 8 L of normal saline, four units of packed red blood cells, and two units of fresh-frozen plasma. The patient received four additional units of fresh-frozen plasma postoperatively. The patient lost vital signs 4 hours after operation. An attempt was made at resuscitation, as per advanced cardiac life support guidelines; however, the patient expired.

An autopsy report was obtained. The cause of death was determined to be intestinal necrosis and peritonitis due to multiple gunshot wounds of the buttocks with perforation of the intestine. There were four penetrating gunshot wounds of

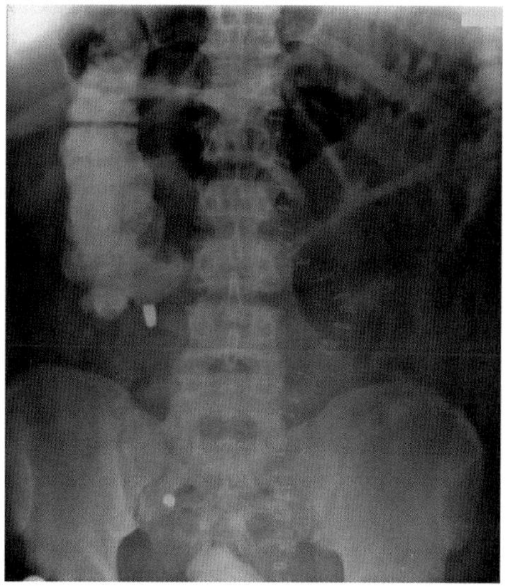

Figure 4: Note that the right upper quadrant bullet has now embolized to the left lower quadrant of the abdomen.

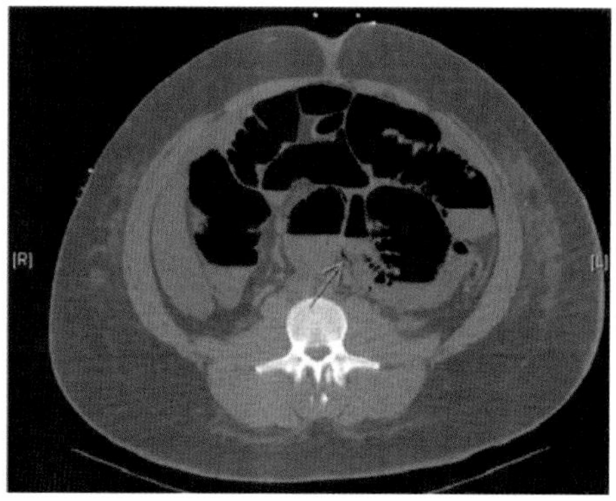

Figure 5: Note the pneumatosis intestinalis now present.

the buttocks. One of these caused perforation of the peritoneal cavity and intestine, which lead to marked peritonitis and resultant intestinal necrosis. The collective wound tracks of the penetrating GSWs passed throughout the soft tissue of the buttocks in a back-to-front direction. Only one wound track entered the peritoneal cavity. This track ended in the lumen of the intestine. It was associated with marked yellow-red fibrinous exudates, which surrounded the right liver, spleen, mesothelial surfaces of the peritoneal cavity, and patches of the remaining serosal surfaces of the small and large intestines.

Three bullets were recovered postmortem. A grey-discolored, small-caliber bullet was recovered from the intraperitoneal track. A small-caliber, yellow, metal-jacketed bullet was recovered from the left pelvic bone at the sacroiliac joint. A similar-appearing bullet was recovered from the anteromedial right thigh.

The pleural cavities each contained approximately 200 mL of clear yellow fluid and were free of adhesion. The stomach contained 150 mL of dark red liquid and had a red mucosa. The remaining intestines had alternating sections of smooth,

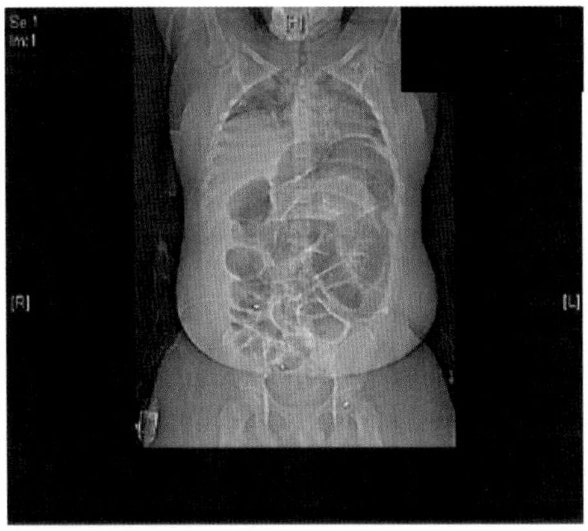

Figure 6: Note the extensive lung and bowel pathology. The bullet in question is still lodged in the left lower quadrant.

tan, edematous mucosa with areas of dusky red discoloration. The colon wall was markedly edematous and without perforating defects. There were moderate adhesions between the bowel loops. Lung microscopy revealed moderate acute bronchioloalveolar pneumonia. The liver was found to have centrilobular ischemia. The serosal surface of the small and large intestines showed mixed chronic and acute inflammatory infiltration. The muscularis layers of the small intestine had hemorrhagic necrosis with focal preservation of the overlying mucosal epithelium.

3. Discussion

Embolism by definition refers to the migration of solid, liquid, or gaseous substance from its point of origin to a distant site. The solid particle can be missile, thrombus, or even a medical device. The liquid can be amniotic fluid. The gaseous substance could be a nitrogen or atmospheric air bubble [3, 4]. Emboli are propelled through a vessel by the flow of blood, air pressure, or active or passive body movements [5].

The first bullet embolism was reported by Thomas Davis in 1834. This case was subsequently cited later, in 1919, by Bland-Sutton [6]. Most of the reports published in English literature are in the form of isolated case reports. One of the earliest and largest report series was by Mattox et al. in 1979. It comprised 28 cases spanning 12 years and provided one of the most significant contributions to understand this rare phenomenon [7, 8].

Krispin et al. [3] has described trauma caused by ballistics as perforating and penetrating. In case of penetrating trauma, the bullet loses its kinetic energy during its travel along its trajectory and remains within the domains of the body cavity. Bullet embolism occurs when a bullet penetrates the body, its movement is stalled, and then it is carried away from its initial site of lodgement to a distant location.

Bullet emboli, in themselves, are rare phenomena. Most reports are regarding military conflicts or vascular emboli. A study by Rich et al. [9] of 7,500 GSWs during the Vietnam War revealed only 22 cases complicated by foreign body emboli (0.3%). This study shows, in a battlefield environment, the incidence of bullet embolism was exceedingly low. Only 3 cases described a whole bullet vessel embolus. The other cases described mostly fragments from explosive devices.

A 10-year retrospective review by Sandler et al. [10] revealed only 46 cases of GSW that resulted in missile emboli. In 1996, Adegboyega et al. [11] reported only 160 cases of bullet emboli since 1834. Michelassi et al. [12] reviewed 153 cases of bullet emboli that were reported in English literature and were mostly amongst the civilian population. The authors concluded that embolization occurred twice more frequently in the arterial system compared to the venous system. They reported 15.5% occurrence when the aorta was the source of the arterial bullet emboli. The left leg was twice more likely than the right to be involved, which can be explained by the asymmetry of the aortic bifurcation. Twenty percent of these patients with arterial bullet embolism were asymptomatic, while 66.7% had peripheral ischemia. More than 70% of missiles that penetrate into arterial circulation enter via the thoracic or abdominal aorta, according to Slobodan et al. [13]. In odd events, missile emboli have even been reported to enter arterial circulation through the heart [12–17].

Isolated reports of distal arterial embolization from peripheral arteries have also been published [18, 19]. The embolism is anterograde in the majority of cases. Rare cases of retrograde (venovenous) [20–22] and paradoxical [23] emboli have also been reported. Schmelzer et al. [22] and Rich et al. [9] mentioned that arterial missile emboli outnumber venous ones by 4 : 1. Biswas et al. [2] described a unique case in which the autopsy study revealed the bullet entered through the thoracic aorta, flowed through the systemic circulation, and eventually lodged into the right popliteal artery. The embolism in this case might have occurred shortly after the initial injury or in the perioperative resuscitative phase. Other reports have shown that embolization has been delayed for days, weeks, or longer [8, 24–26]. Wales et al. [27] have reported a unique case of a right ventricular bullet embolism that manifested clinically 4 years after initial insult. Cardiac bullet emboli can cause cardiac irritability, delayed embolism [22, 28, 29], and recurrent pericardial effusions and may even interfere with valvular functioning [7].

Clinical manifestations are often attributed to the site of penetration of the vascular system, the injury to other viscera, or the site of the embolization. These can all cause delay in diagnosis, which can result in adverse outcome or even death. The signs and symptoms may not correspond with those expected from the presumed course of the bullet. When a bullet is found in an unexpected location, deviant from the conventional trajectory, embolism should be suspected. Pain, claudication, paresthesia, gangrene, pleural or pericardial effusion, endocarditis, sepsis, cardiac arrhythmias, pseudoaneurysm, or even neuroses and psychoses are some of the delayed presentations [7].

Although the final endpoint of an embolized bullet is unpredictable, some consistent patterns have become elucidated as more cases are reported. A peripheral venous embolus generally terminates in the right side of the heart or in the pulmonary artery. A bullet that enters the right side of the heart will commonly embolize to the pulmonary artery, while pellets or small missiles starting from the left side of the heart are likely to embolize into the middle cerebral arteries.

Kase et al. concluded that the right brain is affected more often (70%) than the left [28].

The flow pattern into the innominate artery, which is the first and largest branch of the aortic arch, is the causative factor. Bullets from the thoracic or abdominal aorta usually lodge into the arterial tree of the lower extremity. Left leg involvement is more likely due to the axis of the left common iliac artery forming a narrower angle (30 degrees) from the aorta than from the right side (45 degrees) [19].

The guns and ammunition used in a trauma are also important to identify, because bullet emboli are more common with smaller, blunt-nosed, short-length, or low-velocity bullets [1]. Patel et al. [8] have concluded that the low incidence of bullet embolism is because two major prerequisites need to be satisfied for a projectile to become an embolus. First, the bullet should have little kinetic energy remaining at the precise instant it enters the blood vessel. Second, the diameter of the bullet must be less than the diameter of the blood vessel it penetrates. Patel et al. [8] reported an embolus incidence of 55% with a 0.22-caliber handgun and 27% with a shotgun. In a review by DiMaio and DiMaio, in 24 cases of bullet embolism where the caliber or type of the gun was known, a small, 0.22-caliber bullet accounted for the majority of emboli [29]. Embolism is rarely caused by high velocity bullets, as evidenced by its low incidence in war literature [30].

Small-caliber bullets are more prone to tumbling, may not pierce blood vessels or intestinal lumens, have a slower velocity, and are able to fit through peripheral blood vessels that are too narrow for large-caliber bullets. These small-caliber bullets possess low kinetic energy at the time of impact. The primary ballistic feature of the short 6.35 mm caliber missile is its small weight (3.2 g) and low initial velocity (240 m/s), which translates into low initial kinetic energy (92 J). Therefore the penetrating power of such a missile is limited. Such bullets are blunt-nosed and thus are less streamlined. They are more retarded by tissues and subsequently lose a greater amount of kinetic energy after penetration into the body. The degree of bluntness of the nose also determines the initial value of the area of interphase between the bullet and the tissue and thus the drag of the bullet. Wobbling and tumbling of a bullet during its passing through the tissues cause even further loss of kinetic energy [13].

The density, elasticity, and strength of the tissue hit by a bullet, as well as the length of the wound tract, can influence the loss of initial kinetic energy, as in our case. The denser the tissue the bullet has to overcome is, the greater the retardation is. This, subsequently, leads to greater loss of kinetic energy. Increased density also shortens the period of gyration, which eventually results in greater retardation and increased energy loss [13].

As discussed earlier, the increase in gun violence in the civilian setting has resulted in more reports of bullet emboli. Most of these cases describe embolism in larger vessels, obstruction of distal systemic vascular tree, or even pulmonary or paradoxical emboli. Shiver et al. describe a case of urethral obstruction due to the passage of a projectile retained in the genitourinary system [31]. Raz et al. [32] and Bozeman and Mesri [33] present cases describing acute urinary retention following late migration of a retained bullet. Smalls and Siram describe a unique case of a wandering bullet in which the bullet caused esophageal injury and lodged in the stomach [34]. DiMaio [35], in an article about the application of pathology to crime investigation, has cited a case of bullet migration from the stomach to the intestines. DiMaio has described two interesting cases of bullets expelled through the oral orifice.

In the first case, a spent bullet from an entry point in the back was recovered from the oral cavity, while the second described a missile from a chest wound that halted within the lungs and was coughed up by the victim [34]. One must also consider that "lost" bullets may have actually passed uneventfully through the gastrointestinal tract, as reported by Morrow et al. [36].

A bullet becoming lodged in the intestine is an extremely rare event even though bullet injuries constitute the majority of perforating abdominal trauma and a large part of penetrating trauma [3, 37–39]. Although rarely reported, gastrointestinal embolization should be taken into consideration when searching for a missile in the abdomen during an exploratory laparotomy. In a case in which a bullet halts within the intestines, lack of awareness of the spatial location may result in futile seeking of the missile in the abdominal cavity.

Sometimes a penetrating bullet that punctures the abdominal cavity has enough kinetic energy to perforate the intestines and stop after striking the vertebral column, abdominal musculature, or even just beneath the skin [3]. However, in some rare cases of low-velocity ammunition, the bullet course ends within hollow viscus such as the small or large intestine. Such cases are extremely rare and seldom reported.

In the present case, the bullet had penetrated the small bowel through a small laceration and moved from its initial location as evident from the initial CT scan to a different location seen in subsequent imaging. The migration can be attributed to a peristalsis or even palpation and manipulation of the bowel during the surgical exploration. The bullet was never expelled from the body by defecation, probably due to decreased bowel movement as a component of the ileus and peritonitis that followed the undetected perforation.

Along with low-velocity, small-caliber bullets, bullet fragments or pellets are also prone to embolization. This explains the scenario in our case where a 0.22-caliber was fired probably from a distance of 10–20 feet, which resulted in kinetic energy sufficient to penetrate the intestinal lumen but not enough to exit it. The fact that the patient was morbidly obese and the entry site was the gluteal region slowed the kinetic energy of the projectile. The bullet was also small enough to cause an intestinal entry wound and minute enough to subsequently become sealed enough to be missed on open exploration. The bullet's movement compounded the initial problem of missed location.

Therefore, in rare instances where a bullet is not immediately located, it is important to determine the initial bullet trajectory before its path was possibly changed in the body. To determine this, first the relation of the location of the victim to the shooter must be determined. Thereafter, the axis of the gun barrel must be ascertained. Factors postulated to be responsible for determining distant lodgment sites are (I) power of the missile, (II) caliber and shape, (III) site of penetration into the vascular bed, (IV) effect of gravity especially in the low-pressure venous system, (V) respiratory activity, (VI) force of blood flow, (VII) position of the victim at the moment of penetration of the embolus into the circulation, and (VIII) relative size and angle of the arterial branches [5, 7, 40, 41].

All projectiles can potentially carry bacteria into the wound. In addition they can cause introduction of skin flora, clothing, and foreign particles, any of which can act as a nidus of infection independently [42]. A unique case of *Clostridium difficile* subacute bacterial endocarditis was reported by Bilsker et al. [43]. It was attributed to a bullet that penetrated the left ventricle and subsequently the right subclavian artery.

The argument for bullet extraction after bowel injury includes a decreased risk of sepsis. Sarmiento et al. [44] found that after abdominal GSW, if colon wounds occurred and the bullet was retained, the incidence of shock was higher than if the bullet was removed and surrounding soft tissue debrided. It was also found that if the missile entered the colon but exited spontaneously (in this study the exit was not via embolism in any of the cases, but rather through-and-through penetration), the resultant internal tract should be subjected to a thorough washout and removal of damaged tissue.

Another consideration, which Sari et al. [45] discuss, is elevated blood lead from gunshot injuries that result in ingestion. It was found that the gastrointestinal tract is efficient in absorbing lead from retained bullets. In these instances, there is rapid elevation of blood lead immediately after injury. This level persists even three years after incident.

A very high index of suspicion is of utmost importance to identify a missile embolus. Accounting for all bullets and all bullet wounds allows for a basic reconstruction of each bullet's trajectory, thus identifying organs and tissues at risk of damage. If the number of entry wounds does not equal the number of exit wounds or the clinical signs or symptoms and radiologic imaging do not correlate with the injury, the possibility of bullet embolism should be entertained. Unexplained clinical findings should also trigger the suspicion of missile embolism.

Although the bullet rule is a helpful concept, there are well-documented exceptions to the rule. Two bullets fired in unison as tandem bullets from a handgun entering the body through the same entrance wound, but leaving two bullets in situ, although exceedingly unusual, have been documented [46]. Another example is a bullet that ricochets within the calvarium, entering and exiting from the same point [47].

4. Conclusion

Migratory intraluminal bullets may produce complex and confusing scenarios in patients with GSWs, often resulting in diagnostic and therapeutic dilemmas. This case is a glowing example how a bullet embolism initially unaccounted for eventually influenced the course and outcome of a trauma patient. Given the grave outcome of a missed small bowel injury, an additional confounding variable such as an intraluminal bullet migration presents a truly formidable challenge for even the most experienced trauma surgeon.

This case emphasizes that the true path of a bullet or fragment cannot be always ascertained based on the site of the entrance wound. However, when the suspicion of a bullet embolism has been raised, the missing projectile should be thoroughly accounted for by a thorough and meticulous search and the resultant damage addressed even if the patient is asymptomatic on initial presentation. The real purpose of the bullet rule is to remind clinicians to look for additional injuries and to be diligent in the evaluation of patients who have suffered gunshot wounds.

The consequence of a missed bullet embolism may prove fatal, as our case illustrates.

Acknowledgments

The authors would like to thank April Duckworth, M.D., and Judith Lussier, P.A., for their invaluable assistance with this case report.

References

[1] M. E. Schroeder, H. I. Pryor II, A. K. Chun, R. Rahbar, S. Arora, and K. Vaziri, "Retrograde migration and endovascular retrieval of a venous bullet embolus," *Journal of Vascular Surgery*, vol. 53, no. 4, pp. 1113–1115, 2011.

[2] S. Biswas, H. Cadot, and S. Abrol, "Gunshot wound of the thoracic aorta with right popliteal artery embolization: a case report of bullet embolism with review of relevant literature," *Case Reports in Emergency Medicine*, vol. 2013, Article ID 198617, 5 pages, 2013.

[3] A. Krispin, K. Zaitsev, and J. Hiss, "The elusive slug: bullet intestinal 'embolism,'" *Forensic Science, Medicine, and Pathology*, vol. 6, no. 4, pp. 288–292, 2010.

[4] V. Kumar, K. A. Abbas, and F. Nelson, *Robbins and Cotran's Pathologic Basis of Disease*, Eited by R. S. Cortan, Elsevier Saunders, Philadelphia, Pa, USA, 2005.

[5] B. G. Brogdon, *Forensic Radiology*, CRC Press, Boca Raton, Fla, USA, 1998.

[6] J. Bland-Sutton, "A lecture on missiles as emboli," *The Lancet*, vol. 193, no. 4993, pp. 773–775, 1919.

[7] K. L. Mattox, A. C. Beall Jr., C. L. Ennix, and M. E. DeBakey, "Intravascular migratory bullets," *The American Journal of Surgery*, vol. 137, no. 2, pp. 192–195, 1979.

[8] K. R. Patel, L. E. Cortes, L. Semel, P. V. P. Sharma, and R. H. Clauss, "Bullet embolism," *Journal of Cardiovascular Surgery*, vol. 30, no. 4, pp. 584–590, 1989.

[9] N. M. Rich, G. J. Collins Jr., C. A. Andersen, P. T. McDonald, L. Kozloff, and J. J. Ricotta, "Missile emboli," *Journal of Trauma*, vol. 18, no. 4, pp. 236–239, 1978.

[10] G. Sandler, N. Merrett, C. Buchan, and A. Biankin, "Abdominal shotgun wound with pellet embolization leading to bilateral

lower limb amputation: case report and review of the literature of missile emboli over the past 10 years," *Journal of Trauma*, vol. 67, no. 6, pp. E202–E208, 2009.

[11] P. A. Adegboyega, N. Sustento-Reodica, and A. Adesokan, "Arterial bullet embolism resulting in delayed vascular insufficiency: a rationale for mandatory extraction," *Journal of Trauma*, vol. 41, no. 3, pp. 539–541, 1996.

[12] F. Michelassi, A. Pietrabissa, M. Ferrari, F. Mosca, T. Vargish, and H. H. Moosa, "Bullet emboli to the systemic and venous circulation," *Surgery*, vol. 107, no. 3, pp. 239–245, 1990.

[13] S. Slobodan, N. Slobodan, and A. Djordje, "Popliteal artery bullet embolism in a case of homicide: a case report and review of the tangible literature," *Forensic Science International*, vol. 139, no. 1, pp. 27–33, 2004.

[14] F. Abdo, M. Massad, M. Slim et al., "Wandering intravascular missiles: report of five cases from the Lebanon war," *Surgery*, vol. 103, no. 3, pp. 376–380, 1988.

[15] J. M. Vincent and M. D. DiMaio, *Gunshot Wounds: Practical Aspects of Firearms, Ballistics, and Forensic Techniques*, Elsevier, Amsterdam, The Netherlands, 2nd edition, 1985.

[16] M. Todoric, N. Cvorovic, R. Ilic, A. Simic, G. Kronja, and J. Jablanov, "Arterial embolism caused by penetration and migration of a bullet through the thoracic aorta," *Vojnosanitetski Pregled*, vol. 51, no. 1, pp. 65–69, 1994.

[17] P. Shen, R. Mirzayan, T. Jain, J. McPherson, and E. E. Cornwell III, "Gunshot wound to the thoracic aorta with peripheral arterial bullet embolization: case report and literature review," *Journal of Trauma*, vol. 44, no. 2, pp. 394–397, 1998.

[18] F. Bongard, S. M. Johs, T. A. Leighton, and S. R. Klein, "Peripheral arterial shotgun missile emboli: diagnostic and therapeutic management—case reports," *Journal of Trauma*, vol. 31, no. 10, pp. 1426–1431, 1991.

[19] J. J. Shannon Jr., N. M. Vo, P. E. Stanton Jr., and M. Dimler, "Peripheral arterial missile embolization: a case report and 22-year literature review," *Journal of Vascular Surgery*, vol. 5, no. 5, pp. 773–778, 1987.

[20] S. J. A. Sclafani and W. G. Mitchell, "Retrograde venous bullet embolism," *Journal of Trauma*, vol. 21, no. 8, pp. 656–657, 1981.

[21] M. D. Tripp, J. Tisnado, D. R. Bezirdjian, and S.-R. Cho, "Retrograde venous bullet embolization: a rare occurrence," *Canadian Association of Radiologists Journal*, vol. 38, no. 4, pp. 292–293, 1988.

[22] V. Schmelzer, G. Mendez-Picon, and A. S. Gervin, "Case report: transthoracic retrograde venous bullet embolization," *Journal of Trauma*, vol. 29, no. 4, pp. 525–527, 1989.

[23] M. Schurr, S. McCord, and M. Croce, "Paradoxical bullet embolism: case report and literature review," *Journal of Trauma*, vol. 40, no. 6, pp. 1034–1036, 1996.

[24] P. N. Symbas and N. Harlaftis, "Bullet emboli in the pulmonary and systemic arteries," *Annals of Surgery*, vol. 185, no. 3, pp. 318–320, 1977.

[25] R. L. Fisk, A. Addetia, E. T. Gelfand, C. H. Brooks, and J. Dvorkin, "Missile migration from lung to heart with delayed systemic embolization," *Chest*, vol. 72, no. 4, pp. 534–535, 1977.

[26] B. Levi, C. R. Sainsbury, and D. L. Scharf, "Delayed shotgun pellet migration to the right ventricle," *Clinical Cardiology*, vol. 8, no. 6, pp. 367–371, 1985.

[27] L. Wales, D. P. Jenkins, and P. L. C. Smith, "Delayed presentation of right ventricular bullet embolus," *Annals of Thoracic Surgery*, vol. 72, no. 2, pp. 619–620, 2001.

[28] C. S. Kase, R. L. White, T. L. Vinson, and R. P. Eichelberger, "Shotgun pellet embolus to the middle cerebral artery," *Neurology*, vol. 31, no. 41, pp. 458–461, 1981.

[29] V. J. DiMaio and D. J. DiMaio, "Bullet embolism: six cases and a review of the literature," *Journal of Forensic Sciences*, vol. 17, no. 3, pp. 394–398, 1972.

[30] A. M. Jones, N. J. Graham, and J. R. Looney, "Arterial embolism of a high-velocity rifle bullet after a hunting accident. Case report and literature review," *The American Journal of Forensic Medicine and Pathology*, vol. 4, no. 3, pp. 259–264, 1983.

[31] S. A. Shiver and B. Z. Reynolds, "Urethral obstruction due to the passage of a retained projectile into the genitounrinary system," *The American Journal of Emergency Medicine*, vol. 26, no. 7, pp. 842.e1–842.e2, 2008.

[32] O. Raz, Y. Shilo, K. Stav, and D. Leibovici, "Late migration of a retained bullet into the urinary bladder presenting with acute urinary retention," *Israel Medical Association Journal*, vol. 9, no. 6, pp. 484–485, 2007.

[33] W. P. Bozeman and J. Mesri, "Acute urinary retention from urethral migration of a retained bullet," *Journal of Trauma*, vol. 53, no. 4, pp. 790–792, 2002.

[34] N. M. Smalls and S. M. Siram, "The wandering bullet," *Journal of the National Medical Association*, vol. 80, no. 6, pp. 678–682, 1988.

[35] V. J. M. DiMaio, *Bullet Emboli in Gunshot Wounds: Practical Aspects of Firearms, Ballistics, and Forensic Techniques*, CRC Press, Boca Raton, Fla, USA, 1999.

[36] J. S. Morrow, C. E. Haycock, and E. Lazaro, "The 'Swallowed bullet' syndrome," *Journal of Trauma*, vol. 18, no. 6, pp. 464–466, 1978.

[37] J. A. Asensio, H. Arroyo Jr., W. Veloz et al., "Penetrating thoracoabdominal injuries: ongoing dilemma—which cavity and when?" *World Journal of Surgery*, vol. 26, no. 5, pp. 539–543, 2002.

[38] T. M. Schmelzer, G. Mostafa, O. L. Gunter Jr., H. J. Norton, and R. F. Sing, "Evaluation of selective treatment of penetrating abdominal trauma," *Journal of Surgical Education*, vol. 65, no. 5, pp. 340–345, 2008.

[39] D. Demetriades, P. Hadjizacharia, C. Constantinou et al., "Selective nonoperative management of penetrating abdominal solid organ injuries," *Annals of Surgery*, vol. 244, no. 4, pp. 620–628, 2006.

[40] M. Khalifeh, G. Khoury, H. Hajj, R. Steir, S. Khoury, and G. Abi-Saad, "Penetrating missile embolisation," *European Journal of Vascular Surgery*, vol. 7, no. 4, pp. 467–469, 1993.

[41] P. A. Ward and A. Suzuki, "Gunshot wound of the heart with peripheral embolization: a case report with review of literature," *Journal of Thoracic and Cardiovascular Surgery*, vol. 68, no. 3, pp. 440–446, 1974.

[42] C. S. Bartlett, "Clinical update: gunshot wound ballistics," *Clinical Orthopaedics and Related Research*, no. 408, pp. 28–57, 2003.

[43] M. S. Bilsker, E. J. Bauerlein, and M. L. Kamerman, "Bullet embolus from the heart to the right subclavian artery after gunshot wound to the right chest," *The American Heart Journal*, vol. 132, no. 5, pp. 1093–1094, 1996.

[44] J. M. Sarmiento, P. Yugueros, A. F. Garcia, and B. G. Wolff, "Bullets and their role in sepsis after colon wounds," *World Journal of Surgery*, vol. 21, no. 6, pp. 648–652, 1997.

[45] M. Sari, S. Baylancicek, and S. Inanli, "Atypical penetrating laryngeal trauma: a bullet in the larynx," *European Journal of Emergency Medicine*, vol. 14, no. 4, pp. 230–232, 2007.

[46] A. J. Bentley, A. Busuttil, B. Clifton, and P. Sibbald, "Homicidal tandem bullet wound of the chest," *The American Journal of Forensic Medicine and Pathology*, vol. 18, no. 1, pp. 56–59, 1997.

[47] T. C. Grey, "The incredible bouncing bullet: projectile exit through the entrance wound," *Journal of Forensic Sciences*, vol. 38, no. 5, pp. 1222–1226, 1993.

8

Norepinephrine as a Potential Aggravator of Symptomatic Cerebral Vasospasm: Two Cases and Argument for Milrinone Therapy

F. A. Zeiler,[1] J. Silvaggio,[1] A. M. Kaufmann,[1] L. M. Gillman,[2] and M. West[1]

[1] *Section of Neurosurgery, University of Manitoba, GB-1 820 Sherbrook Street, Winnipeg, MB, Canada R3A 1R9*
[2] *Section of Critical Care, Department of Medicine, University of Manitoba, Room GC425, 820 Sherbrook Street, Winnipeg, MB, Canada R3T 2N2*

Correspondence should be addressed to F. A. Zeiler; umzeiler@cc.umanitoba.ca

Academic Editor: Kurt Lenz

Background. During hypertensive therapy for post-subarachnoid hemorrhage (SAH) symptomatic vasospasm, norepinephrine is commonly used to reach target blood pressures. Concerns over aggravation of vasospasm with norepinephrine exist. *Objective.* To describe norepinephrine temporally related deterioration in neurological examination of two post-SAH patients in vasospasm. *Methods.* We retrospectively reviewed two charts of patients with delayed cerebral ischemia (DCI) post-SAH who deteriorated with norepinephrine infusions. *Results.* We identified two patients with DCI post-SAH who deteriorated during hypertensive therapy with norepinephrine. The first, a 43-year-old male presented to hospital with DCI, failed MABP directed therapy with rapid deterioration in exam with high dose norepinephrine and MABP of 140–150 mm Hg. His exam improved on continuous milrinone and discontinuation of norepinephrine. The second, a 39-year-old female who developed DCI on postbleed day 8 responded to milrinone therapy upfront. During further deterioration and after angioplasty, norepinephrine was utilized to drive MABP to 130–140 mm Hg. Progressive deterioration in examination occurred after angioplasty as norepinephrine doses escalated. After discontinuation of norepinephrine and continuation of milrinone, function dramatically returned but not to baseline. *Conclusions.* The potential exists for worsening of DCI post-SAH with hypertensive therapy directed by norepinephrine. A potential role exists for vasodilation and inotropic directed therapy with milrinone in the setting of DCI post-SAH.

1. Introduction

Delayed cerebral ischemia (DCI) post-subarachnoid hemorrhage (SAH) poses significant challenges to the treating physician. Current standard therapy consists of hypertensive directed measures in order to ensure preservation of cerebral blood flow to risk territories and is titrated typically to the neurological examination [1–3]. In addition to this, maintenance of euvolemia is also a cornerstone of therapy [2]. In order to achieve the desired level of hypertension, a variety of inotropic and vasoconstrictive vasopressors have been utilized in the literature.

Despite our best attempts at preservation of cerebral blood flow with hypertensive therapy, some patients progress to develop cerebral infarcts with a range of morbidity and mortality depending on infarct location and extent [3].

Despite maximal therapy, some patients will fail hypertensive direct therapy for DCI post-SAH. However, with the use of peripheral vasoconstrictive substances to achieve desired mean arterial blood pressure (MABP) goals, one could question their effect on aggravating the cerebral vasoconstriction and having a negative impact on the neurological exam. To date, animal literature points towards cerebral vasoconstriction with the administration of norepinephrine [4–6]. Autopsy evidence suggests a dose dependant vasoconstrictive effect on proximal cerebral vessels with norepinephrine administration [7]. Furthermore, norepinephrine levels are known to be elevated in the cerebral spinal fluid of SAH patients and have been postulated as a potential mediator of cerebral vasospasm post-SAH [8]. Similarly, healthy human controls have displayed cerebral vasospasm via transcranial Dopplers (TCDs) when given intravenous norepinephrine [9]. Thus, norepinephrine may not be a safe choice for MABP directed therapy in post-SAH symptomatic cerebral vasospasm.

Within this paper we describe two cases of DCI post-SAH with worsening neurological examination temporally related to elevation of norepinephrine doses during hypertensive therapy. These effects were ameliorated via discontinuation of norepinephrine and continuing intravenous phosphodiesterase inhibitor (PDEI) based therapy with milrinone.

2. Case Presentations

2.1. Case 1. A 43-year-old male with no significant past medical history presents to hospital with a 4-day history of headache, lethargy, and diplopia. Computed tomography (CT) of the brain demonstrated a Fisher grade 4 SAH; clinically he was Hunt and Hess grade 2 SAH. CT-angiography displayed a left posterior communicating artery aneurysm and left middle cerebral artery (MCA) vasospasm.

Clinically he had a partial oculomotor nerve palsy on the left and a significant headache. He was admitted, with plans for clipping of the aneurysm in the morning. Nimodipine prophylaxis was started. On postbleed day 5, he was seen on morning rounds neurologically unchanged, awaiting surgery. Within 30 minutes he developed progressive dysphasia, both receptive and expressive, with right hemineglect. Repeat CT head failed to display signs of aneurysmal rebleed. He received 2.5 liters of crystalloid and was transferred to the intensive care unit (ICU) for hypertensive therapy prior to going to the operative room (OR). Norepinephrine was started at 0.02 mcg/kg/min and titrated to 0.16 mcg/kg/min to achieve MABP of 130 mm Hg, as measured with the arterial line transducer zeroed at the tragus. Significant deterioration followed this titration of norepinephrine, progressing to right hemiplegia and aphasia.

The patient was then taken to the OR and the aneurysm was clipped successfully. Intraoperatively significant left MCA vasospasm was noted. The vessels were wiped with papaverine soaked gel foam. Mean arterial pressures were maintained between 130 and 140 mm Hg intraoperatively, with no hypotensive episodes noted in the anesthesia records.

Postoperatively in the ICU, the patient awoke with right hemiplegia, right homonymous hemianopsia, and aphasia while achieving the target MABP of 150 mm Hg with norepinephrine at 0.68 mcg/kg/min. It was elected to stop norepinephrine and start intravenous milrinone therapy 45 minutes after emergence from his general anesthetic. A 5 mg bolus of milrinone over 10 minutes was given, followed by a continuous infusion of 0.75 mcg/kg/min. Within 30 minutes of discontinuing the norepinephrine and starting milrinone all deficits, except the third nerve palsy, resolved. His MABP at this time was 95 mm Hg.

On postbleed day 6, after 24 hours of milrinone therapy and a stable neurological examination, he developed acute sensory extinction on the right side and hemianopsia. Milrinone was rebolused, and the infusion was increased to 1.5 mcg/kg/min with partial improvement in symptoms within 40 minutes. Mean arterial pressures at this time were 120 mm Hg. Given only a partial response to milrinone escalation, norepinephrine was restarted with a goal MABP of 140 mm Hg, and interventional neuroradiology was called for angioplasty. While waiting for angioplasty, the norepinephrine was titrated to 0.46 mcg/kg/min with progressive deterioration in the neurological examination leading to hemiplegia.

The angioplasty of a severely spastic left proximal MCA and anterior cerebral artery (ACA) was conducted without incident. The degree of spasm in these arterial segments was noted to be worse compared to previous CT-angiography. Distal small vessel spasm in the left MCA territory was noted as well during angioplasty.

After angioplasty he remained hemiparetic, with hemianopia and dysphasia, while the norepinephrine remained infusing with the goal of achieving MABP of 140 mm Hg. With no improvement in the next 48 hours, the norepinephrine was discontinued, while milrinone was continued at 1.5 mcg/kg/min with MABP around 90 to 110 mm Hg. The patient improved over the following hours after discontinuation of norepinephrine. Milrinone was then titrated down by 0.25 mcg/kg/day increments.

Currently, on postbleed day 25 he only has a partial third cranial nerve palsy and mild expressive language issues. Euvolemia was targeted throughout his entire course. No cardiac output monitoring was conducted throughout the patient's ICU stay.

2.2. Case 2. A 39-year-old female with a past medical history significant for polio, leaving her wheelchair bound secondary to lower extremity involvement, was admitted for a history of acute onset headache and mild confusion. She had a CT of the brain demonstrating a Fisher grade 4 SAH; clinically she was Hunt and Hess grade 2 SAH. Her CT-angiography demonstrated a right MCA aneurysm. She was taken to the OR for microsurgical clipping of the aneurysm and external ventricular drain (EVD) placement.

Postoperatively the patient did initially well. No focal deficits were noted postoperatively other than a partial left abducens palsy related to fluctuations in intracranial pressure (ICP).

On postbleed day 7 a follow-up CT-angiogram was performed displaying right MCA and ACA vasospasm, but the patient was clinically unaffected at that time. On postbleed day 8, significant diuresis and cerebral salt wasting were noted. On postbleed day 9 the patient developed left upper motor neuron (UMN) facial weakness and left arm paresis. She was taken to ICU for management of her DCI.

Milrinone therapy was initiated. Five milligrams of milrinone was bolused over 10 minutes, followed by a continuous infusion at 0.75 mcg/kg/min. She improved within 20 minutes to baseline. On postbleed day 11 she deteriorated again in a similar fashion. Milrinone was then rebolused, and the infusion was increased to 1.5 mcg/kg/min, leading to neurological improvement with minor residual pronator drift.

On postbleed day 13, neurological deterioration occurred again with now left UMN facial weakness and left arm paresis. Norepinephrine was started at 0.02 mcg/kg/min to target MABP of 140 mm Hg and interventional radiology was called for angioplasty. The proximal MCA and ACA were noted to be severely spastic and were the targets of angioplasty. These vessels appear as narrowed, compared to preangioplasty CT-angiography. Distal small vessel spasm was unchanged. The angioplasty occurred without incident and a good angiographic result was obtained.

Neurologically after angioplasty the patient's left arm was plegic. Norepinephrine was increased to 0.22 mcg/kg/min to target MABP of 150 mm Hg. Occasional episodes of improvement were seen in the left arm but not sustained. Episodes of symptomatic pulmonary edema began to develop during this phase of her treatment. An MRI was conducted displaying watershed diffusion weighted changes in the ACA/MCA and MCA/posterior cerebral artery (PCA) territories. There was some perfusion/diffusion mismatch noted, and thus aggressive MABP therapy was continued for these potentially salvageable areas. No improvement occurred over the following 72 hours.

Norepinephrine was then discontinued on postbleed day 16, with milrinone therapy running at 1.5 mcg/kg/min. The norepinephrine was discontinued given concerns over potential aggravation of cerebral vasoconstriction and the presence of maintained MABP goals on milrinone alone. No cardiac output monitoring was conducted during the patient's ICU stay. Within 12 hours of discontinuing norepinephrine, the patients left arm went from plegic to 4/5 strength in biceps, with 2-3/5 strength throughout the other muscles. Her left UMN facial weakness almost completely resolved during this time frame. Milrinone was then titrated off over the following day, as described in the first case.

Currently, on postbleed day 22 the patient has the same examination with mild left UMN facial weakness and the paretic left arm.

3. Discussion

Cerebral vessels are known to be innervated by nerves containing norepinephrine and 5-hydroxytryptamine (5-HT) [4]. Norepinephrine has been demonstrated in both animal and human autopsy specimens, to induce a dose mediated vasoconstrictive effect on cerebral vasculature [7].

Norepinephrine mediates vasoconstriction of cerebral vessels via two mechanisms. First, at low serum concentrations the alpha adrenergic mediated effects of norepinephrine lead to vasoconstriction. Second, at high concentrations, low-affinity sites [7] or gamma adrenoreceptor [8, 9] may be stimulated by norepinephrine leading to a much more pronounced cerebral vasoconstriction. These effects are seen in the proximal large cerebral vessels greater than in the smaller distal vessels [7].

In the setting of aneurysmal SAH, both serum and CSF norepinephrine levels have been demonstrated to be elevated [10, 11]. These serum [11] and CSF levels [10] seem to rise correlating with the severity of SAH and may be related to symptomatic cerebral vasospasm or just a marker of disease severity.

During hypertensive therapy for DCI post-SAH, a variety of vasopressors have been utilized, with norepinephrine displaying the most predictable hemodynamic response in traumatic brain injury as identified in recent literature [12–14]. However there are concerns of cerebral vasoconstriction with norepinephrine administration, as outlined above. Within the two cases described, we were able to temporally relate worsening of the neurological examination with escalating norepinephrine doses during the treatment of their DCI. Though no objective radiographic markers of worsening cerebral vasospasm were identified (other than during angioplasty in Case 1), the deterioration of the neurological examination was dramatic and partially/entirely reversible with discontinuation of the norepinephrine infusions. With the absence of cardiac output monitoring and objective measures of cerebral blood flow, we can only suggest the temporally related decompensation was potentially related to norepinephrine induced vasoconstriction. Furthermore, the potential utility of the PDEI milrinone via continuous intravenous infusions was displayed in both of these cases.

A few important points can be taken from both of these cases. First, MABP directed therapy for DCI postaneurysmal SAH can be challenging. It is not uncommon, as seen in both cases, that there exists a balancing act between symptomatic improvement with pharmacological alterations in cerebral blood flow and inducing systemic hemodynamic complications, such as pulmonary edema. Second, there seemed to be a norepinephrine dose related temporal change in both patients' neurological examinations. One patient displayed this deterioration with escalating norepinephrine both on and off milrinone therapy. The second patient displayed this effect while being on milrinone. Caution should be taken however, since the deteriorations seen may reflect either failure of hypertensive therapy (i.e., refractory DCI) or hypertension induced posterior reversible encephalopathy syndrome (PRES) related to escalating norepinephrine doses. Given the temporal relation between deterioration/improvement and norepinephrine doses, with neuroimaging failing to demonstrate features of PRES, we feel medication induced vasoconstriction is a real possibility. Third, this potential norepinephrine mediated deterioration is seemingly reversible to some extent, as seen when both patients had improvement in their neurological examination with discontinuation of norepinephrine. However, this improvement is clouded by the fact that both were on high dose intravenous infusions of milrinone at the time. Finally, the role of vasodilator therapy utilizing PDEI, such as milrinone, via continuous intravenous infusions is still undefined, though, in the two cases described and in existing literature [15], continuous infusions of milrinone have been shown to lead to neurological improvement in DCI post-SAH. The concerns over aggravation of cerebral vasospasm do not exist with milrinone, as they do with norepinephrine. Thus, maybe vasodilator therapies should be the front line for DCI post-SAH. Further study in this area is warranted.

There are significant limitations to our study. First, we only have two cases and this hardly is proof of concept that norepinephrine leads to worsening of DCI in SAH. This is further exemplified by the numerous other cases treated at both our institution and others, utilizing MABP directed therapy with norepinephrine, which have failed to display this response. This raises the point of a potential genetic driver of cerebrovascular response to particular vasopressors. Genetic polymorphisms within adrenoreceptors have been increasingly linked to hypertension and cardiovascular disease [16]. For example, the alpha 2B adrenergic insertion/deletion polymorphism has demonstrated greater degrees of peripheral vasoconstriction when stimulated with an alpha 2 agonist, dexmedetomidine, compared to controls [17]. Furthermore, this polymorphism has been linked to sudden cardiac death, presumably related to coronary vasospasm [18]. Similarly, alterations in the beta 2 adrenoreceptor have been linked to refractory hypertension, related to impaired vasodilatory effects when stimulated. Endothelin-1, angiotensin II, and nitric oxide-cGMP pathway polymorphisms have also been linked to altered adrenergic vascular reactivity and are associated with hypertension [16]. All of the mentioned polymorphisms could contribute to undesired cerebrovascular reactivity to adrenergic stimulation with vasopressor agents. However, insufficient data exists in the literature to date to make further comments on this. Second, the only data that we have to implicate norepinephrine in worsening cerebral vasospasm is the direct temporal relationship between administration of this drug and deterioration of the neurological examination. Only during angioplasty in Case 1 was the potential for worsening of proximal vasospasm, compared to CT-angiography, made. Though we suspect that this deterioration is related to worsening vasospasm, given the outlined mechanisms of action of norepinephrine on cerebral vasculature, we have no objective imaging evidence of this. The deterioration in these two cases could very well be a demonstration of failure of norepinephrine therapy in DCI or PRES (as previously mentioned), as opposed to worsening vasoconstriction related to norepinephrine. Potentially functional MRI or even Xenon enhanced CT would have shed more light on the matter. Similarly, cerebral microdialysis and cerebral blood flow catheters may have added some useful information about local metabolic changes with alterations in norepinephrine dosing. Finally, even though the response to intravenous PDEI therapy in these two cases was dramatic, it in no way proves superiority or equivalency to standard hypertensive therapy for DCI postaneurysmal SAH. Furthermore, with the absence of cardiac output monitoring during milrinone therapy in these cases, our goal with treatment was to titrate the medication doses to clinical improvement in the neurological examination, as per previously described protocols [15]. It is unknown what the particular hemodynamic changes were during this therapy, which may shed light on more objective targets with milrinone based therapy. Further prospective study with invasive/noninvasive determination of cardiac index during milrinone therapy for DCI is required.

In the setting of DCI post-SAH, hypertensive therapy with norepinephrine may lead to deterioration related to failure of therapy or medication induced vasoconstriction. Overall, we believe that norepinephrine carries the potential for aggravating DCI in certain patients. Prospective studies utilizing genetic profiling, multimodal intracranial monitoring, and neuroimaging need to be conducted in order to determine the effects of various vasopressors on cerebral metabolism and blood flow in post-SAH vasospasm. The role of milrinone in such cases, and for post-SAH vasospasm in general, carries potential and but has yet to be fully determined.

4. Conclusions

Hypertensive directed therapy for DCI post-SAH may not lead to symptomatic improvement and potentially may lead to neurological deterioration. Genetic drivers of cerebrovascular response to vasopressors may dictate potential neurological improvement during hypertensive therapy, and further prospective study is warranted utilizing genotyping, multimodal monitoring, and advanced neuroimaging. The role for intravenous vasodilators in post-SAH vasospasm has yet to be determined but is promising.

Authors' Contribution

J. Silvaggio, A. M. Kaufmann, and L. M. Gillman contributed equally to this work.

References

[1] M. N. Diringer, "Management of aneurysmal subarachnoid hemorrhage," *Critical Care Medicine*, vol. 37, no. 2, pp. 432–440, 2009.

[2] M. N. Diringer and Y. Axelrod, "Hemodynamic manipulation in the neuro-intensive care unit: cerebral perfusion pressure therapy in head injury and hemodynamic augmentation for cerebral vasospasm," *Current Opinion in Critical Care*, vol. 13, no. 2, pp. 156–162, 2007.

[3] A. M. Bauer and P. A. Rasmussen, "Treatment of intracranial vasospasm following subarachnoid hemorrhage," *Frontiers in Neurology*, vol. 5, article 72, 2014.

[4] J. Lincoln, "Innervation of cerebral arteries by nerves containing 5-hydroxytryptamine and noradrenaline," *Pharmacology & Therapeutics*, vol. 68, no. 3, pp. 473–501, 1995.

[5] Y. Liu, X. Yang, H. Gong et al., "Assessing the effects of norepinephrine on single cerebral microvessels using optical-resolution photoacoustic microscope," *Journal of Biomedical Optics*, vol. 18, no. 7, Article ID 076007, 2013.

[6] R. D. Lobato, J. Marin, M. Salaices, F. Rivilla, and J. Burgos, "Cerebrovascular reactivity to noradrenaline and serotonin following experimental subarachnoid hemorrhage," *Journal of Neurosurgery*, vol. 53, no. 4, pp. 480–485, 1980.

[7] J. W. Duckworth, G. C. Wellman, C. L. Walters, and J. A. Bevan, "Aminergic histofluorescence and contractile responses to transmural electrical field stimulation and norepinephrine of human middle cerebral arteries obtained promptly after death," *Circulation Research*, vol. 65, no. 2, pp. 316–324, 1989.

[8] G. D. S. Hirst and T. O. Neild, "Evidence for two populations of excitatory receptors for noradrenaline on arteriolar smooth muscle," *Nature*, vol. 283, no. 5749, pp. 767–768, 1980.

[9] G. D. S. Hirst and T. O. Neild, "Localization of specialized noradrenaline receptors at neuromuscular junctions on arterioles of the guinea-pig," *Journal of Physiology*, vol. 313, pp. 343–350, 1981.

[10] T. Shigeno, "Norepinephrine in cerebrospinal fluid of patients with cerebral vasospasm," *Journal of Neurosurgery*, vol. 56, no. 3, pp. 344–349, 1982.

[11] A. B. Loach and C. R. Benedict, "Plasma catecholamine concentrations associated with cerebral vasospasm," *Journal of the Neurological Sciences*, vol. 45, no. 2-3, pp. 261–271, 1980.

[12] D. Pfister, S. P. Strebel, and L. A. Steiner, "Effects of catecholamines on cerebral blood vessels in patients with traumatic brain injury," *European Journal of Anaesthesiology*, vol. 25, no. 42, pp. 98–103, 2008.

[13] L. A. Steiner, A. J. Johnston, M. Czosnyka et al., "Direct comparison of cerebrovascular effects of norepinephrine and dopamine in head-injured patients," *Critical Care Medicine*, vol. 32, no. 4, pp. 1049–1054, 2004.

[14] S.-N. Kroppenstedt, U.-W. Thomale, M. Griebenow et al., "Effects of early and late intravenous norepinephrine infusion on cerebral perfusion, microcirculation, brain-tissue oxygenation, and edema formation in brain-injured rats," *Critical Care Medicine*, vol. 31, no. 8, pp. 2211–2221, 2003.

[15] M. Lannes, J. Teitelbaum, M. del Pilar Cortés, M. Cardoso, and M. Angle, "Milrinone and homeostasis to treat cerebral vasospasm associated with subarachnoid hemorrhage: the Montreal Neurological Hospital protocol," *Neurocritical Care*, vol. 16, no. 3, pp. 354–362, 2012.

[16] D. Henrion, J. Benessiano, M. Iglarz, I. Philip, and B. I. Levy, "Genetic determinants of vascular reactivity," *Current Hypertension Reports*, vol. 4, no. 1, pp. 41–48, 2002.

[17] P. Talke, C. Stapelfeldt, E. Lobo, R. Brown, M. Scheinin, and A. Snapir, "Alpha-2B adrenoceptor polymorphism and peripheral vasoconstriction," *Pharmacogenetics and Genomics*, vol. 15, no. 5, pp. 357–363, 2005.

[18] J. A. Laukkanen, T. H. Mäkikallio, J. Kauhanen, and S. Kurl, "Insertion/deletion polymorphism in α_2-adrenergic receptor gene is a genetic risk factor for sudden cardiac death," *American Heart Journal*, vol. 158, no. 4, pp. 615–621, 2009.

9

Spontaneous Dissection of the Renal Artery in Vascular Ehlers-Danlos Syndrome

Filipa Pereira,[1] Teresa Cardoso,[2] and Paula Sá[1]

[1]*Serviço de Anestesiologia, Centro Hospitalar do Porto, Largo Professor Abel Salazar, 4099-001 Porto, Portugal*
[2]*Unidade de Cuidados Intensivos Polivalente, Centro Hospitalar do Porto, Largo Professor Abel Salazar, 4099-001 Porto, Portugal*

Correspondence should be addressed to Filipa Pereira; filipapdspereira@gmail.com

Academic Editor: Matej Podbregar

Ehlers-Danlos syndrome (EDS) is a rare heterogeneous group of connective tissue disorders. The vascular type (vEDS) is an autosomal dominant disorder caused by heterozygous mutations in the *COL3A1* gene predisposing to premature arterial, intestinal, or uterine rupture. We report a case of a 38-year-old woman with a recent diagnosis of vEDS admitted in the Emergency Department with a suspicion of a pyelonephritis that evolved to a cardiopulmonary arrest. A fatal retroperitoneal hematoma related with a haemorrhagic dissection of the right renal artery was found after emergency surgery. This case highlights the need to be aware of the particular characteristics of vEDS, such as a severe vascular complication that can lead to a fatal outcome.

1. Introduction

Ehlers-Danlos syndrome (EDS) is a rare heterogeneous group of connective tissue disorders [1]. The estimated prevalence varies between 1/5000 and 1/25000 [1, 2].

The *vascular type* (vEDS), formerly known as EDS type IV [3], is an autosomal dominant disorder caused by heterozygous mutations in the *COL3A1* [4]. Vascular EDS compromises 5–10% of all cases of EDS [4, 5]. The clinical hallmark of vEDS is excessive tissue fragility predisposing to premature arterial, intestinal, or uterine rupture, rarely observed in other forms of EDS [4, 6]. vEDS is also marked clinically by a characteristic facial appearance with decreased subcutaneous fat, a narrow nose, and thin lips and thin skin with visible superficial veins and prominent cutaneous bruising. Patients can also present premature aging of distal extremities (acrogeria) and joint hypermobility [5, 7]. However, these phenotype characteristics can be subtle and may not be diagnosed until postmortem examination [4, 5]. Furthermore, the natural course of vEDS and the clinical phenotype of patients are influenced by the type of COL3A1 variant [8].

A full differential diagnosis must be considered when the presenting signs and symptoms suggest vEDS. This includes *Marfan syndrome*, *Loeys-Dietz syndrome*, kyphoscoliotic types of EDS, idiopathic isolated arterial aneurysms, and autosomal dominant polycystic kidney disease. Clinical features, radiologic findings, and genetic characterization allow the clinical diagnosis and management [9–11].

Approximately 25% of patients with the vEDS experience the first complication by the age of 20, while 80% of patients have at least one complication by the age of 40 [6]. The median survival described in literature varies between 48 and 50 years [4, 6].

Treatment of complications associated with vEDS favours minimal noninvasive interventions. Invasive methods should be used only when necessary, primarily to save the patients' life [12].

We report a case of a 38-year-old woman with vEDS, who died during emergency surgery due to a severe vascular complication.

2. Case Presentation

A 38-year-old woman was admitted in the Emergency Department (ED) with a sudden onset of severe lower back pain, fever, nausea, and vomiting. The patient had a history of

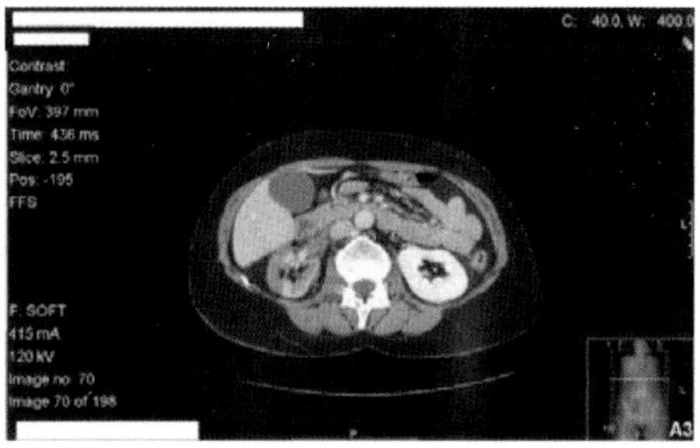

Figure 1: Abdominal Computer Tomography (CT) scan showing diffuse reduction in the parenchymal thickness of the right kidney and multiloculated fluid collection of about 10 centimetres (cm), involving the anterior part and the upper pole of the right kidney and the ipsilateral renal artery.

repeated urinary infections and renal lithiasis. She was being studied in the genetic department because of her history of infertility and spontaneous abortions and also because of the history of sudden deaths in her family (including her father). Therefore, she was diagnosed recently as having vEDS with a mutation in *COLA31* gene, but the specific defect was not mentioned in her genetic report.

On admission, her physical examination revealed translucid skin, thinned nose, and joint hypermobility of the lower limbs.

She had haemoglobin (Hg) of 13 g/dL, leukocytosis (16 × 10^9/L), an elevated C-reactive protein (54 mg/dL), and inactive urinary sediment.

The renal ultrasound showed perirenal fluid and signs of nephritis but without obstruction.

The Abdominal Computer Tomography (CT) scan (Figure 1) showed a diffuse reduction in the parenchymal thickness of the right kidney and multiple areas of *striatum* nephrogram, suggesting an inflammatory/infectious process (pyelonephritis). It also showed a multiloculated fluid collection of about 10 centimetres (cm), involving the anterior part and the upper pole of the right kidney and the ipsilateral renal artery, which appeared tapered and with a reduced calibre.

In between several exams, she was found unconscious in the clinical observation area of the ED and was taken to the Emergency Room (ER) in pulmonary arrest that rapidly evolved to cardiac arrest, from which she recovered with advanced life support in 10 minutes.

After initial stabilization in the ER, it was assumed that this clinical situation was due to a renal abscess, as shown in CT scan. A renal abscess drainage in the operating room was immediately proposed for her.

On arrival to the OR, she presented again in cardiopulmonary arrest in a nonshockable rhythm (pulseless electrical activity). Advanced life support (ALS) was started immediately.

The decision to perform an exploratory laparotomy, while in ALS manoeuvres, was taken and a team of vascular and urologic surgeons started together the procedure.

During surgery, a massive retroperitoneal hematoma was found, being largest at the left side. The infrarenal aorta was isolated but was found pulseless and empty. With the clamping of the supra- and infrarenal aorta no active haemorrhage was identified.

ALS manoeuvres were stopped 30 minutes after the beginning of surgery in the light of these findings and lack of any clinical response to massive transfusion measures.

Request for a clinical autopsy was obtained.

Autopsy Findings. The victim was a normally developed 38-year-old woman with apparent age superior to her real age. The skin of her knees was flaccid and pigmented and she had an articular hypermobility.

Internal findings included a hematoma in the top and posterior face of the right kidney which extended until the exterior of the renal capsule. There were multiple thrombosed renal vessels of medium and large calibre in the renal hilum, some of which presented a haemorrhagic dissection between the intimal and media arterial walls, sometimes with thrombosed pseudo lumens.

In all vascular territories the arterial walls presented morphological alterations of the intimal and media layers, namely, duplication and disruption of the internal elastic lamina, intimal nodular proliferation, and a media layer with thickening and thinning areas.

In These characteristics were suggestive of intimal and media fibromuscular dysplasia.

3. Discussion

Vascular EDS is a very challenging disorder. Therefore, it is important to suspect a severe vascular complication in a patient with a history of vEDS that presents in the ED with unspecific symptoms. These patients should be investigated promptly to rule out life-threatening situations due to vascular complications involving the vascular system, gastrointestinal tract, or gravid uterus [2, 6]. The vascular type of EDS describes a defect in the synthesis of type III procollagen and is the most severe form. Rupture of a previously nondilated artery is a common occurrence that results in considerable mortality and morbidity. Less commonly, an artery can dissect or dilate in either focal or diffuse form.

Therefore, patients with vEDS have a reduced life expectancy due to severe vascular complications. In a series of 31 patients, 61% present with at least one life-threatening vascular complication before the age of 40 [13].

An acute low back/flank pain is a common complaint in young adult presented to the ED and is usually due to a musculoskeletal or genitourinary tract cause. In our patient the exams showed an inflammatory/infectious process which was a likely diagnosis according to her past medical history of renal lithiasis. However, her recent diagnosis of vEDS was initially neglected and only because of a rapid hemodynamic deterioration was a surgical approach decided. There was a lack of communication among the medical staff, as the doctors responsible for the patient in the ED did not find her past medical history of vEDS important for this situation and this was not transmitted to the doctor responsible for the Emergency Room (ER) or to the radiologist responsible for the report of her abdominal CT scan. It is extremely important for radiologists to know if the patient has a collagen vascular disease when ordering the exam. There has to be more awareness about this syndrome among doctors and health staff working on the ED so that such situations can be minimized and a suspicious attitude could be adopted by every personnel that takes care of patients with vEDS. We have to remember that the incidence of this disease is very low (5% of all EDS patients) which means that most surgeons will never, or perhaps only once, meet a patient with the disease [12].

Patients with vEDS have unpredictable clinical courses and management is always challenging as they have high operative mortality rates. Therefore, we will never know if the course of our patient would have been different if a more suspicious attitude took place and all of the team responsible for the patient knew the disease and the complications involved. Nevertheless, we have to be aware of a severe vascular complication when receiving a vEDS patient in the ED.

A *disease specific passport* would be very helpful in these kinds of diseases where severe complications could be present and special attention and care are needed when these patients are in the ED. In the case reported, it would have been very helpful and could have alerted the physicians to have a more careful approach in patient's evaluation and care.

The autopsy revealed a retroperitoneal hematoma related with a haemorrhagic dissection of the right renal artery. This was probably due to the vascular malformation of fibromuscular dysplasia type. Although fibromuscular dysplasia is a different entity, patients with vEDS may have stenosis of renal and visceral arteries that mimic fibromuscular dysplasia. The diagnosis of these conditions relies on associated phenotypic traits and genetic tests: acrogeric dysmorphy, distal joint laxity, and tiny skin elasticity in vEDS, confirmed by detection of *COL3A1* gene mutations [14].

Regarding the treatment in vEDS, the most recent literature points to a rate of 29% mortality due to open and endovascular procedures less than the rates published in older studies [12, 13]. All invasive procedures should be avoided as far as possible as surgery can lead to vascular catastrophes and even death [13, 15]. A conservative approach or minimal invasive procedures should be preferred in these cases. Furthermore, the excessive rate of arterial complications in the past in endovascular procedures is believed to be related to large-diameter sheaths and devices used in prior decades. However, the prognosis after treatment is poor and invasive methods should be used only when necessary to save the patient's life [12].

There is no validated medical therapy in primary prevention of cardiovascular events in presymptomatic vEDS patients. The only medical therapy available is celiprolol, a $\beta 1$-adrenoreceptor antagonist with a $\beta 2$-adrenoreceptor agonist action. The only multicenter randomized trial by Ong et al., 2010, showed an effective prevention of major complications in patients with vEDS, with a reduction in arterial events (rupture or dissection) by three times compared with no treatment. Nevertheless, there is no indication that the benefit of celiprolol is a class effect and the question of beta blocker treatment remains open [16].

In summary, vEDS is associated with severe vascular complications in relatively young patients. We presented a case of a patient with vEDS with a fatal outcome and a misleading diagnosis after a spontaneous dissection of the renal artery.

References

[1] M. Zilocchi, T. A. Macedo, G. S. Oderich, T. J. Vrtiska, P. R. Biondetti, and A. W. Stanson, "Vascular Ehlers-Danlos syndrome: imaging findings," *American Journal of Roentgenology*, vol. 189, no. 3, pp. 712–719, 2007.

[2] P. Morais, A. Mota, C. Eloy et al., "Vascular Ehlers-Danlos Syndrome: a case with fatal outcome," *Dermatology Online Journal*, vol. 17, no. 4, article 1, 2011.

[3] P. Beighton, A. De Paepe, B. Steinmann, P. Tsipouras, and R. J. Wenstrup, "Ehlers-danlos syndromes: revised nosology, Villefranche, 1997," *American Journal of Medical Genetics*, vol. 77, no. 1, pp. 31–37, 1998.

[4] D. P. Germain, "Ehlers-Danlos syndrome type IV," *Orphanet Journal of Rare Diseases*, vol. 2, no. 1, article 32, 2007.

[5] E. J. Mortani Barbosa, R. E. Pyeritz, H. Litt, and B. Desjardins, "Vascular Ehlers-Danlos syndrome presenting as rapidly progressive multiple arterial aneurysms and dissections," *American Journal of Medical Genetics, Part A*, vol. 155, no. 12, pp. 3090–3094, 2011.

[6] L. B. E. Shields, C. M. Rolf, G. J. Davis, and J. C. Hunsaker III, "Sudden and unexpected death in three cases of Ehlers-Danlos syndrome type IV," *Journal of Forensic Sciences*, vol. 55, no. 6, pp. 1641–1645, 2010.

[7] A. de Paepe and F. Malfait, "The Ehlers-Danlos syndrome, a disorder with many faces," *Clinical Genetics*, vol. 82, no. 1, pp. 1–11, 2012.

[8] M. Frank, J. Albuisson, B. Ranque et al., "The type of variants at the COL3A1 gene associates with the phenotype and severity of vascular Ehlers-Danlos syndrome," *European Journal of Human Genetics*, 2015.

[9] B. Callewaert, F. Malfait, B. Loeys, and A. de Paepe, "Ehlers-Danlos syndromes and Marfan syndrome," *Best Practice and Research: Clinical Rheumatology*, vol. 22, no. 1, pp. 165–189, 2008.

[10] L. van Laer, H. Dietz, and B. Loeys, "Loeys-dietz syndrome," *Advances in Experimental Medicine and Biology*, vol. 802, pp. 95–105, 2014.

[11] A. Abayazeed, E. Hayman, M. Moghadamfalahi, and D. Cain, "Vascular type Ehlers-Danlos Syndrome with fatal spontaneous rupture of a right common iliac artery dissection: case report and review of literature," *Journal of Radiology Case Reports*, vol. 8, no. 2, pp. 63–69, 2014.

[12] D. Bergqvist, M. Björck, and A. Wanhainen, "Treatment of vascular Ehlers-Danlos syndrome: a systematic review," *Annals of Surgery*, vol. 258, no. 2, pp. 257–261, 2013.

[13] G. S. Oderich, J. M. Panneton, T. C. Bower et al., "The spectrum, management and clinical outcome of Ehlers-Danlos syndrome type IV: a 30-year experience," *Journal of Vascular Surgery*, vol. 42, no. 1, pp. 98–106, 2005.

[14] P.-F. Plouin, J. Perdu, A. la Batide-Alanore, P. Boutouyrie, A.-P. Gimenez-Roqueplo, and X. Jeunemaitre, "Fibromuscular dysplasia," *Orphanet Journal of Rare Diseases*, vol. 2, article 28, 2007.

[15] Y. Iida, Y. Obitsu, H. Komai, and H. Shigematsu, "Successful coil embolization for rupture of the subclavian artery associated with Ehlers-Danlos syndrome type IV," *Journal of Vascular Surgery*, vol. 50, no. 5, pp. 1191–1195, 2009.

[16] K.-T. Ong, J. Perdu, J. de Backer et al., "Effect of celiprolol on prevention of cardiovascular events in vascular Ehlers-Danlos syndrome: a prospective randomised, open, blinded-endpoints trial," *The Lancet*, vol. 376, no. 9751, pp. 1476–1484, 2010.

10

Takotsubo Cardiomyopathy in the Setting of Tension Pneumothorax

Michael Gale,[1] Pablo Loarte,[2] Brooks Mirrer,[1,3] Thierry Mallet,[1] Louis Salciccioli,[4] Alison Petrie,[5] and Ronny Cohen[1,3]

[1]*Division of Cardiology, Department of Medicine, Woodhull Medical Center, 760 Broadway, Suite 3B320, Brooklyn, NY 11206, USA*
[2]*Department of Medicine, Yale-New Haven Hospital, 20 York Street, CB2041, New Haven, CT 06510, USA*
[3]*NYU School of Medicine, 550 First Avenue, New York, NY 10016, USA*
[4]*Division of Cardiology, Department of Medicine, SUNY Downstate Medical Center, 450 Clarkson Avenue, Brooklyn, NY 11203, USA*
[5]*Saint George's University School of Medicine, 3500 Sunrise Highway, Great River, NY 11739, USA*

Correspondence should be addressed to Ronny Cohen; ronny.cohen@nychhc.org

Academic Editor: Chiara Lazzeri

Background. Takotsubo cardiomyopathy is defined as a transient left ventricular dysfunction, usually accompanied by electrocardiographic changes. The literature documents only two other cases of Takotsubo cardiomyopathy in the latter setting. *Methods.* A 78-year-old female presented to the ED with severe shortness of breath, hypertension, and tachycardia. On physical exam, heart sounds (S1 and S2) were regular and wheezing was noticed bilaterally. We found laboratory results with a WBC of 20.0 (103/μL), troponin of 16.52 ng/mL, CK-mb of 70.6%, and BNP of 177 pg/mL. The patient was intubated for acute hypoxemic respiratory failure. A chest X-ray revealed a large left-sided tension pneumothorax. Initial echocardiogram showed apical ballooning with a LVEF of 10–15%. A cardiac angiography revealed normal coronary arteries with no coronary disease. After supportive treatment, the patient's condition improved with a subsequent echocardiogram showing a LVEF of 60%. *Conclusion.* The patient was found to have Takotsubo cardiomyopathy in the setting of a tension pneumothorax. The exact mechanisms of ventricular dysfunction have not been clarified. However, multivessel coronary spasm or catecholamine cardiotoxicity has been suggested to have a causative role. We suggest that, in our patient, left ventricular dysfunction was induced by the latter mechanism related to the stress associated with acute pneumothorax.

1. Introduction

Takotsubo cardiomyopathy (TCM) is a unique transient form of cardiomyopathy frequently precipitated by a stressful event and has a clinical presentation similar to that of a myocardial infarction. This syndrome was first described by Sato et al. in 1990 [1] and has been increasingly reported in the literature. Various terminologies have been used, such as apical ballooning syndrome, stress-induced cardiomyopathy, and broken heart syndrome. However, Sharkey et al. [2] proposed the universal use of Takotsubo cardiomyopathy, which is now generally accepted.

The typical clinical features of TCM include chest pain and dyspnea [3, 4]. Postmenopausal women who recently went through a stressful event are most commonly affected [5]. Electrocardiographic findings may include transient ST-segment elevation and laboratory findings, a modest rise in cardiac troponin levels [3]. In the typical or most common variant, there is hypokinesis or akinesis of the mid and apical segments of the left ventricle and sparing of the basal ventricular segments seen on echocardiogram or left ventriculogram [3].

Uniquely, coronary angiography reveals no evidence of obstructive coronary disease or plaque rupture. Various criteria need to be met in order to make the diagnosis of TCM. They were recently revised and termed the Mayo Clinic Criteria [3, 4] (see *the Current Mayo Clinic Criteria for Takotsubo Cardiomyopathy*). Complications such as congestive heart failure have been reported. However the overall prognosis of TCM is good, as spontaneous recovery is found in most patients who are treated supportively.

Current Mayo Clinic Criteria for Takotsubo Cardiomyopathy [2, 3] are as follows.

(1) Transient hypokinesia, akinesia, or dyskinesia in the left ventricular mid segments with or without apical involvement; regional wall motion abnormalities that usually extend beyond a single epicardial vascular distribution; and frequently, but not always, a stressful trigger.

(2) The absence of obstructive coronary disease or angiographic evidence of acute plaque rupture. (*Some patients with TCM can exhibit some degree of coronary artery disease.*)

(3) New ECG abnormalities (ST-segment elevations and/or T-wave inversion) or modest elevation in cardiac troponin.

(4) Absence of pheochromocytoma and myocarditis.

The pathophysiology has not been clearly described. Catecholamine cardiotoxicity remains the most common explanation [3]. Broad arrays of clinical conditions have been reported as triggers of TCM and investigating these may improve our understanding of the pathophysiology. The triggers include severe emotional stress, physical stress including central nervous system pathology, severe illness, drug use/withdrawal, and severe pain [3, 4]. Here we report a case of TCM in the setting of a severely painful tension pneumothorax.

2. Case Report

A 78-year-old female with a past medical history of diabetes mellitus type II, hypertension, osteoporosis, and asthma was brought into the emergency department by ambulance with severe shortness of breath. She was afebrile, tachypneic (respiratory rate of 28 rpm), with an elevated blood pressure of 185/105 mmHg and heart rate of 111 beats per minute. Her chest X-ray revealed a large left-sided tension pneumothorax. Because of impending respiratory failure, she was intubated and placed on mechanical ventilation. A chest tube was inserted with subsequent reexpansion of the left lung. The patient was admitted to the intensive care unit for monitoring. Cardiac biomarker, troponin I, was found to be elevated at 16.529 ng/mL (reference range: ≤0.1 ng/mL). Serial Electrocardiograms (ECGs) done over the course of 12 hours demonstrated sinus bradycardia, alternating with sinus tachycardia and normal sinus rhythm. Anterior Q waves were seen, along with dynamic T-wave changes and transient ST-segment elevation was also noted in the lateral leads. Transthoracic echocardiogram revealed global left ventricular hypokinesis sparing the basal segments, apical ballooning, and severe systolic dysfunction with an estimated left ventricular ejection fraction (LVEF) of 13% (Figure 1).

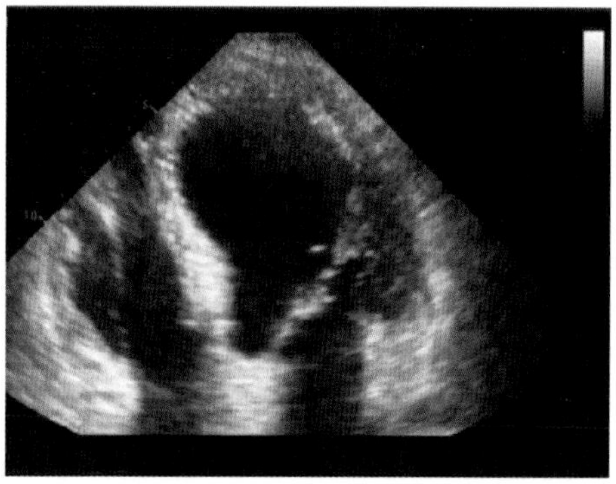

FIGURE 1: Echocardiogram with severely decreased EF of 13% and possible stress cardiomyopathy. PAP systolic 40 mmHg. Apical ballooning involving all left ventricular (LV) wall.

The patient was treated with aspirin, clopidogrel, a statin, and Ramipril and was subsequently transferred to another facility for cardiac catheterization. Coronary angiography revealed normal left and right coronary artery systems and no evidence of coronary artery disease (Figure 2). She was treated supportively and her condition improved over the next few weeks. A transthoracic echocardiogram performed 12 days later revealed no left ventricular dilation, resolved wall motion abnormality, and a significantly improved LVEF of 60%.

3. Discussion

The prevalence of TCM has been estimated to range from 1.7 to 2.2 percent of cases presenting with suspected acute coronary syndrome (ACS) [5–9]. TCM is much more common in elderly women with 80–100% of cases being female [10–13] and the mean age of presentation being 61 to 76 years [12]. Our patient fits these demographics, as she is an elderly postmenopausal female who was originally thought to be suffering from stress-induced acute coronary syndrome.

The clinical presentation of TCM is similar to that of an acute ST-segment elevation myocardial infarction (STEMI) [4, 6, 10, 14], with the most common presenting symptoms being acute substernal chest pain, dyspnea, nausea, and vomiting [4, 6]. We were unable to elicit these classic symptoms from our patient as she was sedated and intubated. The ECG and laboratory values were the clues that prompted cardiac concern.

The most common ECG finding in TCM is ST-segment elevation. Pawlak et al. compared the presentation between women who present with STEMI or TCM and found that the ST-segment was elevated in 70% of the TCM cases [14]. Other ECG findings included ST-segment depression (9.7%) and dynamic T-wave changes (17%) [14]. Other reported late ECG findings include development of diffuse T-wave inversion, prolongation of the QT interval, and rare, transient development of pathological Q waves [3, 10]. Our patient demonstrated the majority of these ECG changes, with transient ST-segment elevation, dynamic T-wave changes,

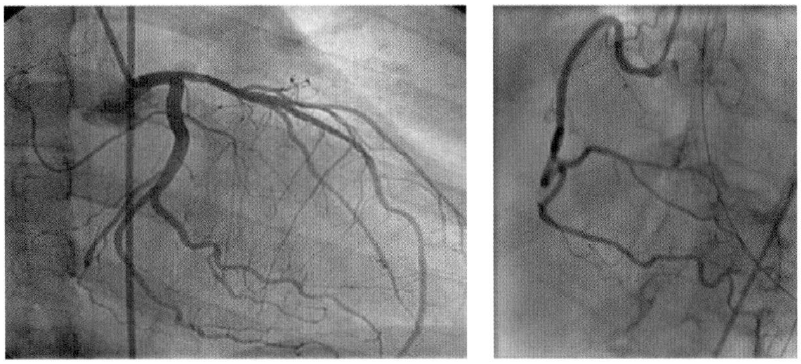

(a) Left coronary artery (b) Right coronary artery

FIGURE 2: Cardiac catheterization revealing normal coronary arteries.

pathological Q waves in leads I and aVL, and borderline QT prolongation.

Additionally, cardiac biomarkers are found to be modestly elevated in TCM. Pawlak et al. found that the median troponin I values for TCM patients are 2.99 ± 5.36 ng/mL compared to a median value of 42.70 ± 64.79 ng/mL in the STEMI patients [14]. Our patient had a peak troponin I value of 16.529 ng/mL, which is higher than the median value found in the literature, but significantly lower than the median value found in the patients having a STEMI. The Mayo Clinic Criteria describe a "modest" rise of cardiac biomarkers [3].

Echocardiography and left ventriculography demonstrate the characteristic regional wall motion abnormalities that define TCM. In the most common and classic variant there is hypokinesis or akinesis of the mid and apical segments of the left ventricle and sparing of the basal systolic function with the wall motion abnormality typically extending beyond the distribution of a single coronary artery [3]. LVEF is significantly reduced, mimicking an acute MI. In the study done by Pawlak et al., it was found that both patients suffering from a STEMI and TCM had a lower LVEF at initial presentation; however, follow-up echocardiograms demonstrated a significantly higher LVEF in the TCM patients than those who had STEMI [14]. Our patient's echocardiogram performed 12 days later demonstrated resolved wall motion abnormalities, no apical ballooning, and a normal LVEF of 60%, consistent with the transient nature of TCM.

4. Risk Factors and Pathogenesis

The unique feature of TCM is the occurrence of a preceding emotional or physical stressful event. In one study done at the Mayo Clinic, 98% of cases were found to have a preceding trigger [12, 15]. Documented emotional triggers are vast and include but are not limited to death or severe illness of a loved one, receiving bad news, divorce, relocation, and natural disasters [3]. Reported physical stressors are also very nonspecific and include surgery (cholecystectomy, hysterectomy), severe illness (asthma, chronic obstructive airway exacerbation, acute cholecystitis, pseudomembranous colitis, cocaine use, opiate withdrawal, and thyrotoxicosis), iatrogenic cases (dobutamine stress echo, exercise stress test), and severe pain (bone fracture, renal colic, pulmonary embolism, and pneumothorax) [3, 4]. Our patient presented in severe pain associated with a tension pneumothorax.

The exact mechanisms of transient left ventricular dysfunction have been disputed with the most commonly discussed possible one being catecholamine cardiotoxicity and the second most common being multivessel coronary spasm [16]. Other proposed factors include a genetic predisposition [17] or a protective role of estrogen as postmenopausal females are most likely at risk [18]. In the present patient, evidence of coronary vascular spasm was excluded by the negative coronary angiogram performed at the time of ST-segment elevation. As mentioned before, this patient is postmenopausal and family history of TCM was not elicited. It is our belief that the TCM in this patient was induced by an increase in catecholamines caused by the stress and pain resulting from tension pneumothorax. A review literature revealed that only one case of TCM triggered by a pneumothorax had been reported [19].

5. Diagnosis

The diagnosis of TCM should be considered in the differential diagnosis of a patient presenting with suspected acute coronary syndrome (ACS), especially postmenopausal females. The Mayo Clinic Criteria for the diagnosis of TCM (see *the Current Mayo Clinic Criteria for Takotsubo Cardiomyopathy*) are very helpful to evaluate and aid in management for patients with a suspicion of TCM [3]. Our patient met all four Mayo Clinic Criteria and was confirmed to have TCM.

Diagnosis is established with ECG and echocardiogram, with the latest one being the most practical imaging technique. Cardiac magnetic resonance (CMR), although not used in this case, is an emerging tool which can be used for differentiating TCM from myocardial infarction. CMR can evaluate possible ischemic damage and more accurately visualize the extent of ventricular dysfunction [3]. The only con is its limited availability and low tolerance in a number of patients making this study more like a complimentary imaging study able to provide additional information in a subset of patients with a nonclear clinical course [20].

6. Treatment and Prognosis

Although optimal management of TCM has not been established and spontaneous recovery of the cardiac function follows, it is important to treat the patient for possible ACS. At time of presentation, TCM will mimic ACS, and initial management should be directed towards management and support as if it is an acute myocardial infarction (AMI). Once the diagnosis of TCM is confirmed, with supportive care, cardiac recovery usually takes no longer than 4 to 8 weeks [3]. As mentioned previously it took our present patient less than 2 weeks to recover spontaneously with supportive therapy alone.

A number of complications have been seen in the acute phase of the disease and some studies have reported an in-hospital mortality of around 2%. Some recurrence has been documented also [19].

7. Conclusion

Takotsubo cardiomyopathy is a distinct reversible cardiomyopathy resulting from the effects of stress. Since it generally mimics ACS it should be included in the differential diagnosis of ACS, especially if the patient is a postmenopausal female. It is important to identify the presence of emotional or physical stressors, including conditions that can cause severe pain such as tension pneumothorax in the case described. This diagnosis can only be made after proof of recovery has been obtained, stressing the need to carefully explain to our patients the importance of clinical follow-up.

Authors' Contribution

The authors listed originally prepared all materials. The authors listed have contributed to, read, and approved the paper.

References

[1] H. Sato, H. Tateishi, T. Uchida, K. Dote, M. Ishihara, and K. Sasaki, "Tako-tsubo-like left ventricular dysunction due to multivessel coronary spasm," in *Clinical Aspect of Myocardial Injury: From Ischemia to Heart Failure*, K. Kodama, K. Haze, and M. Hori, Eds., pp. 56–64, Kagakuhyoronsha, Tokoyo, Japan, 1990.

[2] S. Sharkey, J. Lesser, M. Maron, and B. Maron, "Why not just call it Tako-Tsubo cardiomyopathy," *Journal of the American College of Cardiology*, vol. 57, no. 13, pp. 1496–1497, 2011.

[3] A. Prasad, A. Lerman, and C. S. Rihal, "Apical ballooning syndrome (Tako-Tsubo or stress cardiomyopathy): a mimic of acute myocardial infarction," *American Heart Journal*, vol. 155, no. 3, pp. 408–417, 2008.

[4] K. A. Bybee, T. Kara, A. Prasad et al., "Systematic review: Transient left ventricular apical ballooning: a syndrome that mimics ST-segment elevation myocardial infarction," *Annals of Internal Medicine*, vol. 141, no. 11, pp. 858–865, 2004.

[5] M. Gianni, F. Dentali, A. M. Grandi, G. Sumner, R. Hiralal, and E. Lonn, "Apical ballooning syndrome or takotsubo cardiomyopathy: a systematic review," *European Heart Journal*, vol. 27, no. 13, pp. 1523–1529, 2006.

[6] S. Azzarelli, A. R. Galassi, F. Amico et al., "Clinical characteristics and thrombolysis in myocardial infarction frame counts in women with transient left ventricular apical ballooning syndrome," *American Journal of Cardiology*, vol. 94, no. 3, pp. 343–346, 2004.

[7] K. Ito, H. Sugihara, S. Katoh, A. Azuma, and M. Nakagawa, "Assessment of Takotsubo (ampulla) cardiomyopathy using 99mTc-tetrofosmin myocardial SPECT-comparison with acute coronary syndrome," *Annals of Nuclear Medicine*, vol. 17, no. 2, pp. 115–122, 2003.

[8] Y. J. Akashi, K. Nakazawa, M. Sakakibara, F. Miyake, H. Musha, and K. Sasaka, "123I-MIBG myocardial scintigraphy in patients with 'takotsubo' cardiomyopathy," *Journal of Nuclear Medicine*, vol. 45, no. 7, pp. 1121–1127, 2004.

[9] K. Matsuoka, S. Okubo, E. Fujii et al., "Evaluation of the arrhythmogenecity of stress-induced 'takotsubo cardiomyopathy' from the time course of the 12-lead surface electrocardiogram," *The American Journal of Cardiology*, vol. 92, no. 2, pp. 230–233, 2003.

[10] K. Tsuchihashi, K. Ueshima, T. Uchida et al., "Transient left ventricular apical ballooning without coronary artery stenosis: a novel heart syndrome mimicking acute myocardial infarction," *Journal of the American College of Cardiology*, vol. 38, no. 1, pp. 11–18, 2001.

[11] S. W. Sharkey, J. R. Lesser, A. G. Zenovich et al., "Acute and reversible cardiomyopathy provoked by stress in women from the United States," *Circulation*, vol. 111, no. 4, pp. 472–479, 2005.

[12] Y. J. Akashi, D. S. Goldstein, G. Barbara, and T. Ueyama, "Takotsubo cardiomyopathy a new form of acute, reversible heart failure," *Circulation*, vol. 118, no. 25, pp. 2754–2762, 2008.

[13] V. Kurowski, A. Kaiser, K. von Hof et al., "Apical and midventricular transient left ventricular dysfunction syndrome (Takotsubo cardiomyopathy): frequency, mechanisms, and prognosis," *Chest*, vol. 132, no. 3, pp. 809–816, 2007.

[14] M. Pawlak, M. Roik, J. Kochanowski et al., "Comparison of on-admission ST-segment elevation tako-tsubo patients and myocardial infarction women: in-hospital course and long-term follow-up," *Kardiologia Polska*, vol. 70, no. 3, pp. 233–240, 2012.

[15] I. S. Wittstein, "Acute stress cardiomyopathy," *Current Heart Failure Reports*, vol. 5, no. 2, pp. 61–68, 2008.

[16] M. Fiol, A. Carrillo, A. Rodriguez, J. Herrero, and J. García-Niebla, "Left ventricular ballooning syndrome due to vasospasm of the middle portion of the left anterior descending coronary artery," *Cardiology Journal*, vol. 19, no. 3, pp. 314–316, 2012.

[17] G. Kumar, D. R. Holmes Jr., and A. Prasad, "'Familial' apical ballooning syndrome (Takotsubo cardiomyopathy)," *International Journal of Cardiology*, vol. 144, no. 3, pp. 444–445, 2010.

[18] T. Ueyama, T. Hano, K. Kasamatsu, K. Yamamoto, Y. Tsuruo, and I. Nishio, "Estrogen attenuates the emotional stress-induced cardiac responses in the animal model of Tako-Tsubo (Ampulla) cardiomyopathy," *Journal of Cardiovascular Pharmacology*, vol. 42, supplement 1, pp. S117–S119, 2003.

[19] Y. J. Akashi, M. Sakakibara, and F. Miyake, "Reversible left ventricular dysfunction 'takotsubo' cardiomyopathy associated with pneumothorax," *Heart*, vol. 87, no. 2, article e1, 2002.

[20] R. Citro, A. Lyon, P. Meimoun et al., "Standard and advanced echocardiography in takotsubo (stress) cardiomyopathy: clinical and prognostic implications," *Journal of the American Society of Echocardiography*, vol. 28, no. 1, pp. 57–74, 2015.

11

Rapid Resolution of Acute Fulminant Myocarditis after IVIG and Steroid Treatment

Michael Barrie,[1] Lucas McKnight,[2] and Pallavi Solanki[3]

[1] *Department of Emergency Medicine, The Ohio State University Wexner Medical Center, Columbus, OH 43210, USA*
[2] *Department of Internal Medicine and Department of Pediatrics, The Ohio State University Wexner Medical Center, Columbus, OH 43210, USA*
[3] *Division of Cardiovascular Medicine, Department of Internal Medicine and The Dorothy M. Davis Heart and Lung Research Institute, The Ohio State University Wexner Medical Center, Columbus, OH 43210, USA*

Correspondence should be addressed to Pallavi Solanki, pallavi.solanki@osumc.edu

Academic Editors: K. Chergui, G. Klinger, and P. Kopterides

We report a case of a 59-year-old woman who presented with worsening dyspnea which rapidly progressed to severe heart failure. Coronary arteries showed no obstruction. Supportive measures stabilized the patient's hemodynamics. Initially intravenous solumedrol was given, but when the patient's condition continued to deteriorate, intravenous immunoglobulin (IVIG) was added to the treatment regimen and her condition improved. Studies show no benefit to using immunosuppressive agents in viral myocarditis, but benefits have been demonstrated in other etiologies. Patients presenting with acute fulminant myocarditis with unknown etiology that continue to deteriorate with aggressive heart failure treatment may benefit from steroids and IVIG.

1. Introduction

Myocarditis describes a group of heterogeneous disease processes that all involve inflammation of the myocardium. Diagnosis can be challenging due to nonspecific symptoms. Initiating causes include infectious causes and noninfectious etiologies such as toxins or primary immunologic processes. Acute myocarditis refers to the initial insult where pathogens or toxins invade the myocardium and directly cause myocyte damage. The innate immune response to the insult can release previously hidden autoantigens, which then trigger a subacute autoimmune responses in susceptible individuals [1]. This immunologic understanding has led to the use of immunosuppressive therapies, including steroids and intravenous immunoglobulin (IVIG), to treat fulminant myocarditis in addition to supportive heart failure treatment [2]. However, the efficacy of IVIG and steroids to prevent long-term systolic dysfunction remains controversial. We report a case of a middle-aged female with acute fulminant myocarditis who recovered rapidly after treatment with IVIG and steroids.

2. Case Report

A 59-year-old woman with no prior cardiac history presented in the springtime to an outside hospital with one month of progressive fatigue, palpitations, and exertional chest pain. Past medical history included chronic lumbar and cervical disc disease with cervical vertebral body fixation ten years previously, with continued chronic pain. Current medications were unknown at presentation. She was found to have elevated cardiac enzymes, a new left bundle branch block (LBBB), and new onset atrial fibrillation on electrocardiogram (ECG) (Figure 1).

These findings prompted evaluation with a left heart catheterization and coronary angiography to evaluate for acute coronary syndrome. Angiography showed nonobstructive coronary artery disease. Transthoracic echocardiogram showed biventricular heart failure with global hypokinesis with left ventricular ejection fraction (LVEF) of 30%. She was treated for suspected myopericarditis with nonsteroidal anti-inflammatory drugs (NSAIDs) and diuresis. Atrial fibrillation was treated with a loading dose of intravenous

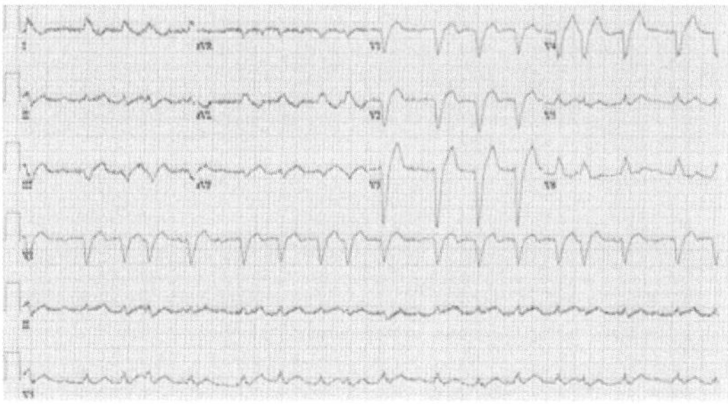

Figure 1: ECG on presentation demonstrating new onset atrial fibrillation and LBBB.

amiodarone. However, she continued to decompensate and developed respiratory distress and hypotension refractory to vasopressors.

She was transferred to our hospital and was found to be in acute cardiogenic shock with acute pulmonary edema suggestive on chest plain films (Figure 2). She was started on inotropes, continuous Lasix infusion, was intubated, and had an IABP placed at bedside. Transthoracic echocardiogram showed LVEF <20% without significant valvular pathology or regurgitation with normal ventricular size, LVED 4.1 cm (Figure 3). Right heart catheterization was consistent with cardiogenic shock. Cardiac magnetic resonance imaging (MRI) was deferred due to the presence of cervical and lumbar orthopedic hardware. She received solumedrol 1 gram intravenous due to clinical suspicion for acute myocarditis. The LBBB and atrial fibrillation resolved after two hours of solumedrol. On hospital day (HD) 2 she remained on mechanical ventilation, continued inotropic support with dobutamine and milrinone, and continued afterload reduction with an IABP. An EMB showed aggressive myocarditis with predominant monocytes and neutrophils with rare eosinophils (Figure 4). She was continued on intravenous solumedrol 250 mg every six hours. IABP was weaned, but she developed ventricular bigeminy. This prompted administration of IVIG 40 g via intravenous bolus in attempt to prevent myocarditis progression. This management led to hemodynamic stability, normal cardiac electrical activity, improved organ perfusion, and pulmonary edema resolution. IVIG treatments were given daily and discontinued after four doses. Gradually diuretics were discontinued, inotropes were weaned, and IV steroids were transitioned to oral prednisone that was tapered over 5 days. Serum studies were negative for bacterial or viral antibodies that would suggest recent infection. These studies included serum or blood antigens for *Streptococcus pneumonia*, *Borrelia burgdorferi*, *Chlamydia pneumonia*, *C. trachomatis*, *C. psittaci*, legionella, *Trypanosoma cruzi*, *M. tuberculosis*, toxoplasma, hepatitis B/C, EBV, CMV, HIV1/2, coxsackie panel, adenovirus, mycoplasma, influenza A/B, RSV A/B, metapneumo virus, parainfluenza 1–3, and Parvovirus B19. On HD 7 she was extubated and weaned to room air. Repeat cardiac echocardiography showed a normal ejection fraction with complete resolution of severe biventricular failure (Figure 3) and chest X-ray confirmed resolution of pulmonary edema.

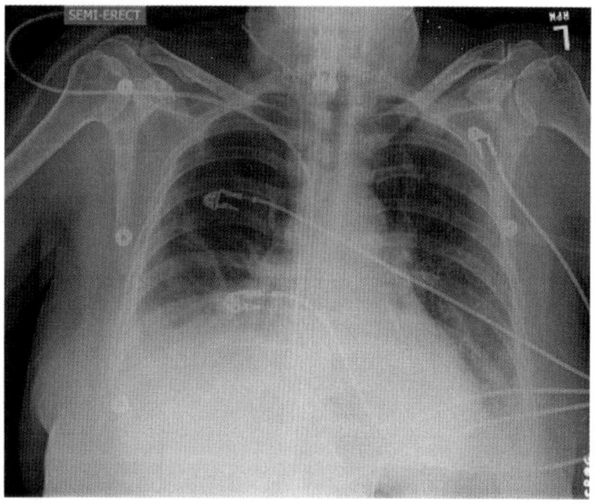

Figure 2: Chest plain film on presentation demonstrating likely pulmonary edema without cardiomegaly.

On HD 10, she was discharged home without dyspnea or chest pain. Last echo showed LVEF 60% with normal ventricular size and EKG normalized (Figure 5).

3. Discussion

Myocarditis is a rare disease with a wide spectrum of clinical presentation, ranging from anginal chest pains to fulminant heart failure and death [1]. Diagnosis can be challenging and specific etiology elusive. Excluding postmortem exam, the gold standard diagnosis of myocarditis requires endomyocardial biopsy (EMB). Class I indications for biopsy only include those with acute severe heart failure requiring inotropic or mechanical support, symptomatic ventricular tachycardia, high degree heart block, or those that fail to respond to standard therapy [3]. For patients who do not meet these criteria for EMB, cardiac MRI is a valuable alternative diagnostic tool to distinguish between different patterns of pathology and help guide diagnosis [4]. In our patient, we deferred MRI because we could not exclude the presence of ferromagnetic orthopedic hardware. Determining etiology of myocarditis is important, as many primary immune processes improve with targeted therapies.

Treatment for acute fulminant myocarditis is primarily supportive following evidence-based recommendations [1]. The use of an intra-aortic balloon pump or other methods of left-ventricular mechanical support have been shown to improve outcomes [5]. Some clinicians use high dose steroids and IVIG to treat the underlying inflammatory pathology in myocarditis. However, immunologic based therapies have remained controversial for most types of myocarditis. While several studies have shown benefits of steroids and IVIG in myocarditis, randomized controlled trials have failed to show a benefit [1]. Patients with acute dilated cardiomyopathy who were treated with IVIG had similar LVEF 12 months after treatment compared to those given placebo [6]. However, most patients show significant improvement with supportive measures alone [7]. Also, there are many limitations inherent in available studies. The Dallas

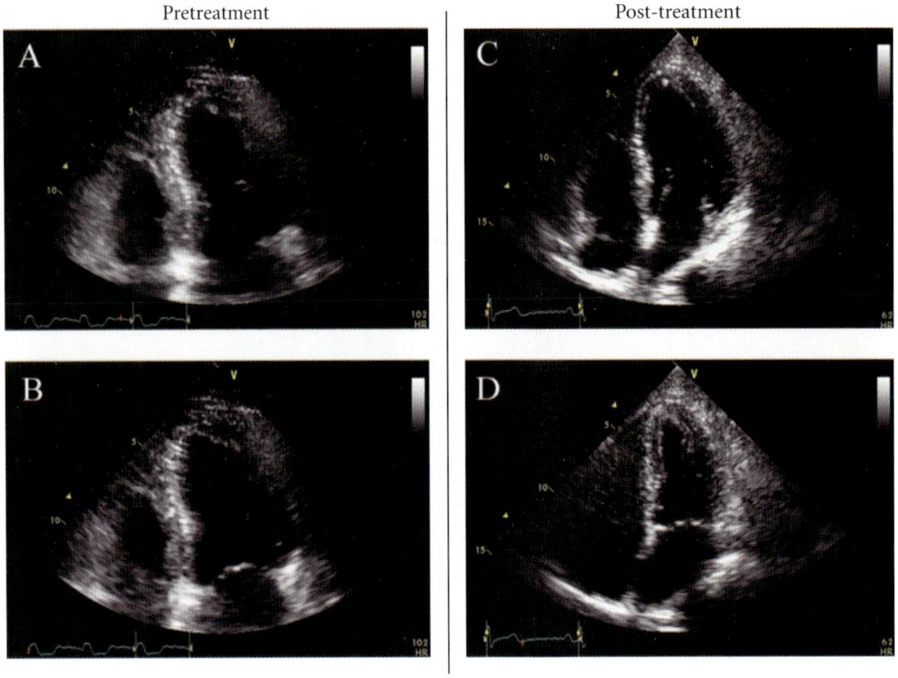

FIGURE 3: Transthoracic echocardiogram before and after treatment with IVIG and steroids. Apical 4-chamber view with pretreatment end diastole (A) and end systole (B) demonstrating severe global systolic dysfunction, LVEF <20%. The repeat transthoracic echocardiogram before treatment prior to discharge end diastole (C) and end systole (D) demonstrating a near complete resolution of ventricular systolic dysfunction.

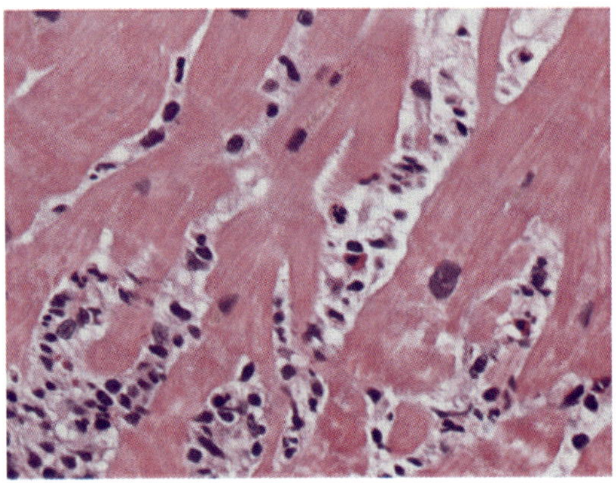

FIGURE 4: Right ventricular biopsy demonstrating interstitial inflammatory cell infiltrate in the myocardium, H&E stained with ×400 magnification. Most infiltrating cells are mononuclear cells, admixed with occasional eosinophils.

criteria may misdiagnose myocarditis and many current trials lack appropriate molecular biologic analysis of EMB to diagnose specific etiology [1]. In the context of these limitations, there is no clear support for immunosuppressive therapy in patients with known viral myocarditis. Evidence does support the use of immunosuppressive therapy in those with giant cell myocarditis, sarcoidosis, and primary autoimmune disease such as lupus [1, 8, 9]. It is often difficult to rapidly diagnose these etiologies. Thus, some clinicians initiate steroids with or without IVIG when patients clinically decompensate despite advanced cardiopulmonary support in an effort to treat cryptogenic primary immune processes. Although IVIG treatment is controversial and its use cannot be routinely recommended, it is possible that in select cases when myocarditis has been proven and there is no response to intensive supportive measures, IVIG may be considered.

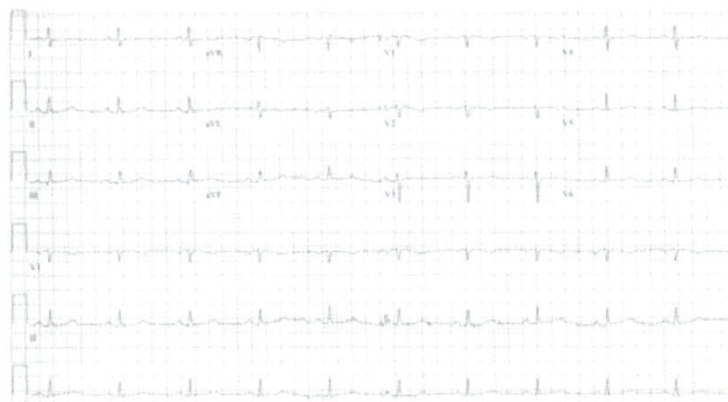

FIGURE 5: ECG after discharge shows sinus rhythm and no LBBB.

References

[1] I. Kindermann, C. Barth, F. Mahfoud et al., "Update on myocarditis," *Journal of the American College of Cardiology*, vol. 59, no. 9, pp. 779–792, 2012.

[2] S. Goland, L. S. Czer, R. J. Siegel et al., "Intravenous immunoglobulin treatment for acute fulminant inflammatory

cardiomyopathy: series of six patients and review of literature," *Canadian Journal of Cardiology*, vol. 24, pp. 571–574, 2008.

[3] L. T. Cooper, K. L. Baughman, A. M. Feldman et al., "The role of endomyocardial biopsy in the management of cardiovascular disease: a scientific statement from the American Heart Association, the American College of Cardiology, and the European Society of Cardiology. Endorsed by the Heart Failure Society of America and the Heart Failure Association of the European Society of Cardiology," *Journal of the American College of Cardiology*, vol. 50, pp. 1914–1931, 2007.

[4] H. Abdel-Aty, P. Boyé, A. Zagrosek et al., "Diagnostic performance of cardiovascular magnetic resonance in patients with suspected acute myocarditis: comparison of different approaches," *American College of Cardiology Foundation*, vol. 45, no. 11, pp. 1815–1822, 2005.

[5] M. Mirabel, C. E. Luyt, P. Leprince et al., "Outcomes, long-term quality of life, and psychologic assessment of fulminant myocarditis patients rescued by mechanical circulatory support," *Critical Care Medicine*, vol. 39, no. 5, pp. 1029–1035, 2011.

[6] D. M. McNamara, R. Holubkov, R. C. Starling et al., "Controlled trial of intravenous immune globulin in recent-onset dilated cardiomyopathy," *Circulation*, vol. 103, no. 18, pp. 2254–2259, 2001.

[7] R. E. McCarthy, J. P. Boehmer, R. H. Hruban et al., "Long-term outcome of fulminant myocarditis as compared with acute (nonfulminant) myocarditis," *The New England Journal of Medicine*, vol. 342, no. 10, pp. 690–695, 2000.

[8] L. T. Cooper Jr., J. M. Hare, H. D. Tazelaar et al., "Usefulness of immunosuppression for giant cell myocarditis," *American Journal of Cardiology*, vol. 102, no. 11, pp. 1535–1539, 2008.

[9] H. Nunes, O. Freynet, N. Naggara et al., "Cardiac sarcoidosis," *Seminars in Respiratory and Critical Care Medicine*, vol. 31, no. 4, pp. 428–441, 2010.

12

Ibuprofen-Induced Hypokalemia and Distal Renal Tubular Acidosis: A Patient's Perceptions of Over-the-Counter Medications and their Adverse Effects

Mark D. Salter[1,2]

[1] The University of Sydney, NSW 2006, Australia
[2] Emergency Medicine Department, Nepean Hospital, P.O. Box 63, Penrith, NSW 2751, Australia

Correspondence should be addressed to Mark D. Salter; the12thman82@hotmail.com

Academic Editors: G. Klinger, C. Lazzeri, and G. Pichler

We highlight a case of distal renal tubular acidosis secondary to ibuprofen and codeine use. Of particular interest in this case are the patient's perception of over-the-counter (OTC) medication use, her own OTC use prior to admission, and her knowledge of adverse reactions or side effects of these medications prior to taking them.

1. Introduction

Ibuprofen is a nonsteroidal anti-inflammatory drug (NSAID) which is available over-the-counter (OTC) as a nonprescription drug. It is used widely as an antipyretic and analgesic. Our patient had hypokalemia secondary to type one, distal renal tubular acidosis (dRTA), after long-term ibuprofen and codeine use. The combination of biochemical abnormalities including hypokalemia, hyperchloremic metabolic acidosis, hypophosphatemia, and urine pH >5.5 was consistent with those found in our patient [1–3].

The mechanism behind ibuprofen-induced renal tubular acidosis is not well understood and is believed to involve the inhibition or deficiency of carbonic anhydrase activity, especially carbonic anhydrase type two, which is the predominant form in the kidneys. Essentially, the hyperchloremic metabolic acidosis is a result of impairment of renal acidification and the hypokalaemia is due to the acidosis impairing proximal sodium reabsorption, causing increased potassium secretion in the distal tubules [4–6].

2. Case Presentation

A 38-year-old patient presents with myalgia, evolving paralysis, and vomiting for 3 weeks on a background of iron deficiency anaemia, migraines, and gastroesophageal reflux disease. Her only medications were esomeprazole 20 mg and amitriptyline 50 mg. She had been sent in by her GP with moderate hypokalaemia (potassium 2.6 mmol/L, range 3–5 mmol/L) and possible myositis (CK 2500 u/L) after blood tests the prior evening. Her examination demonstrated conjunctiva pallor, minor right upper quadrant, and epigastric tenderness. Neurological exam showed generalised upper and lower limbs flaccid weakness (grade 3/5 proximally and 4/5 distally) with normal sensation and cranial nerve examination. Repeat blood tests demonstrated a hyperchloremic metabolic acidosis, hypokalemia (potassium 2.1 mmol/L), a mild transaminitis, an inflammatory response (WCC 27.1 × 10^9/L and procalcitonin 108 ug/L with normal CRP), and a creatinine kinase 26,100 u/L. This was in the context of normal renal function (urea 5.4 mmol/L and creatinine 85 umol/L). Urinary myoglobin was 266,900 ug/L, pH 9, and spot urinary potassium 22 mmol/L (overall >20 mmol over a 24-hour period). ECG showed mild ST depression without U waves and a CT-Abdomen was essentially normal. All biochemistry was consistent with type 1 distal renal tubular acidosis (dRTA) with rhabdomyolysis (Table 1) and a possible differential of undifferentiated myositis. She was reviewed by an emergency registrar, two emergency consultants, a surgical registrar, a medical registrar and an intensive care registrar

Table 1: Biochemistry results on presentation.

	Numbers
Venous blood gas	
pH	7.25
pO_2 (mmHg)	29
pCO_2 (mmHg)	33
HCO_3 (mmol/L)	14
Base excess (mmol/L)	−12
Full blood count	
Hb (g/L)	109
WCC ($\times 10^9$/L)	27.1
Platelets	573
Haematocrit	0.36
Procalcitonin (ug/L)	108
CRP (mg/L)	5
ESR (mm/hr)	9
Electrolytes	
Na^+ (mmol/L)	141
K^+ (mmol/L)	2.1
Cl^- (mmol/L)	115
HCO_3 (mmol/L)	15
Urea (mmol/L)	5.4
Creatinine (umol/L)	85
Anion gap (mmol/L)	13
Thyroid function tests	
TSH (mIU/L)	1.51
T4 (pmol/L)	14
Liver function tests	
Bilirubin (umol/L)	9
Albumin (g/L)	39
AST (U/L)	413
ALT (U/L)	159
GGT (U/L)	27
ALP (U/L)	134
Calcium/magnesium/phosphate	
Ca^{2+} (mmol/L)	2.28
Mg^{2+} (mmol/L)	1.05
PO_4^{2-} (mmol/L)	0.63
Creatinine kinase U/L	26,135
Urine tests	
Urine Na^+ (mmol/L)	105
Urine K^+ (mmol/L)	22
Urine pH	9
Urine protein (g/L)	0.61
Urine creatinine (mmol/L)	2
Urine osmolality (mmol/kg)	218
Urine myoglobin (ug/L)	266.900
Urine protein/creat. ratio (mg/mmol creat.)	299

and denied any nonsteroidal anti-inflammatory or laxative use when asked specifically about these medications with these exact words. She was taken to ICU and had both oral and intravenous potassium replacement totalling 430 mmol over the next 36 hours with intermittent use of sodium bicarbonate to maintain urine alkalinisation. Remarkably, 8 hours after ICU admission she complained of a previously undisclosed dental problem and admitted to a second intensive care registrar that she was taking 1.2–2 g of nurofen (ibuprofen) and 8 fiorinal dental capsules (paracetamol 500 mg, codeine phosphate 10 mg, and doxylamine succinate 2 mg) daily for the past five weeks. This combination of ibuprofen and codeine is likely the cause of the dRTA. With cessation of ibuprofen and codeine, adequate replacement, and other supportive therapy, our patient was discharged from ICU after 48 hours.

3. Discussion

What made this case stand out for us was not the significant medical process occurring for the patient but the perceptions of our patient in regard to her ibuprofen and codeine use. We realised after exhaustive review that because she did not understand them to be relevant to her ongoing condition and that she did not consider these tablets "medications" because they were OTC and easily accessible. She unknowingly missed the link between their use and her subsequent decline in health, and by not reporting their use, her ongoing care was compromised.

The importance of patient's perceptions surrounding nonprescription medications and what constitutes a medication is poorly understood within the medical community. As physicians we assume that our patients' understanding of the medications they are taking would prevent them from being used inappropriately and that they recognise that nonprescription medications may also have detrimental effects. There is ample evidence in the literature to show how misuse or prolonged use of these medications can cause substantial morbidity and mortality, with paracetamol and NSAIDs among those being regularly reported to cause liver failure, hypokalaemia, and gastrointestinal bleeding and perforation [7–9].

The literature on this subject also points towards the general public's lack of understanding of ibuprofen adverse effects, and other OTC medications adverse effects, as a whole. This includes the potential harms and serious side effects of these medication types which may occur without the patients linking the cause and effect. Wilcox et al. in two collated surveys of patients taking OTC and prescription NSAIDs showed that ibuprofen was the most frequent NSAID analgesic used due to being an OTC medication. Over 60% were unaware of the potential adverse effects of this drug and more than a quarter used more than the recommended daily dose [10]. This finding was strengthened in a survey of 183 patients by Ngo et al. which found that 65% of people did not seek medical advice prior to ibuprofen use, 66% had never read the manufacturer's printed warning instructions on potential interactions or adverse reactions, and 71% had used it for over 1 year [11]. Of note, a study in Northern Ireland in regard to patients' perceptions of OTC medications, including the misuse or abuse of these preparations found that over 86% would always follow the product directions and were very aware of the potential for abuse and adverse effects of the OTC medications they were using. This finding is in direct contrast to most of the published literature and is likely an outlier [12]. It has also been shown that in general patients had poor knowledge of the potential side effects of their medication but could still identify these problems as they occurred, unlike our patient who did not make the connection between her use and the hypokalaemia-induced dRTA [13].

Interestingly, our patient did not directly report the use of nurofen or fiorinal dental capsules as her belief was that their use was as a short-term analgesic for a preexisting dental problem. She did not anticipate their harmful effects over a prolonged period and finally reported their use as an incidental disclosure after suffering from her preexisting but unreported dental pain in the intensive care unit. Of significant importance in this case was the fact that she had multiple patient-doctor interactions, was asked about regular medication use on multiple occasions, and, despite this, was only asked for generic use of ibuprofen rather than brand names, like nurofen. This highlighted the importance of specific questioning if a class of medication is suspected to be causing the clinical illness. It has been shown that patients are willing and generally happy to disclose their OTC medication use if asked and will readily try OTC medications on physician advice [14]. These findings and many patients' lack of understanding of potential adverse effects of the OTC medications they use have previously been demonstrated in paediatric settings, especially regarding cough and cold syrups [15].

This case illustrated the need for physicians to be more suspicious of OTC medication use and the possible adverse reactions associated with them. It also shows that we as physicians should not be afraid to enquire about their use and to educate our patients on the adverse effects of these drugs when used correctly or abused. Taylor et al. highlighted in their small study that if the framing of discussion into the risk of adverse effects of OTC medications was done in a positive way, then this increased the likelihood of the patient taking the medication and adhering to the directions on the label, despite previous adverse effects with the same or similar drugs [16].

4. Conclusion

This case highlighted a typeI dRTA secondary to ibuprofen and codeine use and demonstrated that patient perceptions of OTC medications and their adverse reaction profile dictated the level of clinical suspicion of the treating physicians. Multiple studies in the literature demonstrate that patients may not perceive these medications as drugs that treating physicians should be aware of at the time of review and likely do not fully comprehend the adverse reactions when taking them. We have shown that education about OTC medications and their adverse effects is a positive development in patient care and that suspicion of use must be followed with specific rather than broad interrogation. We have further shown that in an age of multiple patient-doctor interactions we must always take care to illicit information at the level of the patient we are reviewing.

References

[1] A. P. Lambert and C. Close, "Life-threatening hypokalaemia from abuse of Nurofen Plus," *Journal of the Royal Society of Medicine*, vol. 98, no. 1, p. 21, 2005.

[2] B. T. Dyer, J. L. Martin, J. L. Mitchell, N. C. Sauven, and B. G. Gazzard, "Hypokalaemia in ibuprofen and codeine phosphate abuse," *International Journal of Clinical Practice*, vol. 58, no. 11, pp. 1061–1062, 2004.

[3] J. L. Ng, D. J. R. Morgan, N. K. M. Loh et al., "Life-threatening hypokalaemia associated with ibuprofen-induced renal tubular acidosis," *Medical Journal of Australia*, vol. 194, no. 6, pp. 313–316, 2011.

[4] J. M. Purkerson and G. J. Schwartz, "The role of carbonic anhydrases in renal physiology," *Kidney International*, vol. 71, no. 2, pp. 103–115, 2007.

[5] J. Rodríguez Soriano, "Renal tubular acidosis: the clinical entity," *Journal of the American Society of Nephrology*, vol. 13, no. 8, pp. 2160–2170, 2002.

[6] M. G. Cogan and F. C. Rector Jr., "Proximal reabsorption during metabolic acidosis in the rat," *The American Journal of Physiology*, vol. 242, no. 5, pp. F499–F507, 1982.

[7] A. M. Larson, J. Polson, R. J. Fontana et al., "Acetaminophen-induced acute liver failure: results of a United States multicenter, prospective study," *Hepatology*, vol. 42, no. 6, pp. 1364–1372, 2005.

[8] S. C. Smolinske, A. H. Hall, S. A. Vandenberg, D. G. Spoerke, and P. V. McBride, "Toxic effects of nonsteroidal anti-inflammatory drugs in overdose. An overview of recent evidence on clinical effects and dose-response relationships," *Drug Safety*, vol. 5, no. 4, pp. 252–274, 1990.

[9] C. P. Godshalk, J. K. Roush, R. B. Fingland, D. Sikkema, and M. W. Vorhies, "Gastric perforation associated with administration of ibuprofen in a dog," *Journal of the American Veterinary Medical Association*, vol. 201, no. 11, pp. 1734–1736, 1992.

[10] C. M. Wilcox, B. Cryer, and G. Triadafilopoulos, "Patterns of use and public perception of over-the-counter pain relievers: focus on nonsteroidal antiinflammatory drugs," *Journal of Rheumatology*, vol. 32, no. 11, pp. 2218–2224, 2005.

[11] S. N. T. Ngo, I. Stupans, W. S. Leong, and M. Osman, "Appropriate use of non-prescription ibuprofen: a survey of patients' perceptions and understanding," *International Journal of Pharmacy Practice*, vol. 18, no. 1, pp. 63–65, 2010.

[12] M. Wazaify, E. Shields, C. M. Hughes, and J. C. McElnay, "Societal perspectives on over-the-counter (OTC) medicines," *Family Practice*, vol. 22, no. 2, pp. 170–176, 2005.

[13] L. Hughes, C. Whittlesea, and D. Luscombe, "Patients' knowledge and perceptions of the side-effects of OTC medication," *Journal of Clinical Pharmacy and Therapeutics*, vol. 27, no. 4, pp. 243–248, 2002.

[14] C. P. Bradley, A. Riaz, R. S. Tobias, J. E. Kenkre, and D. Y. Dassu, "Patient attitudes to over-the-counter drugs and possible professional responses to self-medication," *Family Practice*, vol. 15, no. 1, pp. 44–50, 1998.

[15] V. L. Gunn, S. H. Taha, E. L. Liebelt, and J. R. Serwint, "Toxicity of over-the-counter cough and cold medications," *Pediatrics*, vol. 108, no. 3, p. e52, 2001.

[16] J. Taylor, M. Seyed-Hosseini, and D. Quest, "Framing the risk of an OTC medication side effect," *Canadian Pharmacists Journal*, vol. 144, no. 1, pp. 34–39, 2011.

13

Fatal H1N1-Related Acute Necrotizing Encephalopathy in an Adult

Yu-Jin Lee,[1] D. Scott Smith,[2] Vivek A. Rao,[3] Robert D. Siegel,[4] Jon Kosek,[5] Carol A. Glaser,[6] and Alexander C. Flint[3]

[1] *Department of Human Biology, Stanford University, Stanford, CA 94305, USA*
[2] *Department of Infectious Disease and Geographic Medicine, Kaiser Permanente, Redwood City, CA 94063, USA*
[3] *Department of Neuroscience, Kaiser Permanente, Redwood City, CA 94063, USA*
[4] *Department of Microbiology and Immunology, Stanford University, Stanford, CA 94305, USA*
[5] *Department of Pathology, Veterans Affairs Palo Alto Health Care System, Palo Alto, CA 94304, USA*
[6] *Center for Infectious Diseases, California Department of Public Health, Richmond, CA 94804, USA*

Correspondence should be addressed to Alexander C. Flint, alexander.c.flint@kp.org

Academic Editors: K. Klouche, P. Kopterides, and Z. Molnar

Acute necrotizing encephalopathy (ANE) is a severe neurological complication of influenza infection, including H1N1 influenza. Many cases of ANE have been reported in the pediatric literature, but very few cases have been described in adults. The cause of ANE remains unknown—the influenza virus is not known to be neurotropic, and evidence of direct viral involvement of the central nervous system (CNS) has not been demonstrated in the limited cases of ANE in which pathological specimens have been obtained. Here we report a fatal case of ANE from H1N1 influenza infection in an adult. Neuroimaging and postmortem analysis both showed widespread brain edema, necrosis, and hemorrhage, but molecular studies and postmortem pathology revealed no evidence of direct viral involvement of the CNS. This case of fatal ANE in an adult is consistent with the hypothesis generated from pediatric cases that the host immune response, and not direct viral invasion of the CNS, is responsible for pathogenesis of ANE.

1. Introduction

Acute necrotizing encephalopathy (ANE) is a rare central nervous system (CNS) complication of influenza that is characterized by altered mental status and seizures, and often leads to profound disability or death [1]. ANE associated with influenza A was originally reported in pediatric patients of Asian descent [1], but subsequent reports worldwide indicate that ANE is not limited to a particular race/ethnicity [2–4] and can occur, albeit rarely, in adults [5–8]. During the 2009 influenza A (H1N1) pandemic, many pediatric ANE cases were reported but adult cases were uncommon [7, 9]. In this report, we present the first case of H1N1 encephalopathy progressing to brain death in an adult patient. The radiographic and pathologic findings in this fatal adult case of ANE are consistent with reports from pediatric cases. Molecular analyses of cerebrospinal fluid (CSF) and brain tissue from this case support the hypothesis that ANE occurs as a result of secondary immune-related mechanisms rather than direct invasion of the CNS by the influenza virus.

2. Clinical Case

A 27-year-old woman with a history of obesity and asthma was admitted to hospital with a diagnosis of H1N1 influenza A pneumonia and acute respiratory distress syndrome (ARDS). After a prodrome of nonproductive cough and chest tightness, she presented to the emergency department with worsened shortness of breath and subsequently required intubation and mechanical ventilation for hypoxic respiratory failure. On the day of admission, a nasopharyngeal sample was positive for influenza A by reverse transcriptase-polymerase chain reaction (RT-PCR). She had not received seasonal influenza or 2009 H1N1 pandemic flu vaccinations prior to her illness.

Antiviral therapy with oseltamivir was administered for a 10-day initial course. Given a persistently positive RT-PCR for influenza A in 3 samples over 3 weeks and worsening of her ARDS despite the course of oseltamivir, she subsequently received the investigational antiviral agent peramivir intravenously after consent was obtained from her family. The patient's severe ARDS required treatment with a course of intravenous methylprednisolone and neuromuscular paralysis to facilitate appropriate mechanical ventilation. On day 11 of her hospitalization, the patient developed acute oliguric renal failure and required hemodialysis for several weeks. Tracheostomy was performed approximately one month into her hospitalization.

Five weeks into her hospitalization, as her sedation was lightened in the context of improved oxygen requirements, the patient was found to have altered mental status and quadriparesis. The next day, she became unarousable with nonreactive pupils, absent corneal reflexes, and absent motor response to noxious stimuli. An unenhanced head computed tomography (CT) showed diffuse cerebral white matter edema, with posterior fossa edema causing effacement of the fourth ventricle and obstructive hydrocephalus. The CT also showed a small intraparenchymal hemorrhage in the left occipital lobe. The patient was urgently transferred to the Neuroscience Intensive Care Unit at our Neurosurgical Center, where a ventriculostomy was placed.

Magnetic resonance imaging (MRI) of the brain illustrated diffuse abnormal T2/FLAIR hyperintensities with swelling in the gray matter and subcortical white matter throughout the bilateral cerebral hemispheres, cerebellum, brainstem, and thalami (Figures 1(a)–1(d)). There was also evidence of edema in the bilateral lentiform nuclei and posterior limb of the internal capsules. There were signs of tonsillar herniation and upward cerebellar herniation. Diffuse leptomeningeal enhancement and patchy parenchymal enhancement were present throughout the bilateral cerebellar hemispheres, right basal ganglia, and the left ventromedial thalamus. Multiple areas of microhemorrhage were seen on gradient echo sequences at the gray-white junction in the cerebrum and cerebellum. The CT and MRI findings were consistent with a diagnosis of ANE [1].

Cerebrospinal fluid (CSF) obtained from the patient's ventriculostomy showed 7 white blood cells per microliter (97% polymorphonuclear leukocytes, 3% lymphocytes), protein level of 78 mg per deciliter, and glucose level of 65 mg per deciliter. Molecular analyses of the CSF and serum samples were negative for the virus.

After treatment of the patient's obstructive hydrocephalus by ventriculostomy, no clinical improvement was observed. Given the possibility of an inflammatory or parainfectious etiology for the patient's acute necrotizing meningoencephalitis, treatment with intravenous immunoglobulin was begun and steroid therapy was restarted. Despite these treatments, her neurological examination continued to deteriorate and the patient progressed to brain death.

Postmortem examination revealed evidence of severe influenza pneumonia and advanced interstitial pneumonitis with fibrosis. The brain showed extensive and widespread edema, necrosis, and hemorrhage (Figures 1(e)–1(f)). Multiple brain regions demonstrated diffuse edema, venous congestion, and multifocal areas of hypoxic ischemic neuronal injury. The internal capsule and basis pontis demonstrated intravascular fibrin thrombi surrounded by cellular debris with early necrosis. Beta-amyloid precursor (beta-APP) immunostains in these regions demonstrated widespread axonal injury associated with the vascular lesions. The thalamus showed venous congestion and parenchymal hemorrhage without associated inflammation. The corpus callosum had small necrotic foci with a macrophage response and also showed evidence of marked axonal injury on the beta-APP immunostains. The cerebellar hemispheres were necrotic with associated hemorrhage (Figure 1(e)), and the basilar leptomeninges were congested.

Molecular analyses of multiple samples of postmortem brain tissue were negative for the virus.

3. Discussion

We describe an adult patient with fatal acute necrotizing encephalopathy (ANE) associated with 2009 H1N1 influenza infection. The findings on neuroimaging and postmortem examination in this case support the concept that ANE is a clinically recognizable form of severe necrotizing encephalopathy that has similar characteristics in adults and children. Molecular analysis of CSF and brain tissue support the hypothesis that ANE is not caused by direct invasion of brain by the influenza virus, but instead may represent a consequence of the immune response to the virus [10].

In addition to respiratory illness, influenza virus infections can be associated with a number of different neurological complications [7]. Among the neurological syndromes reported, the most devastating is ANE, which presents as a rapid neurological decline following influenza infection [10]. ANE is associated with high morbidity and mortality [7]. The term ANE was first coined by Mizuguchi following reports of encephalopathy associated with influenza infection in East Asia [1]. Initially described as a neurological syndrome in pediatric patients of Asian descent, influenza-associated ANE is now recognized worldwide[39]. Although ANE appears to have a predilection for the pediatric age group, a small number of cases in adults have also been reported [5–7]. The characteristic neuroimaging findings of ANE are bilateral, multifocal lesions in the thalami, cerebral and cerebellar deep white matter, brainstem tegmentum, and putamen [1, 10]. Common clinical signs and symptoms include altered mental status, seizures, ophthalmoparesis, quadriparesis, and delayed parkinsonism among survivors. During the 2009 H1N1 pandemic, a wide range of neurological complications were reported in association with influenza infection, including ANE in several pediatric cases and in some adults [3, 4, 7, 8, 11–14].

Neuroimaging in ANE characteristically shows abnormalities in the subcortical and cerebellar white matter, with microhemorrhages and abnormal enhancement [1, 10]. Our patient's MRI showed edema throughout the bilateral cerebral hemispheres, cerebellum, brainstem, and thalami.

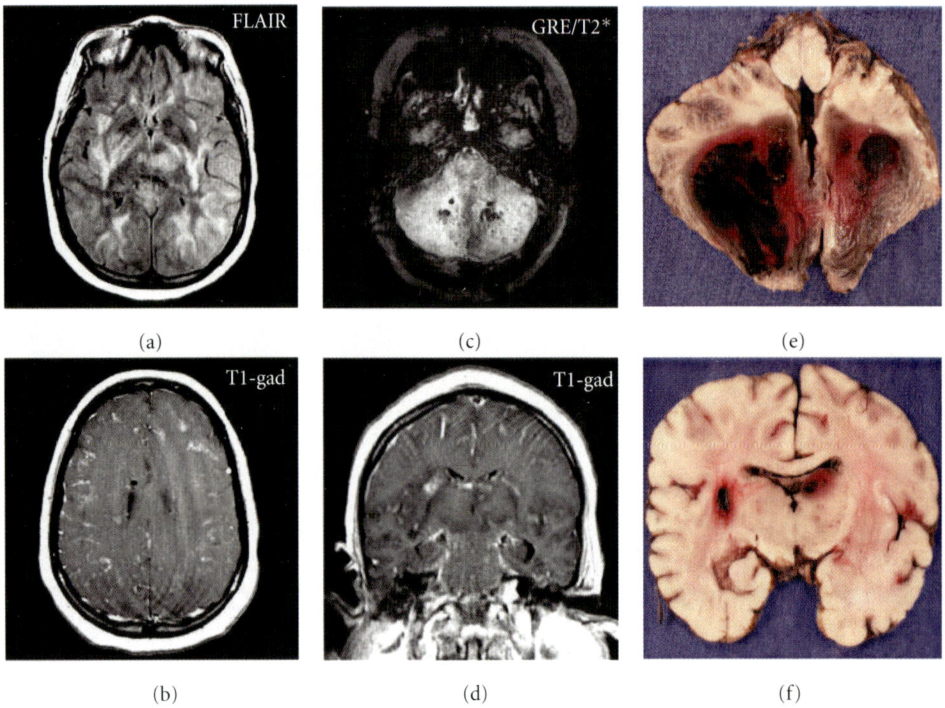

Figure 1: (a) FLAIR MRI sequence demonstrates widespread abnormal signal in the subcortical white matter, internal capsule, putamen, globus pallidus, and thalamus bilaterally. (b) T1 post-gadolinium axial MRI sequence demonstrates diffuse leptomeningeal enhancement over the convexities bilaterally and foci of parenchymal enhancement within the cortex bilaterally. (c) Gradient echo (GRE/T2*) MRI sequence demonstrates hemorrhage in the deep cerebellar white matter bilaterally (mottled black signal, representing magnetic susceptibility). (d) T1 post-gadolinium coronal MRI sequence demonstrates basal leptomeningeal enhancement surrounding the brainstem. (e) Postmortem axial section through the brainstem and cerebellum demonstrates severe bilateral hemorrhage and necrosis of the cerebellar hemispheres. (f) Postmortem coronal section demonstrates widespread but patchy areas of hemorrhage and necrosis in the deep gray nuclei bilaterally and the cerebral hemispheres bilaterally.

The gradient echo (GRE) sequence showed microhemorrhages at the gray-white junction in the cerebrum and cerebellum. Postmortem brain sections illustrated hemorrhage and necrosis in both the cerebral and cerebellar hemispheres. These findings were consistent with a diagnosis of ANE and support the hypothesis that characteristic neuroimaging findings in ANE are seen in both pediatric and adult cases [1].

The influenza virus has not been detected in the CNS in ANE cases analyzed to date, including in CSF and brain tissue samples from pediatric cases [2–4, 11, 15] and only in CSF samples from adult cases [5, 7]. In our patient, RT-PCR for influenza virus was negative on both CSF and brain tissue, and postmortem analysis showed no evidence for viral invasion of the CNS such as cellular inclusions. Our postmortem pathological analysis and molecular biological analysis results thus provide further evidence that direct viral invasion of the CNS may not be involved in the pathogenesis of ANE [2, 11]. The lack of viral detection in CSF and brain tissue in this adult patient further supports the notion that ANE is not a fundamentally different condition in pediatric and adult patients. However, it should be noted that the RT-PCR may have been negative as a result of the interval between the initial influenza infection and the time CSF and brain samples were obtained. It is difficult to know at what point this patient developed the neurological complications, but it is likely that it was relatively early in her hospital course. ANE usually occurs within a few days of the onset of respiratory illness [1, 5, 9]. Because she required neuromuscular paralysis for ventilatory management of her ARDS, daily sedation interruptions to facilitate neurologic evaluation were not possible.

This case typifies the rare but devastating complication of ANE associated with influenza (H1N1) infection. In the wake of the recent 2009 H1N1 pandemic, awareness of this rare but significant complication is important. In order for early detection of ANE, closer neurological monitoring of patients with ARDS is necessary. Given the mounting evidence that this dramatic syndrome is not caused by direct viral invasion of the CNS, better understanding of the pathophysiology of this severe inflammatory condition is needed so that appropriate prevention or treatment measures may be applied.

Funding

The authors declare that there are no sources of funding to disclose.

References

[1] M. Mizuguchi, J. Abe, K. Mikkaichi et al., "Acute necrotising encephalopathy of childhood: a new syndrome presenting with multifocal, symmetric brain lesions," *Journal of Neurology Neurosurgery and Psychiatry*, vol. 58, no. 5, pp. 555–561, 1995.

[2] S. D. Mastroyianni, D. Gionnis, K. Voudris, A. Skardoutsou, and M. Mizuguchi, "Acute necrotizing encephalopathy of childhood in non-Asian patients: report of three cases and literature review," *Journal of Child Neurology*, vol. 21, no. 10, pp. 872–879, 2006.

[3] F. Ormitti, E. Ventura, A. Summa, E. Picetti, and G. Crisi, "Acute necrotizing encephalopathy in a child during the 2009 influenza A(H1N1) pandemia: MR imaging in diagnosis and follow-up," *American Journal of Neuroradiology*, vol. 31, no. 3, pp. 396–400, 2010.

[4] J. B. Lyon, C. Remigio, T. Milligan, and C. Deline, "Acute necrotizing encephalopathy in a child with H1N1 influenza infection," *Pediatric Radiology*, vol. 40, no. 2, pp. 200–205, 2010.

[5] H. Iijima, K. Wakasugi, M. Ayabe, H. Shoji, and T. Abe, "A case of adult influenza A virus-associated encephalitis: magnetic resonance imaging findings," *Journal of Neuroimaging*, vol. 12, no. 3, pp. 273–275, 2002.

[6] A. Gadoth, O. Aizenstein, and A. Mosek, "Influenza A/H1N1 encephalitis," *Neurology*, vol. 75, no. 7, pp. 666–667, 2010.

[7] P. T. Akins, J. Belko, T. M. Uyeki, Y. Axelrod, K. K. Lee, and J. Silverthorn, "H1N1 encephalitis with malignant edema and review of neurologic complications from influenza," *Neurocritical Care*, vol. 13, no. 3, pp. 396–406, 2010.

[8] J. E. Fugate, E. M. Lam, A. A. Rabinstein, and E. F. M. Wijdicks, "Acute hemorrhagic leukoencephalitis and hypoxic brain injury associated with H1N1 influenza," *Archives of Neurology*, vol. 67, no. 6, pp. 756–758, 2010.

[9] A. Haktanir, "MR imaging in novel influenza A(H1N1)-associated meningoencephalitis," *American Journal of Neuroradiology*, vol. 31, no. 3, pp. 394–395, 2010.

[10] M. Mizuguchi, H. Yamanouchi, T. Ichiyama, and M. Shiomi, "Acute encephalopathy associated with influenza and other viral infections," *Acta Neurologica Scandinavica*, vol. 115, supplement 186, pp. 45–56, 2007.

[11] P. Mariotti, R. Iorio, G. Frisullo et al., "Acute necrotizing encephalopathy during novel influenza A (H1N1) virus infection," *Annals of Neurology*, vol. 68, no. 1, pp. 111–114, 2010.

[12] A. Martin and E. P. Reade, "Acute necrotizing encephalopathy progressing to brain death in a pediatric patient with novel influenza a (H1N1) infection," *Clinical Infectious Diseases*, vol. 50, no. 8, pp. e50–e52, 2010.

[13] B. E. Gonzalez and D. G. Brust, "Novel influenza A (H1N1) presenting as an acute febrile encephalopathy in a mother and daughter," *Clinical Infectious Diseases*, vol. 49, no. 12, pp. 1966–1967, 2009.

[14] S. Kitcharoen, M. Pattapongsin, K. Sawanyawisuth, V. Angela, and S. Tiamkao, "Neurologic manifestations of pandemic (H1N1) 2009 virus infection," *Emerging Infectious Diseases*, vol. 16, no. 3, pp. 569–570, 2010.

[15] W. F. Ng, S. C. Chiu, D. S. Y. Lam et al., "A 7 year old boy dying of acute encephalopathy: Com august 2009 case 1," *Brain Pathology*, vol. 20, no. 1, pp. 261–264, 2010.

14

Prone Position Ventilation used during a Transfer as a Bridge to Ecmo Therapy in Hantavirus-Induced Severe Cardiopulmonary Syndrome

R. Cornejo,[1] D. Ugalde,[1] O. Llanos,[1] P. Bisbal,[1] L. De la Barrera,[1] C. Romero,[1] R. Neira,[1] Roberto González,[1] and J. Gajardo[2]

[1] *Unidad de Pacientes Críticos, Departamento de Medicina, Hospital Clínico, Universidad de Chile, Chile*
[2] *Unidad de Pacientes Críticos, Complejo Asistencial Hospital Barros Luco Trudeau, Chile*

Correspondence should be addressed to R. Cornejo; racornej@gmail.com

Academic Editors: R. Alaghehbandan, P. Del Rio, C.-C. Lai, W. Mauritz, and V. Papadopoulos

Background. Transport of critically ill patients is a complex issue. We present a case using prone positioning as a bridge to extracorporeal membrane oxygenation (ECMO), performed by a critical retrieval team from a university hospital. *Case Report.* A 28-year-old male developed fever, progressive respiratory failure, and shock. He was admitted to ICU from a public hospital, and mechanical ventilation was begun, but clinical response was not adequate. ECMO was deemed necessary due to severe respiratory failure and severe shock. A critical retrieval team of our center was assembled to attempt transfer. Prone positioning was employed to stabilize and transfer the patient, after risk-benefit assessment. Once in our hospital, ECMO was useful to resolve shock and pulmonary edema secondary to Hantavirus cardiopulmonary syndrome. Finally, he was discharged with normal functioning. *Conclusion.* This case exemplifies the relevance of a retrieval team and bridge therapy. Prone positioning improves oxygenation and is safe to perform as transport if performed by a trained team as in this case. Preparation and organization is necessary to improve outcomes, using teams and organized networks. Catastrophic respiratory failure and shock should not be contraindications to transferring patients, but it must be done with an experienced team.

1. Introduction

Transport of critically ill patients remains a complex issue; respiratory or hemodynamic instability increases the risks during the procedures required to transfer mechanically ventilated patients between units and particularly between ICUs at different hospitals. Interhospital transportation of critically ill patients is of paramount importance when patients require therapies not available at the hospital of origin, often life-saving measures such as extracorporeal membrane oxygenation (ECMO). In this context patients may require bridging therapy to overcome life-threatening cardiopulmonary failure for a time long enough to reach destination, performed by a specialized team, experienced in those measures.

The aim of this report is to communicate how the assessment and management by a critical care rescue team allowed the transfer of a patient with severe respiratory failure and concomitant circulatory failure in prone positioning and high dose of vasoactive drugs.

2. Case Report

A 28-year-old male, previously healthy, was admitted to a public hospital in Santiago because of respiratory failure and hypotension. He referred a history of 7 days of fever, progressive shortness of breath, abdominal pain, and vomiting. The patient had been camping in the foothills of the Araucanía region of Chile five weeks before the onset of symptoms. At the emergency room the patient was acutely ill with fever of 38.9°C, tachycardia of 146 beats per minute, signs of peripheral hypoperfusion, MAP of 60 mmHg, cyanosis, and tachypnea up to 40 per minute, requiring 100% oxygen to achieve and O_2 saturation of 88%.

He was transferred to the ICU and connected to mechanical ventilation. He developed rapid and progressive respiratory failure achieving PaO_2/FiO_2 ratio 52 mmHg, oxygenation index (OI) 34,6 (employing tidal volume of 6 mL/kg, FiO_2 of 100%, and PEEP 24 cm of water), and hemodynamic instability characterized by high requirements of vasoactive drugs, oligoanuria, and lactacidemia over 5 mmol/L. A pulmonary artery catheter showed a cardiac index of 2.0 L/min/m^2 while receiving norepinephrine at 2 mcg/kg/min and epinephrine 0,3 mcg/kg/min, and the $SvcO_2$ was 55%. Among hematological and biochemical parameters an hematocrit of 50%, thrombocytopenia of 33.000× mm^3, and C-reactive protein of 130 mg/L were found. X-chest ray showed bilateral and diffuse pulmonary infiltrates. After 7 hours of treatment with no evident improvement in general conditions and with the provisory diagnostic of Hantavirus cardiopulmonary syndrome, ECMO was considered the most adequate therapeutic option. As this approach was not available at the ICU, the transfer to the University Hospital ICU was evaluated.

Given the patient unstable condition with O2 saturation of 84% with 100% FiO2, pCO2 67 mmHg, and MAP 60 mmHg receiving the above-mentioned dose of vasoactive drugs, an specialized retrieval team was assembled to assess the patient and carry out the transfer. When this critical care rescue team arrived to the referring ICU the patient was stabilized and prepared for transfer. After draining abundant respiratory secretions, PEEP was lowered and vasopressors adjusted to improve CI, increasing epinephrine, decreasing norepinephrine, and setting the patient in prone position to improve respiratory function. Mechanical ventilation settings were tidal volume of 6 mL/kg, PEEP 16 cm of water, respiratory rate of 32 per minute, and 100% oxygen; the hemodynamic support based on vasoactive drugs was norepinephrine at 0.9 mcg/kg/min and adrenaline 0.7 mcg/kg/min. The team opted for transferring the patient in prone positioning as a bridge therapy to ECMO, due to the severity of shock, ARDS and what appeared to be massive capillary leakage. This decision was made in spite of the severity of the situation, and taking into account that hemodynamic as respiratory functions were partially stabilized. Additionally, the possibility of transferring the patient in ECMO was considered unviable. An ambulance was called in, and the patient was transported in prone position under the management of the critical care rescue team with no incidents or new interventions (Figure 1).

At the arrival at the University Hospital, the O_2 saturation was 88% with 100% FiO_2 and MAP was 72 mmHg without changes in the doses of vasoactive drugs. The patient entered immediately to the operating room for ECMO installation. During the procedure he was unstable hemodynamically and presented a large bleeding and received several transfusions (red blood cells 5 units, fresh frozen plasma 3 units, and platelets 10 units), but the procedure was completed satisfactorily.

The patient was transferred to the ICU, while on ECMO, and high volume hemofiltration was started. Among laboratory parameters a decreased fibrinogen (87 mg/dL), increased serum creatinine of 2.6 mg/dL, arterial lactate of 17 mmol/L,

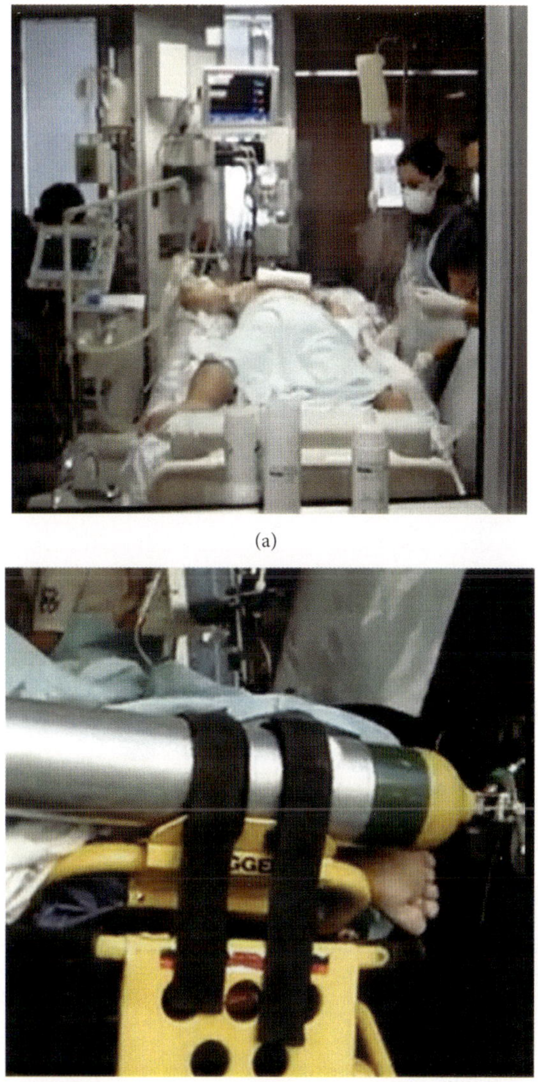

(a)

(b)

FIGURE 1: Prone position transport. Patient after prone positioning and stabilization by the retrieval team on the referring ICU (a) and during transport procedure on the ambulance where the foot orientation evidences the prone position (b).

and thrombocytopenia of 24.000 were found. Hantavirus infection was confirmed by enzyme-linked immunosorbent assay (ELISA). Echocardiography at day 2 on ECMO revealed severe left ventricle systolic dysfunction with an ejection fraction of 26%. However, continuous ultrafiltration therapy was well tolerated, and a day after, vasopressors were suspended. Arterial lactate decreased to 4.8 mmol/L, and central venous saturation was 61%. Left ventricular function improved to an ejection fraction of 53% at day 3. A low dose of dobutamine (2 mcg/kg/min) was continued, and ultrafiltration rate was progressively increased to 250 mL/h.

In the fifth day since admission, ECMO was removed, and the patient continued on mechanical ventilation, achieving a PaO_2/FiO_2 ratio of 180 and OI of 10,5 with PEEP 10 cm of water and FiO_2 of 60%. Four days later he was extubated and supported by noninvasive ventilation. Chest X-ray revealed

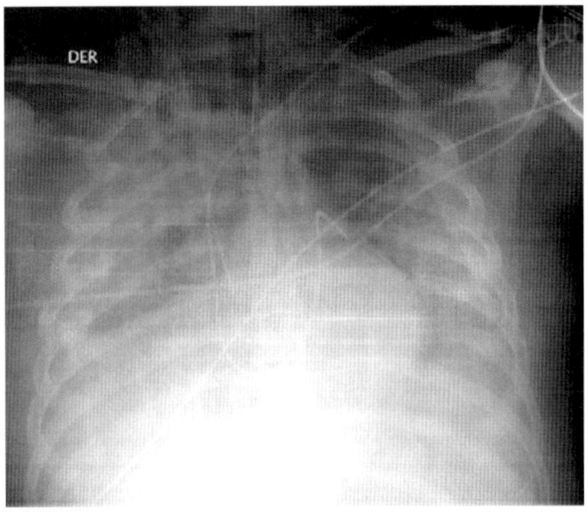

(a)

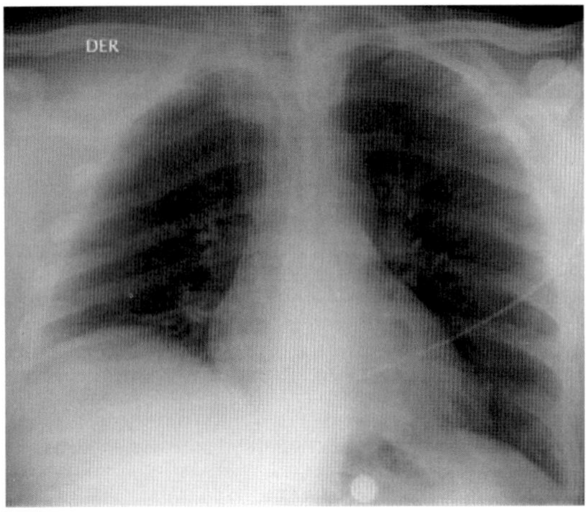

(b)

Figure 2: Chest imaging evolution. Chest X-ray on day 2 shows opaque lung fields (a) with resolution of infiltrates an normalization of aeration a week later (b).

a significant reduction of pulmonary infiltrates (Figure 2). During the following days, the patient evidenced the recovery of his respiratory, cardiovascular, and kidney functions and the normalization of the coagulation disorder. He was transferred to intermediate care and then to the general ward. He was discharged after a month of hospitalization requiring physical rehabilitation with no other dysfunctions and normal cognitive functions, resuming his graduate studies.

3. Discussion

In this case of Hantavirus-induced cardiopulmonary syndrome, catastrophic respiratory failure and severe shock were treated with prone positioning and vasoactive drugs adjustment to stabilize and transfer the patient as a bridge to ECMO therapy. The treatment in the University Hospital using ECMO was required because both respiratory and cardiac failures were considered potentially reversible, and the patient had not responded to conventional therapy. The transfer of this type of patients is associated with a high incidence of potentially life-threatening complications. In this case, the participation of a trained and experienced team of critical care physicians to rescue the patient was determinant in the success of procedure, after stabilizing the patient, and risk-benefit assessment of employing prone position ventilation as a bridge to definitive therapy.

Transport of critically ill patients has increased in the last years; it was particularly important during the 2009 flu pandemic, when the rapid onset of refractory hypoxemia, together with multisystem organ failure, caused that clinical outcomes largely depended on hospitals capacities and clinicians' expertise to apply sophisticated mechanical ventilatory support and adjunct therapies unavailable in all hospitals. When transferring critical patients is decided, the benefits of more specialized care—the usual reason to transfer—must be weighed against risks of morbidity and mortality related to the procedure [1]. The most common complications of transport are hypotension and hypoxemia, frequently seen in the most severely ill patients receiving higher levels of PEEP or FiO_2 [2]. Preparations may render the procedure safer if performed by a dedicated team [3].

Clinicians should notice that the rescue therapies used in this case, prone positioning and ECMO, have the potential to cause harm if not implemented in a coordinated manner by an experienced ICU team. Many hospitals may not have adequate numbers of physicians with this expertise or staffing structures to facilitate timely treatment of complications or technical problem resolution at any time. Attempting a high-risk maneuver to accomplish interhospital transportation of critically ill patients should be ruled out if the team does not have sufficient experience, training, or familiarity implementing prone positioning or ECMO. Both strategies have been used in interhospital transportation without major adverse events [4, 5].

Some countries have addressed this issue with national guidelines, coordinating tertiary ICUs to facilitate adequate access to more intensivist-staffed ICUs and implementing dedicated teams and devices as mobile intensive care units "MICUs" that have shown to improve outcomes making transfers a safe procedure [6].

Transporting mechanically ventilated patients in prone positioning due to life-threatening hypoxemia can be achieved successfully with a trained team [5]. In our experience, patients have been transported in prone between different hospital units, from ICU to the department of radiology not only for computed tomography assessment and studies [7] but also for open lung biopsies in the operating room, without adverse events [8]. Noteworthy, before transporting mechanically ventilated patients in prone positioning outside the ICU, the patients have always been assessed by a trained ICU team, carefully reviewed following a detailed protocol, and the maneuvers performed only by experienced intensive care specialists using previously known equipment, such as ventilator and infusion pumps.

Prone ventilation is a feasible and relatively safe therapy that improves oxygenation in ARDS, reduces the risk of ventilator induced lung injury [9], and improves the survival in patients with severe form of ARDS as suggested previously and recently demonstrated in the large clinical trial PROSEVA [10, 11]. Our team has developed experience in prolonged prone ventilation as a protocolized routine therapy for severe ARDS [12], recently applied during the 2009 flu pandemic [13]. In addition, several procedures are performed in prone positioning in ARDS patients in our unit, as the installation of intravascular devices using ultrasound-guided central catheter insertions in the case of central venous and artery pulmonary catheters, fiber optic bronchoscopy, and transesophageal echocardiography; the latter has been reported in other centers [14, 15].

To the best of our knowledge there are no reports transferring patients with Hantavirus cardiopulmonary syndrome in prone position ventilation as a bridge to ECMO. However, there is an interesting case series transporting critically ill patients with severe respiratory and cardiac failures, performed in prone position ventilation, with no complications [5]. These suggest that prone position ventilation is not a contraindication for transport if performed appropriately.

In case reported here, the severe cardiopulmonary syndrome was caused by Hantavirus. Hantavirus is a rodent borne virus from the Bunyaviridae family; its reservoir is the long-tailed pygmy rice rat (*Oligoryzomys longicaudatus*), endemic to some regions of USA, Argentina, Brazil, Chile, Paraguay, Bolivia, Panama, and Canada. Hantavirus infection can lead to different manifestations. Hantavirus cardiopulmonary syndrome is the most severe form, characterized by fever and progressive symptoms. This condition rapidly evolves to cardiogenic shock and pulmonary edema with severe capillary leak. If adequate support is applied, recovery of the most severe dysfunctions occurs in a few days [16]. Thus, Hantavirus infection is a model of hyperacute multisystem failures that can require ECMO as rescue therapy with potential full recovery. Therefore, transfer to centers in which ECMO is available may constitute the difference between and almost certain death and survival. In this context, prone position ventilation could be a lifesaving tool if employed as a bridge to ECMO if other treatments are insufficient to provide safe limits of oxygenation or is not feasible to implement a transfer on ECMO. The key point is adequate monitorization and management on a case-by-case basis by a specialized retrieval team with expertise on rescue therapies [17].

In conclusion, we found that an unstable patient with Hantavirus cardiopulmonary could be transferred without major complications allowing survival. We acknowledge that this is only a single case, but several series show that the participation of a specialized retrieval team, proper patient stabilization before transport, an ambulance with appropriate intensive care equipment, and interhospital transfers of critically ill patients appear to be feasible. Catastrophic cardiorespiratory failures should not be considered contraindications to attempt transfer to tertiary centers if deemed necessary, and prone position ventilation may be the required bridge to do so.

References

[1] T. J. Iwashyna, "The incomplete infrastructure for interhospital patient transfer," *Critical Care Medicine*, vol. 40, pp. 2470–2478, 2012.

[2] G. Marx, B. Vangerow, H. Hecker et al., "Predictors of respiratory function deterioration after transfer of critically ill patients," *Intensive Care Medicine*, vol. 24, no. 11, pp. 1157–1162, 1998.

[3] W. E. Edge, R. K. Kanter, C. G. M. Weigle, and R. F. Walsh, "Reduction of morbidity in interhospital transport by specialized pediatric staff," *Critical Care Medicine*, vol. 22, no. 7, pp. 1186–1191, 1994.

[4] V. Lindén, K. Palmér, J. Reinhard et al., "Inter-hospital transportation of patients with severe acute respiratory failure on extracorporeal membrane oxygenation—national and international experience," *Intensive Care Medicine*, vol. 27, no. 10, pp. 1643–1648, 2001.

[5] A. Uusaro, I. Parviainen, J. Takala, and E. Ruokonen, "Safe long-distance interhospital ground transfer of critically ill patients with acute severe unstable respiratory and circulatory failure," *Intensive Care Medicine*, vol. 28, no. 8, pp. 1122–1125, 2002.

[6] J. S. Wiegersma, J. M. Droogh, J. G. Zijlstra, J. Fokkema, and J. J. M. Ligtenberg, "Quality of interhospital transport of the critically ill: impact of a Mobile Intensive Care Unit with a specialized retrieval team," *Critical Care*, vol. 15, no. 1, article R75, 2011.

[7] R. A. Cornejo, J. C. Diaz, E. A. Tobar et al., "Effects of prone positioning on lung protection in patients with acute respiratory distresssyndrome," *American Journal of Respiratory and Critical Care Medicine*. In press.

[8] R. Cornejo, O. Llanos, C. Fernández et al., "Organizing pneumonia in patients with severe respiratory failure due to novel A, (H1N1) influenza," *BMJ Case Reports*, 2010.

[9] E. Galiatsou, E. Kostanti, E. Svarna et al., "Prone position augments recruitment and prevents alveolar overinflation in acute lung injury," *American Journal of Respiratory and Critical Care Medicine*, vol. 174, no. 2, pp. 187–197, 2006.

[10] F. Abroug, L. Ouanes-Besbes, F. Dachraoui, I. Ouanes, and L. Brochard, "An updated study-level meta-analysis of randomised controlled trials on proning in ARDS and acute lung injury," *Critical Care*, vol. 15, no. 1, article R6, 2011.

[11] C. Guérin et al., "Prone positioning in severe acute distress syndrome," *The New England Journal of Medicine*, vol. 368, pp. 2159–2168, 2013.

[12] C. M. Romero, R. Cornejo, L. R. Gálvez et al., "Extended prone position ventilation in severe acute respiratory distress syndrome: a pilot feasibility study," *Journal of Critical Care*, vol. 24, pp. 81–88, 2009.

[13] R. Cornejo, E. Tobar, G. Díaz et al., "Systematic approach for severe respiratory failure due to novel a (H1N1) influenza," *Minerva Anestesiologica*, vol. 77, no. 5, pp. 510–521, 2011.

[14] A. Mekontso Dessap, O. Proost, F. Boissier, B. Louis, F. Roche Campo, and L. Brochard, "Transesophageal echocardiography in prone position during severe acute respiratory distress syndrome," *Intensive Care Medicine*, vol. 37, no. 3, pp. 430–434, 2011.

[15] A. Vieillard-Baron, "Acute cor pulmonale in acute respiratory distress syndrome submitted to protective ventilation: incidence, clinical implications, and prognosis," *Critical Care Medicine*, vol. 29, pp. 1551–1555, 2001.

[16] M. R. Crowley, R. W. Katz, R. Kessler et al., "Successful treatment of adults with severe Hantavirus pulmonary syndrome with extracorporeal membrane oxygenation," *Critical Care Medicine*, vol. 26, no. 2, pp. 409–414, 1998.

[17] G. Bellingan, T. Olivier, S. Batson, and A. Webb, "Comparison of a specialist retrieval team with current United Kingdom practice for the transport of critically ill patients," *Intensive Care Medicine*, vol. 26, no. 6, pp. 740–744, 2000.

15

Buried Bumper Syndrome Revisited: A Rare but Potentially Fatal Complication of PEG Tube Placement

Saptarshi Biswas, Sujana Dontukurthy, Mathew G. Rosenzweig, Ravi Kothuru, and Sunil Abrol

Department of General Surgery, Brookdale University Hospital Medical Center, Brooklyn, NY 11212, USA

Correspondence should be addressed to Saptarshi Biswas; saptarshibiswas@comcast.net

Academic Editors: C. Diez, Y. Durandy, H. Kern, and Z. Molnar

Percutaneous endoscopic gastrostomy (PEG) has been used for providing enteral access to patients who require long-term enteral nutrition for years. Although generally considered safe, PEG tube placement can be associated with many immediate and delayed complications. Buried bumper syndrome (BBS) is one of the uncommon and late complications of percutaneous endoscopic gastrostomy (PEG) placement. It occurs when the internal bumper of the PEG tube erodes into the gastric wall and lodges itself between the gastric wall and skin. This can lead to a variety of additional complications such as wound infection, peritonitis, and necrotizing fasciitis. We present here a case of buried bumper syndrome which caused extensive necrosis of the anterior abdominal wall.

1. Introduction

Percutaneous endoscopic gastrostomy (PEG) was first reported in the literature in 1980 as an alternative way to provide tube feeding for patients without a laparotomy [1]. Today, PEG placement is widely accepted as a safe technique to provide long-term enteral nutrition for a variety of patients including those with neurologic deficits and swallowing disorders and those with oropharyngeal or esophageal tumors and various hypercatabolic states like burns, short bowel syndrome, and major traumas [2]. Although considered a safe procedure, immediate and delayed complications have been described with the PEG placement. These complications vary from minor complications like wound infections to major life threatening complications like peritonitis and buried bumper syndrome. BBS is an uncommon but serious complication of PEG, occurring in 0.3–2–4% of patients [3]. We present here a case of BBS followed by a discussion of its etiology, management, and prevention.

2. Case description

A 70-year-old female with multiple comorbidities presented to the ER from the nursing home with symptoms suggestive of septic shock. At the time of admission, the patient was undergoing active treatment for urinary tract infection in the nursing home. Physical examination of the patient revealed respiratory distress and hypotension, so emergency intubation was done and vasopressors started to maintain blood pressure. Empiric broad spectrum antibiotics were initiated for septic shock. Patient was then transferred to the medical intensive care unit for further management.

Patient history revealed that the PEG tube was inserted one year prior due to dysphagia from a stroke. Upon abdominal examination, the PEG tube was in place in the epigastric area with signs of edema and erythema on the right lateral side of the abdomen.

Bullae were spread diffusely across the abdomen (Figure 1), and gastric contents were noted to be leaking around the PEG tube. The patient localized tenderness to palpation, and bowel sounds were normal with no rebound or guarding.

The general surgery team was consulted for PEG tube position and abdominal wall erythema and edema.

Laboratory studies revealed leukocytosis of 18000 cells/cubic mm, hemoglobin of 5.3 g/dl, hematocrit of 15.2%, and an INR greater than 10 as the patient was on regular

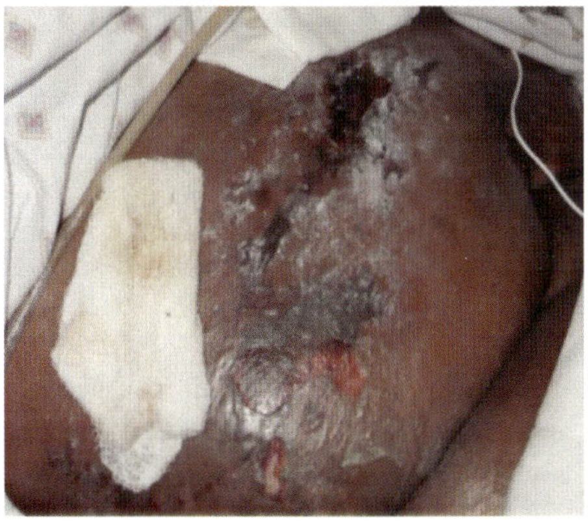

FIGURE 1: Anterior abdominal wall showing edema, erythema, and ruptured bullae over the abdomen.

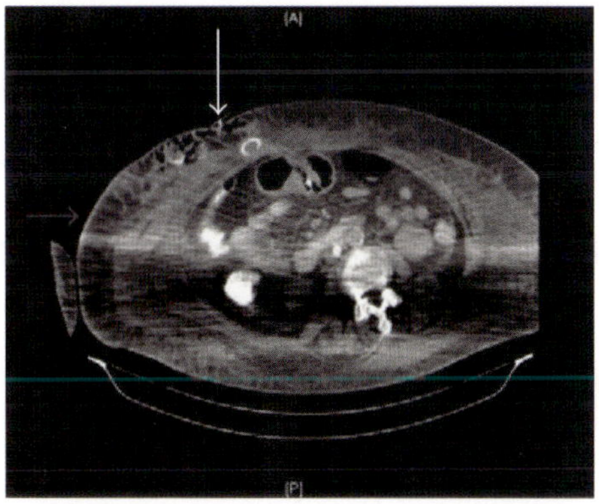

FIGURE 2: CT image of the abdomen. (1) The solid arrow indicates dislodgement of the internal bumper of the PEG tube into the abdominal wall outside the peritoneum. (2) The hollow arrow shows subcutaneous collection of fluid and air in the abdominal wall.

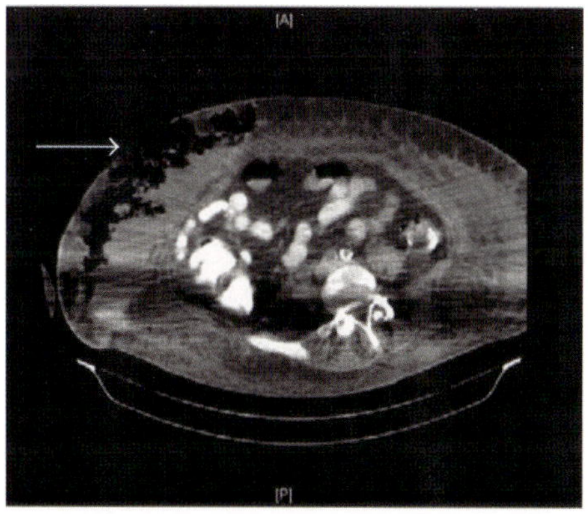

FIGURE 3: CT image of the abdomen. The arrow indicates extensive subcutaneous collection of fluid and air in the abdominal wall.

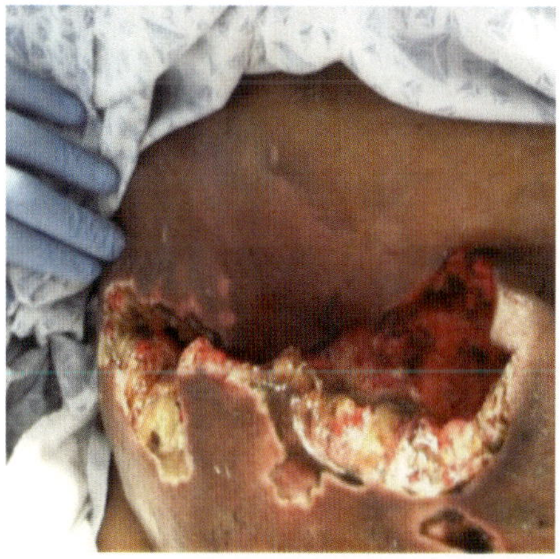

FIGURE 4: Anterior abdominal wall with erythema and edema prior to debridement.

Coumadin for chronic atrial fibrillation. Computed tomography scan of the abdomen and pelvis was recommended to confirm PEG tube position and to evaluate for retroperitoneal hematoma in view of high INR and low hemoglobin. The nursing staff was subsequently instructed to hold feeding through the PEG tube till its position could be confirmed with the CT scan.

CT scan of the abdomen showed dislodgement of the internal button of the gastrostomy tube into the abdominal wall and a large collection measuring 10 × 7.5 × 20 cm. The collection showed equal parts of gas and fluid density in the subcutaneous compartment of the right anterolateral abdominal wall just lateral to the percutaneous gastrostomy tube outside the muscle and peritoneal reflection (Figures 2 and 3).

After explaining the benefits and risks of the surgical procedure for drainage in the operating room, the intervention was denied by the patient's next of kin. Aspiration of the subcutaneous collection by the interventional radiologist was scheduled; however, the plan was withheld due to hemodynamic instability and the risk of transport to the radiology suite. A plan was made for bedside incision, drainage, and debridement of the subcutaneous collection. Vitamin K and FFP was administered for increased INR. After explaining the risks and benefits, informed consent was obtained from the patient's next of kin.

Bedside debridement was performed, and over 600 milliliters of foul smelling brownish fluid was aspirated from the wound (Figures 4 and 5). The fluid and the PEG tube tip were sent for culture and sensitivity. Wound vacuum was inserted and kept in situ for further drainage (Figure 6). The aspirated fluid and PEG tube tip culture and sensitivity revealed Klebsiella Pneumonia and Candida Vulgaris. Despite resuscitative efforts, the patient expired 10 days after debridement from septic shock.

Wound vac was inserted after bedside debridement and drainage. Appropriate antibiotics and antifungals were initiated according to the microbial sensitivity.

3. Discussion

PEG placement complications can be minor ranging from wound infection around the PEG tube to major complications like BBS, necrotizing fasciitis, and colocutaneous fistula. The overall complication rate ranges from 4% to 23.8% of cases [4–7]. Three to 4% of all cases are affected by

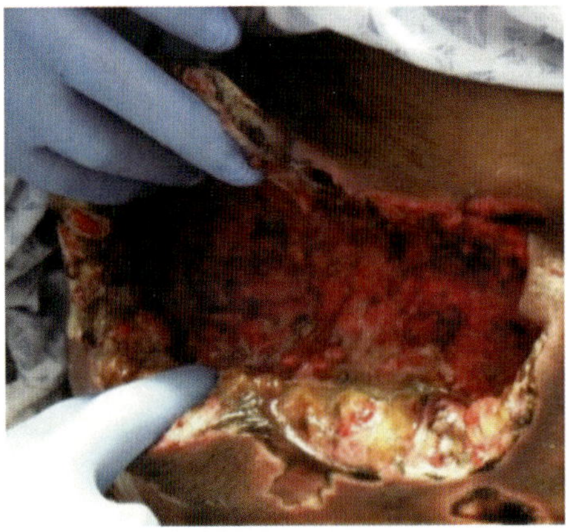

Figure 5: Bedside debridement and pulse lavage of the subcutaneous collection of the anterior abdominal wall.

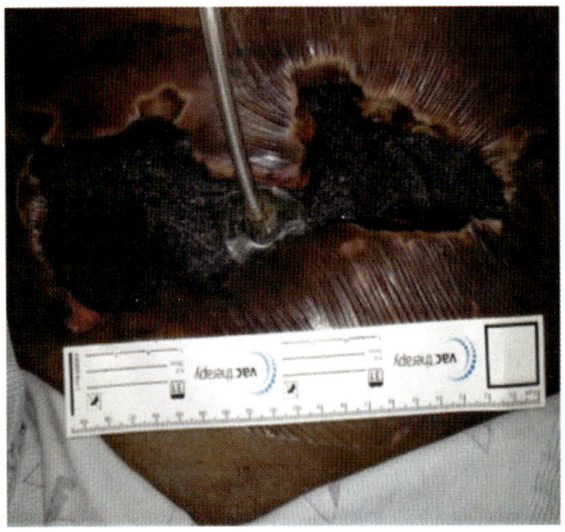

Figure 6: Wound vac after debridement for further drainage.

major complications [4, 6, 8]. The more common minor complications occur between 7.4% and 20.0% of cases [4, 6, 8]. Generally, complications are more likely to occur with elderly patients, especially those with comorbid conditions, as well as those with a past history of aspiration [9]. BBS, first described in 1988, is considered a late and rare complication of PEG placement [10]. It occurs when the internal bumper of the feeding tube erodes into the gastric wall leading to ischemic necrosis and the ultimate migration of the internal bumper and lodging itself between the gastric wall and the skin. A relationship is believed to exist between tightening of the external bolster in an effort to prevent leaking of gastric contents causing increased tension in the tube [3]. Other contributing factors include gastric acid alteration of the internal bumper, PEG tube characteristics such as a hard plastic composition, and inadequate patient care [11].

Although many risk factors like obesity, rapid weight gain, patient manipulation, gauze placement beneath the external bumper instead of over it, chronic cough, tube manipulation by inexperienced personnel, and malnutrition have been associated with BBS, obesity is considered as the single most important risk factor for this syndrome [3]. It can be ascertained that any unnecessary increased tension of the tube can lead to BBS over a period of time. While the earliest reported complication occurred at 8 days after insertion, in a range of 1–50 months the majority of BBS occur with a median of 18 months [9, 12]. Ultimately, the migration of the internal bolster can lead to a loss of feeding access and a variety of other minor and major complications as previously discussed. Patients with this syndrome typically present with leakage around the PEG tube or signs of infection like edema or erythema, an immobile catheter, and abdominal pain or resistance to administer formula infusion. Diagnosis of BBS is made clinically and confirmed endoscopically or with computed tomography [3].

The mainstay of treatment for these patients includes the removal of the buried bumper, even in the asymptomatic patient in order to avoid further complications such as stomach perforation, peritonitis, and infection of the subcutaneous tissue [11]. Various internal techniques including surgery or endoscopic snare retrieval through the mouth can be implemented for tube removal [11, 13]. Often times, simple external traction is possible with a collapsible internal bumper [2]. Additional techniques are currently being described such as using an angioplasty balloon dilator under radiological guidance to avoid surgery [14].

While the current literature lacks strong evidence to support a specific preventive practice, possible considerations have been suggested. Among these are allowing for an additional 1.5–2 cm between the external bumper and the skin, gently rotating and manipulating the PEG in and out daily, and measuring the length of the external portion of the tube in order to recognize migration and avoid unnecessary tube traction [3, 11].

4. Conclusion

BBS is a rare and typically late presenting complication of PEG tube placement. Early recognition of this complication reduces the life threatening consequences involved. A multidisciplinary team approach and patient education are essential efforts for preventing BBS.

Acknowledgments

The authors would like to thank Clarence Ojo, M.D., and Tak-Keung Wong, M.D., for their invaluable assistance with this case report.

References

[1] W. L. Gauderer, J. L. Ponsky, and R. J. Izant Jr., "Gastrostomy without laparotomy: a percutaneous endoscopic technique," *Journal of Pediatric Surgery*, vol. 15, no. 6, pp. 872–875, 1980.

[2] T. Elbaz, S. Rejchrt, T. Douda, J. Cyrany, R. Repak, and J. Bures, "Buried bumper syndrome: an uncommon complication

of percutaneous gastrostomy. Report of three cases," *Folia Gastroenterol Hepatol*, vol. 4, no. 2, pp. 61–66, 2006.

[3] G. H. Pop, "Buried bumper syndrome: can we prevent it?" *Practical Gastroenterology*, vol. 34, no. 5, pp. 8–13, 2010.

[4] D. E. Larson, D. D. Burton, K. W. Schroeder, and E. P. DiMagno, "Percutaneous endoscopic gastrostomy. Indications, success, complications, and mortality in 314 consecutive patients," *Gastroenterology*, vol. 93, no. 1, pp. 48–52, 1987.

[5] L. Rabeneck, N. P. Wray, and N. J. Petersen, "Long-term outcomes of patients receiving percutaneous endoscopic gastrostomy tubes," *Journal of General Internal Medicine*, vol. 11, no. 5, pp. 287–293, 1996.

[6] C. Löser, S. Wolters, and U. R. Fölsch, "Enteral long-term nutrition via percutaneous endoscopic gastrostomy (PEG) in 210 patients: a four-year prospective study," *Digestive Diseases and Sciences*, vol. 43, no. 11, pp. 2549–2557, 1998.

[7] M. A. Lockett, M. L. Templeton, T. K. Byrne, and E. D. Norcross, "Percutaneous endoscopic gastrostomy complications in a tertiary-care center," *American Surgeon*, vol. 68, no. 2, pp. 117–120, 2002.

[8] M. Neeff, V. L. Crowder, N. P. McIvor, J. M. Chaplin, and R. P. Morton, "Comparison of the use of endoscopic and radiologic gastrostomy in a single head and neck cancer unit," *ANZ Journal of Surgery*, vol. 73, no. 8, pp. 590–593, 2003.

[9] T.-H. Lee and J.-T. Lin, "Clinical manifestations and management of buried bumper syndrome in patients with percutaneous endoscopic gastrostomy," *Gastrointestinal Endoscopy*, vol. 68, no. 3, pp. 580–584, 2008.

[10] H. I. Schwartz, R. I. Goldberg, J. S. Barkin, R. S. Phillips, A. Land, and M. Hecht, "PEG feeding tube migration impaction in the abdominal wall," *Gastrointestinal Endoscopy*, vol. 35, no. 2, p. 134, 1989.

[11] Q. Khalil, R. Kibria, and S. Akram, "Acute buried bumper syndrome," *Southern Medical Journal*, vol. 103, no. 12, pp. 1256–1258, 2010.

[12] R. P. Venu, R. D. Brown, B. J. Pastika, and L. W. Erikson Jr., "The buried bumper syndrome: a simple management approach in two patients," *Gastrointestinal Endoscopy*, vol. 56, no. 4, pp. 582–584, 2002.

[13] S. A. McClave and N. S. Jafri, "Spectrum of morbidity related to bolster placement at time of percutaneous endoscopic gastrostomy: buried bumper syndrome to leakage and peritonitis," *Gastrointestinal Endoscopy Clinics of North America*, vol. 17, no. 4, pp. 731–746, 2007.

[14] J. J. Crowley, D. Vora, C. J. Becker, and L. S. Harris, "Radiologic removal of buried gastrostomy bumpers in pediatric patients," *American Journal of Roentgenology*, vol. 176, no. 3, pp. 766–768, 2001.

16

Hyperammonemic Coma in an Adult due to Ornithine Transcarbamylase Deficiency

Daniel L. Roberts,[1] David A. Galbreath,[2] Bhavesh M. Patel,[3] Timothy J. Ingall,[4] Amer Khatib,[5] and Daniel J. Johnson[6]

[1] *Division of Hospital Internal Medicine, Department of Medicine, Mayo Clinic, Phoenix, AZ 85054, USA*
[2] *Kansas City Family Medical Clinic, Kansas City, MO 64114, USA*
[3] *Department of Critical Care Medicine, Mayo Clinic, Phoenix, AZ 85054, USA*
[4] *Department of Neurology, Mayo Clinic, Phoenix, AZ 85054, USA*
[5] *Division of Gastroenterology, Faculty of Medicine, University of Jordan, Amman 11942, Jordan*
[6] *Department of Surgery, Mayo Clinic, Phoenix, AZ 85054, USA*

Correspondence should be addressed to Daniel L. Roberts; roberts.daniel@mayo.edu

Academic Editors: K. Chergui, Y. Durandy, W. J. Ko, Z. Molnar, S. Natoli, J. Starkopf, and M. R. Suchyta

Objective. To report an unusual cause of coma in an adult. *Design.* Case report. *Setting.* University teaching hospital. *Patient.* A previously healthy 53-year-old man initially presented with altered mental status and progressed to coma. He was found to be substantially hyperammonemic and did not improve with lactulose therapy and continuous venovenous hemodialysis. *Results.* Biochemical testing revealed previously undiagnosed ornithine transcarbamylase deficiency, and the patient responded to arginine, sodium phenylacetate, and sodium benzoate. *Conclusion.* Even in adult patients with no known history, inborn errors of metabolism must be considered in the differential diagnosis of unexplained coma. Defects of the urea cycle can present with an unprovoked hyperammonemic coma.

1. Introduction

The differential diagnosis of coma in adults is notoriously broad, but the presence of hyperammonemia narrows it to Reye's syndrome, high-dose chemotherapy, *Proteus* infection, glycine toxicity (after transurethral resection of prostate) [1], liver failure, and late-onset urea cycle defects [2]. Although disorders of the urea cycle are predominantly the purview of the neonatologist, presentations of urea cycle enzyme deficiencies in adults have been reported.

2. Case Report

A fifty-three-year-old man was admitted to an outside hospital with a significantly decreased level of consciousness. He had awoken at night and urinated on the bathroom floor, and the following morning, his wife was unable to fully awaken him. He had reported progressive fatigue over the preceding two weeks, but had otherwise been in his usual state of good health. Specifically, he had no history of fevers, chills, rigors, weight loss, chest pain, shortness of breath, nausea, vomiting, or abdominal pain.

His past medical history was significant only for benign prostatic hypertrophy and hyperlipidemia. He had no history of alcohol abuse, diabetes mellitus, or liver disease. His medications included terazosin, tamsulosin, and a recent methylprednisolone taper for a nonspecific groin rash. He had initiated therapy with simvastatin approximately one month prior to admission. His only recent toxin exposure was the use of a permethrin-based insecticide, and he reported no symptoms during or after this exposure.

On admission to the outside hospital, the patient was afebrile and anicteric with normal vital signs. The neurologic examination revealed that he was only intermittently arousable to verbal stimuli, with the remainder of the exam being

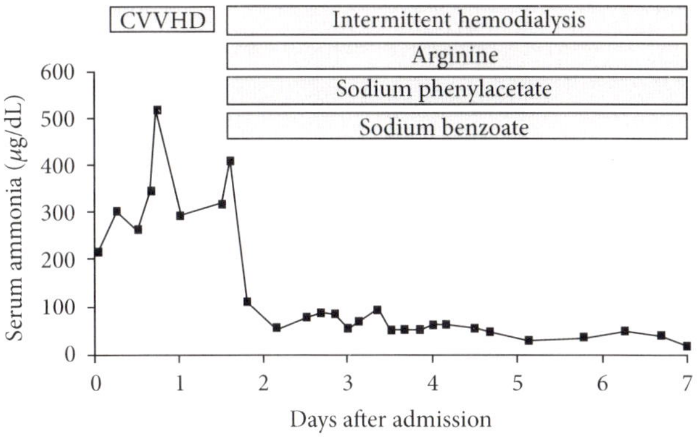

FIGURE 1: The patient's serum ammonia charted against time after admission, with graphic representation of timing of interventions. CVVHD: continuous venovenous hemodialysis.

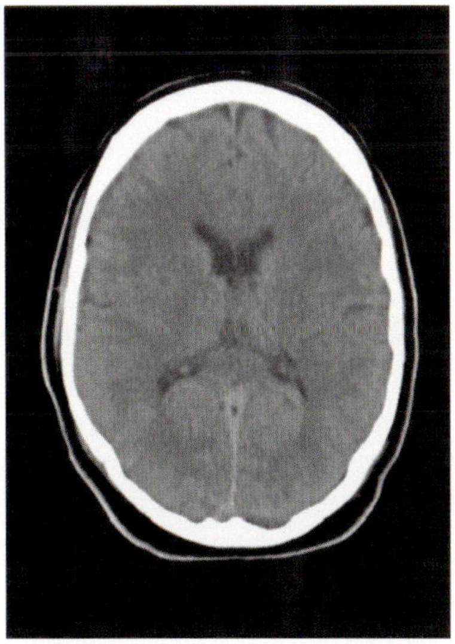

FIGURE 2: CT of the head without contrast reveals evidence of mild cerebral edema.

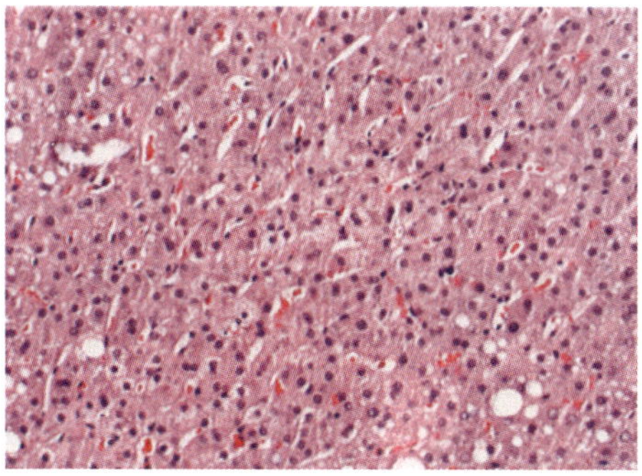

FIGURE 3: Liver biopsy reveals centrilobular steatosis without fibrosis. (Hematoxylin and eosin, 40x.)

nonfocal. A complete blood count, serum electrolytes, serum alcohol, cardiac enzymes, urine drug screen, chest X-ray, CT scan of the head, and MRI/MRA of the brain were normal. His ammonia level was noted to be elevated at 202 umol/L (normal range = 11–35 umol/L). His other liver function tests were as follows: AST = 19 units/L (8–14 units/L), ALT = 70 units/L (7–55 units/L), total bilirubin = 1.4 mg/dL (0.1–1.0 mg/dL), and INR = 1.12. A CT scan of the abdomen revealed fatty infiltration of the hepatic parenchyma, but was otherwise unremarkable. Over the course of his stay, he became less responsive, and his ammonia level failed to normalize despite aggressive lactulose therapy. He was intubated for airway protection and transferred to our institution for further evaluation.

On arrival, the patient withdrew to pain in his lower extremities, with no response in the upper extremities. Pupils were equal and reactive, deep tendon reflexes were normal and symmetric, and his left plantar response was equivocal. His Glasgow Coma Scale score was 10 (E4, V2, M4). His vital signs and the remainder of his physical examination were unremarkable. Initial laboratory data were significant for a leukocytosis (16.6×10^9/L, normal range $3.5–10.5 \times 10^9$/L), hypernatremia (155 mEq/L, 135–145 mEq/L), hypocalcemia (8.8 mg/dL, 8.9–10.1 mg/dL), an AST level of 34 units/L, an ALT level of 50 units/L, an ammonia level of 215 ug/dL, and an INR of 1.21. Alkaline phosphatase and total bilirubin were within normal limits. MRI of his brain and cervical spine was negative and specifically revealed no evidence of spinal cord compression as a cause for his upper extremity weakness. An electroencephalogram (EEG) showed diffuse slowing and triphasic waves consistent with hepatic encephalopathy. Quantitative serum amino acids, urine organic acid screen, and urine heavy metal screen were drawn, while lactulose and respiratory support were continued.

Over the next twelve hours, the patient's ammonia level worsened to 516 ug/dL (Figure 1). Moderate flux continuous venovenous hemodialysis (CVVHD) was initiated, and his ammonia decreased to 291 ug/dL without any observable improvement in his level of consciousness. A repeat CT of his head demonstrated new cerebral edema (Figure 2). A subarachnoid bolt was placed and revealed normal intracerebral pressures. Transcutaneous liver biopsy was obtained, revealing mild-to-moderate centrilobular steatosis without evidence of fibrosis (Figure 3). This was felt to be inconsistent with the diagnosis of Reye's syndrome.

At this time, laboratory data returned revealing a marked elevation in the patient's urine orotic acid and uracil and confirming the diagnosis of ornithine transcarbamylase deficiency. The patient was subsequently treated with an infusion of intravenous arginine with dextrose. On hospital day 2, his ammonia level worsened to 410 ug/dL while on CVVHD, and there was a deterioration of lower extremity withdrawal strength to painful stimuli. He was switched to intermittent hemodialysis. He was also started on intravenous sodium phenylacetate and sodium benzoate. His ammonia level subsequently normalized, and his mental status improved to the point that he was extubated on hospital day 7. When he resumed oral intake, he was started on oral sodium phenylacetate, sodium benzoate, and a protein-restricted diet. His mental status subsequently returned to baseline, and he was discharged home. His simvastatin was restarted by his primary physician with no adverse effects.

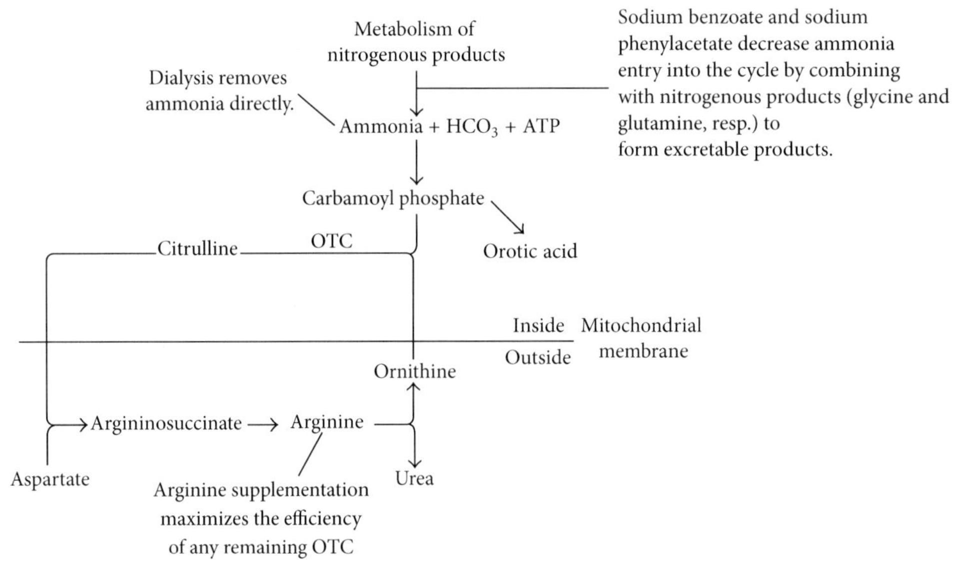

Figure 4: The urea cycle, demonstrating steps at which interventions are targeted in OTCD. ATP: adenosine triphosphate. ASAS: argininosuccinate synthetase. ASAL: argininosuccinate lyase. ARG-1: arginase 1.

The patient's family initially denied any family history of metabolic disorders. However, after some investigations, they subsequently remembered that the patient's maternal second cousin had been diagnosed with OTC deficiency. His relatives were tested for OTC deficiency. The patient currently takes arginine and sodium phenylbutyrate and has not suffered any further complications of his disease over eleven years of followup.

3. Discussion

The urea cycle is the primary metabolic pathway for the excretion of nitrogenous wastes as urea. Ornithine transcarbamylase (OTC) catalyzes the second of the five reactions that make up the cycle (Figure 4). It catalyzes the mitochondrial reaction of ornithine (the end product of the extraction of urea from arginine) with carbamoyl phosphate (the first storage form of ammonia) to produce citrulline. Deficiency of OTC leads to the formation of excess carbamoyl phosphate, some of which is excreted as an orotic acid. When this pathway is overwhelmed, hyperammonemia results. Thus, patients with OTCD tend to have hyperammonemia, elevated levels of orotic acid in the urine, and low plasma citrulline.

OTCD is the most common urea cycle defect, with an estimated incidence of one in 14,000 live births [3]. The OTC gene is located on the short arm of the X chromosome, and its X-linked recessive inheritance makes it the only urea cycle defect not to be inherited in an autosomal recessive manner [4]. Most males with the deficiency die as neonates. However, phenotypic variability has been noted, and cases of patients presenting as adults have been reported [5, 6]. Female heterozygotes are also occasionally noted to manifest symptoms [7, 8].

Symptoms of late-onset OTCD are those of hyperammonemia, and include lethargy, confusion, nausea, vomiting, bizarre behavior, coma, and death. During more severe attacks, intracranial edema and a resulting rapidly fatal course are known complications [9]. Animal models have suggested that this edema may be due to selective astrocytic swelling secondary to hyperammonemia [2].

Hyperammonemia associated with OTCD requires prompt identification and treatment to avoid adverse neurological sequelae and death. Multiple modalities for lowering the serum ammonia level are generally applied simultaneously. On an emergent basis, ammonia can be filtered from the blood via hemodialysis or continuous venovenous hemodiffusion. Lactulose is given simultaneously in a manner similar to that used in hyperammonemia secondary to hepatic failure. Finally, a dextrose infusion is started to provide nonprotein caloric intake and prevent proteolysis.

While these immediate interventions are underway, intravenous sodium benzoate and sodium phenylacetate are given to shunt nitrogen-containing compounds away from the urea cycle [10]. Sodium benzoate conjugates with glycine to form hippuric acid, and sodium phenylacetate conjugates with glutamine to form phenylacetylglutamine. Both end products are readily excreted in the urine. Since adults presenting with OTCD are assumed to have only partial deficiencies, arginine has been given to provide ornithine substrate to react with the resulting excess carbamoyl phosphate and, as a result, to maximize activity of the remaining OTC enzyme. Because patients with OTCD are generally arginine deficient, its replenishment also tends to decrease proteolysis, thus diminishing traffic through the urea cycle. Finally, pyridoxine and folate can be supplemented to drive glycine synthesis and maximize the effectiveness of sodium benzoate [11].

The increased effectiveness of HD over CVVHD in the setting of hyperammonemia due to OTCD (as manifested by this patient) has been previously reported [12].

The specific trigger for this patient's presentation with life-threatening hyperammonemia remains unclear. Typical triggers (increased protein ingestion, infection, perioperative or postpartum state, and anticonvulsant medications) were not noted. No prior reports could be found linking the use of simvastatin or any other HMG Co-A reductase inhibitor with the unmasking of OTCD. Immunosuppressant doses of corticosteroids have been found to trigger attacks of hyperammonemia in OTCD [13], but not at the doses our patient briefly received for his nonspecific dermatitis.

Also poorly understood is the degree and pattern of weakness that he manifested. Although an imaging study suggested mild cerebral edema, invasive intracranial pressure monitoring did not show any evidence of elevated pressures. His neurological recovery was complete.

In summary, late-onset OTCD is uncommon, but it must be considered in the differential diagnosis of hyperammonemia in the setting of relatively normal hepatic enzymes and synthetic function. Although it is frequently fatal, prompt diagnosis and initiation of definitive therapy can be lifesaving.

References

[1] P. T. Hoekstra, R. Kahnoski, M. A. McCamish, W. Bergen, and D. R. Heetderks, "Transurethral prostatic resection syndrome: a new perspective: encephalopathy with associated hyperammonemia," *Journal of Urology*, vol. 130, no. 4, pp. 704–707, 1983.

[2] R. S. Mathias, D. Kostiner, and S. Packman, "Hyperammonemia in urea cycle disorders: role of the nephrologist," *American Journal of Kidney Diseases*, vol. 37, no. 5, pp. 1069–1080, 2001.

[3] B. K. Burton, "Urea cycle disorders," *Clinics in Liver Disease*, vol. 4, no. 4, pp. 815–830, 2000.

[4] M. Trivedi, S. Zafar, M. J. Spalding, and S. Jonnalagadda, "Ornithine transcarbamylase deficiency unmasked because of gastrointestinal bleeding," *Journal of Clinical Gastroenterology*, vol. 32, no. 4, pp. 340–343, 2001.

[5] E. P. DiMagno, J. E. Lowe, P. J. Snodgrass, and J. D. Jones, "Ornithine transcarbamylase deficiency—a cause of bizarre behavior in a man," *The New England Journal of Medicine*, vol. 315, no. 12, pp. 744–747, 1986.

[6] D. E. Choi, K. W. Lee, Y. T. Shin, and K. R. Na, "Hyperammonemia in a patient with late-onset ornithine carbamoyltrasferase deficiency," *Journal of Korean Medical Science*, vol. 27, no. 5, pp. 556–559, 2012.

[7] M. D. Bogdanovic, D. Kidd, A. Briddon, J. S. Duncan, and J. M. Land, "Late onset heterozygous ornithine transcarbamylase deficiency mimicking complex partial status epilepticus," *Journal of Neurology Neurosurgery and Psychiatry*, vol. 69, no. 6, pp. 813–815, 2000.

[8] A. Legras, F. Labarthe, F. Maillot, M. A. Garrigue, A. Kouatchet, and H. Ogier de Baulny, "Late diagnosis of ornithine transcarbamylase defect in three related female patients: polymorphic presentations," *Critical Care Medicine*, vol. 30, no. 1, pp. 241–244, 2002.

[9] O. D. Klein, D. R. Kostiner, K. Weisiger et al., "Acute fatal presentation of ornithine transcarbamylase deficiency in a previously healthy male," *Hepatology International*, vol. 2, no. 3, pp. 390–394, 2008.

[10] G. M. Enns, S. A. Berry, G. T. Berry, W. J. Rhead, S. W. Brusilow, and A. Hamosh, "Survival after treatment with phenylacetate and benzoate for urea-cycle disorders," *The New England Journal of Medicine*, vol. 356, no. 22, pp. 2282–2292, 2007.

[11] W. L. Nyhan and P. T. Ozand, *Atlas of Metabolic Diseases*, Chapman & Hall, London, UK, 1st edition, 1998.

[12] C. Y. Chen, Y. C. Chen, J. T. Fang, and C. C. Huang, "Continuous arteriovenous hemodiafiltration in the acute treatment of hyperammonaemia due to ornithine transcarbamylase deficiency," *Renal Failure*, vol. 22, no. 6, pp. 823–836, 2000.

[13] G. R. Lichtenstein, L. R. Kaiser, M. Tuchman et al., "Fatal hyperammonemia following orthotopic lung transplantation," *Gastroenterology*, vol. 112, no. 1, pp. 236–240, 1997.

17

Management of Cerebellar Tonsillar Herniation following Lumbar Puncture in Idiopathic Intracranial Hypertension

Kenneth R. Hoffman,[1] Sean W. Chan,[1] Andrew R. Hughes,[2] and Stephen J. Halcrow[3]

[1] *Intensive Care Unit, Canberra Hospital, Yamba Drive, Canberra, ACT 2605, Australia*
[2] *Neurology Department, Canberra Hospital, Yamba Drive, Canberra, ACT 2605, Australia*
[3] *Neurosurgical Unit, Canberra Hospital, Yamba Drive, Canberra, ACT 2605, Australia*

Correspondence should be addressed to Kenneth R. Hoffman; kenneth.hoffman@act.gov.au

Academic Editor: Moritoki Egi

Lumbar puncture is performed routinely for diagnostic and therapeutic purposes in idiopathic intracranial hypertension, despite lumbar puncture being classically contraindicated in the setting of raised intracranial pressure. We report the case of a 30-year-old female with known idiopathic intracranial hypertension who had cerebellar tonsillar herniation following therapeutic lumbar puncture. Management followed guidelines regarding treatment of traumatic intracranial hypertension, including rescue decompressive craniectomy. We hypothesize that the changes in brain compliance that are thought to occur in the setting of idiopathic intracranial hypertension are protective against further neuronal injury due to axonal stretch following decompressive craniectomy.

1. Introduction

Idiopathic intracranial hypertension (IIH) causes symptoms and signs of raised intracranial pressure (ICP) without focal neurological signs. It has an overall incidence of 1.6/100,000 per annum [1], an unclear pathogenesis, although it has significantly higher incidence in obese females aged 20–44 at 19/100,000 [2].

Lumbar puncture (LP) is classically contraindicated in the setting of raised ICP due to the risk of cerebellar tonsillar herniation. However, LP is routinely performed both for diagnostic and therapeutic purposes in IIH [3]. It has been postulated that the reason herniation does not occur in this setting is a reduction in brain compliance due to persistently high ICP [4].

To date two case reports of herniation have been reported in IIH following LP, although both of these patients had focal neurological signs on presentation and a fatal outcome [5].

We report a case of herniation following LP in a patient with IIH, her subsequent intensive care management, and clinical course.

2. Case Report

A 30-year-old female with a BMI of 37.9 was diagnosed with IIH seven months prior to this presentation. Her MRI at diagnosis demonstrated 4 mm of cerebellar tonsillar descent (Figure 1) with flattening of the posterior globes, mild distension of the optic nerve sheaths, and a partially empty sella turcica. At the time of diagnosis, her LP revealed an opening pressure of 42 cm H_2O. She was prescribed regular oral acetazolamide and regularly underwent therapeutic drainage of 15 mL of cerebrospinal fluid (CSF) for symptom control without complication. Her opening pressures were consistently between 35 and 50 cm H_2O. MR venogram demonstrated an aplastic left transverse sinus with a right transverse sinus stenosis with extrinsic compression, for which she was being considered for a stenting procedure (Figure 2).

She presented to the emergency department with four days of severe headache, nausea, and vomiting. Her past history included renal tubular acidosis diagnosed two years prior and treated with sodium bicarbonate and electrolyte

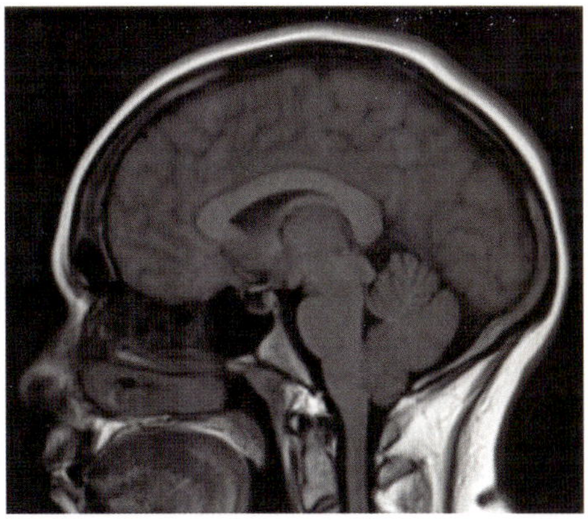

FIGURE 1: Sagittal MRI at diagnosis demonstrated 4 mm of cerebellar tonsillar descent.

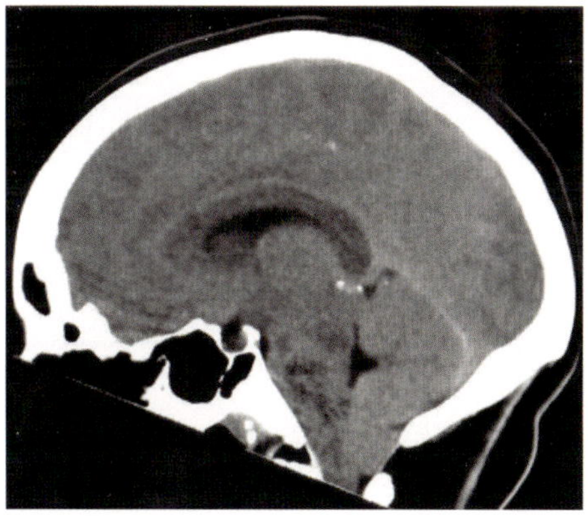

FIGURE 3: Sagittal CT scan demonstrating 10 mm of tonsillar descent with posterior fossa crowding.

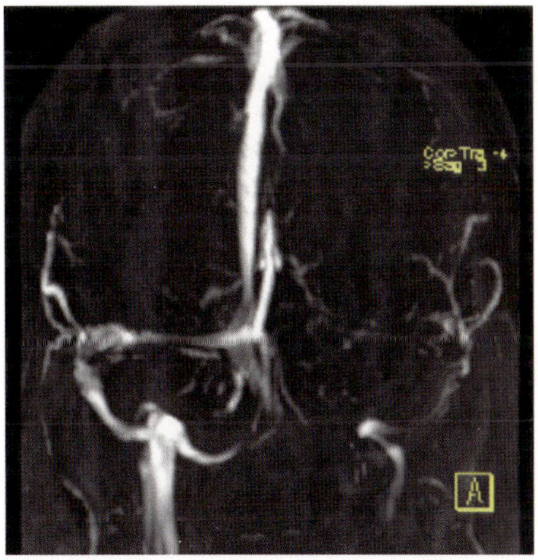

FIGURE 2: Time of flight MR venogram (anterior view) demonstrating aplastic L transverse sinus with R transverse sinus stenosis.

replacement. In the emergency department she had bilateral papilloedema with no new focal neurology. She was normothermic with a CRP of 2.8 mg/L. A therapeutic LP was performed with an opening pressure of 43 cm H_2O. 18 mL of clear CSF was drained and she was admitted to the neurology ward for observation and analgesia.

Overnight she had a medical emergency team (MET) call for hypotension attributed to hypovolemia due to ongoing vomiting, which was treated with intravenous fluids. She had a further MET call overnight for transient visual disturbance and reported being unable to appreciate light/dark and had severe headache. Her pupils were bilaterally dilated but responsive to light. She was alert and interactive and had no motor deficits. The visual changes resolved without intervention and she was taken for a CT venogram, which demonstrated bilateral tentorial herniation with 10 mm of cerebellar tonsillar herniation. There were no features of dural venous thrombosis.

She was reviewed on the morning of day 1 and found to be agitated, Glasgow Coma Scale (GCS) 13 (M6, V4, E3), with a fixed dilated right pupil 7 mm. Her left pupil was 5 mm and reactive. Plantar response was upgoing bilaterally and her neck was hyperextended with extreme pain on neck flexion. Heart rate was 65 bpm and blood pressure was 112/66 mmHg. She was transferred urgently to the intensive care unit (ICU) and intubated for anticipated decline whilst awaiting a CT brain. During the CT scan she became bradycardic with a heart rate of 30 and asystolic pauses, treated with osmotic therapy of 10 mL 20% sodium chloride. Her BP was then recorded as 147/77 mmHg. The CT scan again showed 10 mm of tonsillar descent and an increase in fourth ventricle size with posterior fossa crowding (Figure 3). Her initial LP result showed a mildly elevated white cell count of 7×10^6/L (normal $< 5 \times 10^6$/L) and she was commenced on aciclovir empirically.

She was treated with a further 20 mL of 20% sodium chloride and taken for urgent insertion of an external ventricular drain (EVD), a technically difficult procedure due to small ventricular size, which rapidly improved right pupil reactivity although it remained sluggish. She returned to ICU with the EVD on free drainage 15 cm above the tragus. Her ICP remained persistently high at >45 cm H_2O and the EVD was lowered to 10 cm to allow further drainage. As her pressure on previous LPs was 35–50 cm H_2O, a target of 35 cm H_2O was agreed upon for initial management.

On day 2 she had persistently high ICP >60 cm H_2O despite aggressive management with hyperventilation to $PaCO_2$ of 35 mmHg, osmotic therapy with 20% sodium chloride, deep sedation with morphine and midazolam, and aggressive temperature management, targeting normothermia. Her ICP did not respond to intermittent paralysis; thus a paralytic infusion was not commenced. CT scan demonstrated 12 mm of tonsillar herniation. She was treated with 16 mg dexamethasone and taken for rescue bifrontal decompressive craniectomy. The brain was noted to be grossly swollen, hyperaemic, and herniating with marked cortical venous distension. The craniectomy was insufficient alone to provide cerebral decompression due to the inelasticity of the dura; thus the latter was opened with multiple slits during which a cortical vein was lacerated requiring diathermy. The EVD was removed and a fibre-optic pressure monitor was placed.

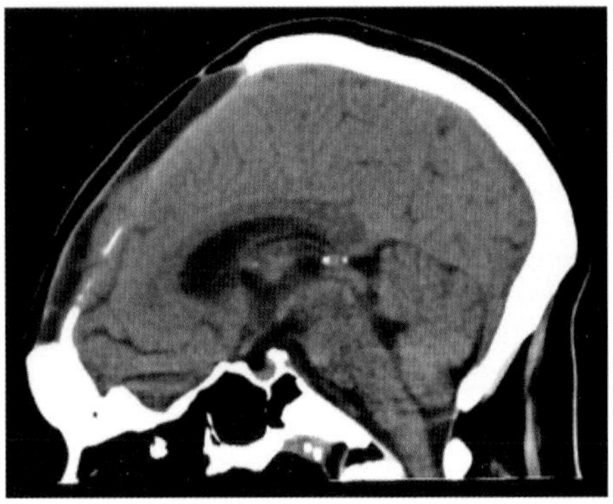

FIGURE 4: Sagittal CT demonstrating normal cerebellar tonsillar position after decompressive craniectomy.

Following this, her ICP remained <10 cm H_2O. Postoperative CT scan showed 8 mm of tonsillar herniation and a significant increase in size of the third ventricle. CSF culture was negative and viral PCR for HSV1, HSV2, enterovirus, and VZV were also negative and her empiric aciclovir was ceased.

On day 3 high dose sedation was ceased with slow recovery including transient diabetes insipidus treated with desmopressin and reintubation for poor sputum clearance. She had a gradual neurological improvement and was discharged to the neurology ward with a GCS 15 and no focal neurology on day 15 of her admission.

Unfortunately she developed CSF rhinorrhoea and pneumocephalus due to a CSF fistula through the frontal air sinus requiring surgical repair. She subsequently developed a venous infarct complicated by seizures and the requirement for intubation for reduced level of consciousness.

After rehabilitation, she was discharged home on day 69 after admission and was able to function independently, although she had not returned to work. At the time of publication she is undergoing neuropsychological testing to evaluate her readiness to return to work. Her cerebellar tonsils had returned to a normal position on a follow-up outpatient CT scan (Figure 4).

3. Discussion

Given the rarity of cerebellar tonsillar herniation in this setting, literature regarding management was not available. Management was thus based upon physiological principles such as the Monro-Kellie hypothesis and consensus between medical teams.

There were several unusual aspects to her presentation. Firstly, she had a known vascular malformation with an aplastic left transverse sinus and stenosis of the right transverse sinus. Vascular abnormalities do not preclude the diagnosis of IIH and have been implicated in the pathogenesis [6]. Resolution of symptoms has been reported in those with dural venous sinus stenting [7], the procedure she was being considered for. She also already had 4 mm of cerebellar tonsillar descent documented on an MRI six months prior to presentation; however criterion for identifying a clearly pathological Chiari 1 malformation is 5 mm [8]. It has previously been suggested that the combination of low lying tonsils and raised ICP potentially contributed to herniation in this setting [5]. Despite mild elevation of her CSF white cell count and empiric treatment with aciclovir, her viral PCR returned negative and her clinical presentation was not consistent with encephalitis.

Prior to her urgent transfer to ICU, there was a high index of suspicion of raised ICP given her fixed dilated pupil. However, at the time she was conscious, moving all limbs, and interactive despite severe pain. This was considered unusual compared with the significantly decreased level of consciousness associated with raised ICP in traumatic brain injury (TBI). It is therefore pertinent to recognize that TBI represents a syndrome comprising both the primary brain injury and secondary rise in ICP with hematoma formation and/or oedema.

There were several differences in this patient compared with the two previously reported cases. Firstly, herniation in IIH usually occurs as a late complication following lumbar peritoneal shunting [9]. This is consistent with the hypothesis that a reduction in pressure gradually restores normal brain compliance [4]. Secondly, in the rare case of herniation following LP the time course has previously been reported as occurring within minutes [5], whereas this case occurred over a period of 14 hours. This may suggest an alternative cause of the rise in ICP, perhaps a rebound phenomenon due to her inability to tolerate oral acetazolamide due to vomiting. Acetazolamide has been demonstrated to significantly reduce intracranial pressure [10].

In the absence of supportive literature, management followed local practice of TBI patients with raised ICP. Medical management initially involved sedation, analgesia, $PaCO_2$ control, targeted temperature management, and intermittent osmotic therapy with 20% sodium chloride. As the above interventions were not able to control her ICP, barbiturate coma was unlikely to be successful, and a surgical option was pursued.

Issues arose however regarding the ICP target once the EVD was inserted given the fact that her usual pressures were between 35 and 50 cm H_2O. An initial target of 35 cm H_2O was decided upon to provide a moderate reduction in pressure, without requiring excessive vasopressor doses to achieve an adequate cerebral perfusion pressure. The goal was to gradually reduce this down to 30 cm H_2O.

The surgical procedure to control her critical intracranial hypertension was performed to provide rapid and life-saving control. It appeared that the aplastic left transverse sinus and consequent anomalous posterior cranial fossa drainage led to grossly hypertrophied cerebellar and circular venous sinuses. Foramen magnum decompression and cerebellar tonsillar disimpaction were considered in addition to bifrontal craniectomy. However, these were not performed acutely because her aberrant venous anatomy presented an unacceptably high risk of uncontrollable venous sinus haemorrhage.

Decompressive craniectomy was performed as a rescue procedure. In a recent trial, worse functional outcomes have been identified in TBI patients with second line decompressive craniectomy [11]. It has been postulated that this is the result of neuronal injury due to axonal stretch with herniation

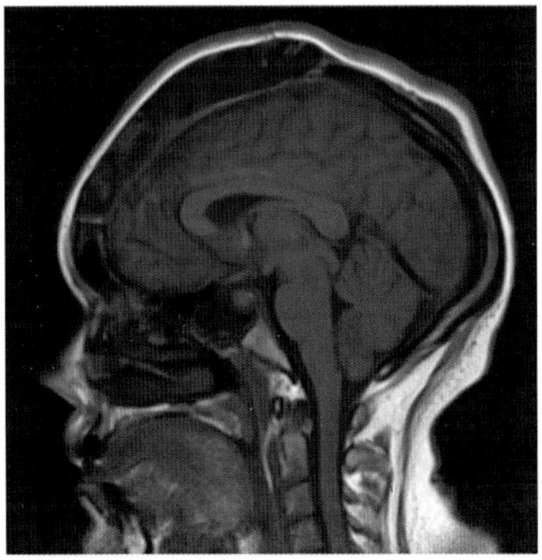

FIGURE 5: Sagittal MRI 3 weeks after decompressive craniectomy.

via the craniectomy site. Given the hypothesis regarding reduced brain compliance in IIH [4] it is possible that this is protective against further neuronal injury due to stretch. In this case, the decompressive craniectomy not only brought her intractable intracranial hypertension under immediate control but also resulted in disimpaction of her cerebellar tonsillar herniation (Figure 5).

4. Conclusion

In this patient with IIH who had cerebellar tonsillar herniation following LP, management similar to traumatic intracranial hypertension was successful. ICP targets in this setting are unknown; however we recommend a moderate reduction compared with baseline pressures as long as focal neurology resolves. Given the rapid improvement in ICP control and favourable neurological outcome, we recommend that decompressive craniectomy be considered, especially given the possible protection against further brain injury from axonal stretch due to reduced brain compliance.

References

[1] B. E. McGeeney and D. I. Friedmanet, "Pseudotumor Cerebri pathophysiology," *Headache: The Journal of Head and Face Pain*, vol. 54, no. 3, pp. 445–458, 2014.

[2] F. J. Durcan, J. J. Corbett, and M. Wall, "The incidence of pseudotumor cerebri. Population studies in Iowa and Louisiana," *Archives of Neurology*, vol. 45, no. 8, pp. 875–877, 1988.

[3] S. R. A. Paruchuri, M. Lawlor, K. Kleinhomer, L. Mason, and C. Johnson, "Risk of cerebellar tonsillar herniation after diagnostic lumbar puncture in pseudotumor cerebri," *Anesthesia and Analgesia*, vol. 77, no. 2, pp. 403–404, 1993.

[4] M. Salman, "Why does tonsillar herniation not occur in idiopathic intracranial hypertension?" *Medical Hypotheses*, vol. 53, no. 4, pp. 270–271, 1999.

[5] H. C. Sullivan, "Fatal tonsillar herniation in pseudotumor cerebri," *Neurology*, vol. 41, no. 7, pp. 1142–1144, 1991.

[6] B. R. Wakerly, M. H. Tan, and E. Y. Ting, "Idiopathic intracranial hypertension," *Cephalgia*, 2014.

[7] R. M. Ahmed, M. Wilkinson, G. D. Parker et al., "Transverse sinus stenting for idiopathic intracranial hypertension: a review of 52 patients and of model predictions," *The American Journal of Neuroradiology*, vol. 32, no. 8, pp. 1408–1414, 2011.

[8] A. O. Aboulezz, K. Sartor, C. A. Geyer, and M. H. Gado, "Position of cerebellar tonsils in the normal population and in patients with Chiari malformation: a quantitative approach with MR imaging," *Journal of Computer Assisted Tomography*, vol. 9, no. 6, pp. 1033–1036, 1985.

[9] F. J. Rowe, "Diplopia and visual impairment as presenting symptoms of shunt failure in association with tonsillar herniation in idiopathic intracranial hypertension," *Strabismus*, vol. 20, no. 4, pp. 181–184, 2012.

[10] M. R. Chaaban, E. Illing, K. O. Riley, and B. A. Woodworth, "Acetazolamide for high intracranial pressure cerebrospinal fluid leaks," *International Forum of Allergy and Rhinology*, vol. 3, no. 9, pp. 718–721, 2013.

[11] D. James Cooper, J. V. Rosenfeld, L. Murray et al., "Decompressive craniectomy in diffuse traumatic brain injury," *The New England Journal of Medicine*, vol. 364, no. 16, pp. 1493–1502, 2011.

18

Beriberi Induced Cardiomyopathy Requiring Salvage Venoarterial Extracorporeal Membrane Oxygenation

Aditya Shah,[1,2] Samir Patel,[2] Sorabh Kothari,[1,2] and Jennifer Denk[2]

[1] *University of Illinois at Chicago, Chicago, IL, USA*
[2] *Advocate Christ Medical Center, Oak Lawn, IL, USA*

Correspondence should be addressed to Aditya Shah; aditya.shah@advocatehealth.com

Academic Editor: Ricardo Oliveira

Beriberi refers to a constellation of symptoms caused primarily by thiamine (vitamin B1) deficiency. An acute and fulminant presentation of this rare condition has been described in the literature as "Shoshin" beriberi which is characterized by catastrophic cardiovascular collapse. Early recognition and treatment lead to dramatic improvements of symptoms. We present a case of thiamine deficiency-induced acute heart failure in a malnourished patient leading to cardiac arrest necessitating VA-ECMO (venoarterial extracorporeal membrane oxygenation) with improvement in heart function secondary to thiamine administration.

1. Introduction

Beriberi refers to a constellation of symptoms caused primarily by thiamine (vitamin B1) deficiency. Beriberi has traditionally been divided into four separate entities, relating to the organ system mainly involved (nervous, cardiovascular, or gastrointestinal) with an additional specification for age (i.e., infantile) [1–5]. The neurologic form has traditionally been referred to as "Dry beriberi," whereas the cardiovascular form is known as "Wet beriberi." An acute and fulminant presentation of this rare condition has been described in the literature as "Shoshin" beriberi which is characterized by catastrophic cardiovascular collapse [6]. This condition requires early recognition and management, often leading to dramatic improvement in symptoms, whereas failure to diagnose and treat can have devastating consequences.

2. Case Report

Our patient was a 33-year-old female who in adolescence and early adulthood was diagnosed with multiple allergies manifesting as erythema, urticaria, and dyspnea. As a result, she consumed an increasingly restrictive diet. Initially, she was diagnosed with a latex allergy; hence she avoided all cross reactants known to be associated with this. At 22 years of age, she was found to have a corn allergy and therefore she eliminated corn and all corn related foods from her diet. Her symptoms subjectively improved after these lifestyle modifications.

5 years before presentation, she experienced unintentional weight loss from her baseline of 61.7 kilograms owing to an extremely restricted diet to a nadir at presentation of 40.8 kilograms. She also endorsed body aches, alopecia, dyspnea, fatigue, headaches, Raynaud's phenomenon, and cold intolerance. She had no pertinent familial, surgical, or social histories.

Our patient's condition declined significantly 1 month before her admission when she was admitted for palpitations, intermittent hematochezia, and worsening shortness of breath. She was found to have dark subcutaneous nodules on her shins, which were diagnosed as erythema nodosum accompanied by Raynaud's phenomenon. She was found to be anemic to 7.3 milligrams/deciliter with leukopenia at 1.9 thousand/microliter. Iron studies yielded mixed results consistent with iron deficiency anemia along with low folate and vitamin B12 levels. For her dyspnea, a contrast enhanced chest computerized tomography scan and lower extremity venous Doppler were done, which were negative with respect to thromboembolic disease. An echocardiogram revealed normal systolic and diastolic function without valvulopathy. Given her leukopenia and anemia, outpatient bone marrow

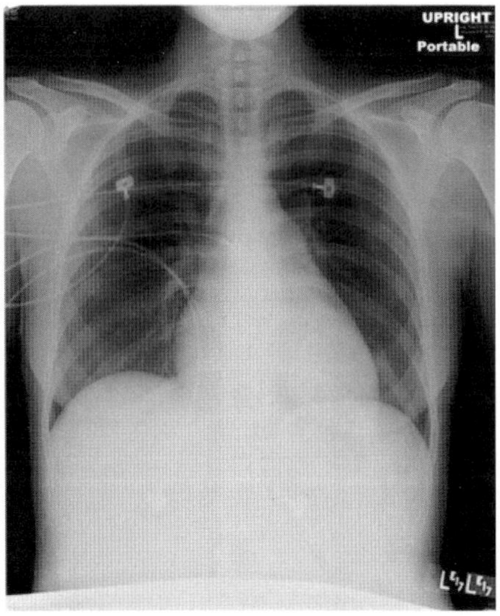

Figure 1: Initial chest X-ray showed no acute findings.

biopsy, esophagogastroduodenoscopy, and colonoscopy were recommended. Celiac disease and autoimmune diagnostics produced negative results. Over the course of the admission, the patient's shortness of breath improved with hemoglobin stabilization.

She was discharged home on ferrous sulfate for her anemia, folic acid supplement, B12 1000 micrograms intramuscularly once a week for four weeks, and scheduled for outpatient follow-up with gastroenterology as well as the hematology service for the diagnosis of mixed anemia.

Approximately 2 weeks after discharge, she represented with shortness of breath, generalized weakness, and pallor. According to the patient's husband, she became debilitated from her dyspnea and generalized weakness which resulted in an inability to walk. In the emergency department, she was afebrile, hypoxic with oxygen saturation of 87 percent on 6-liter nasal cannula, and tachycardic at 120 beats per minute with a blood pressure of 102 millimeters Hg/67 millimeters Hg. On physical exam, the patient appeared in moderate distress, with auscultation of the lungs revealing crackles bilaterally, with bilateral lower extremity subcutaneous nodules and rash.

Chest X-ray initially showed no acute findings (Figure 1). A contrast enhanced chest tomography study was done, which showed a small distal right pulmonary embolus (Figures 2 and 3). An echocardiogram was performed, the parasternal short axis of which showed significant dilation of the right ventricle along with slit-like left ventricle (Figure 4). During positioning of patient to left lateral decubitus position for optimal echocardiographic imaging, the patient sustained a pulseless electrical activity (PEA) cardiac arrest requiring cardiopulmonary resuscitation along with intubation with return of spontaneous circulation after two cycles. She required epinephrine and norepinephrine infusions for hemodynamic support after return of spontaneous circulation.

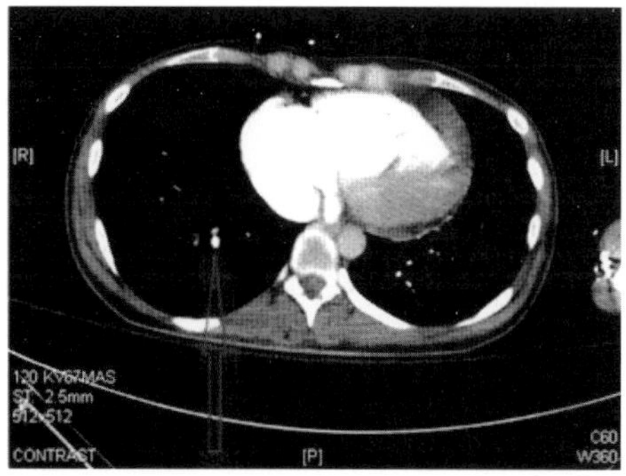

Figure 2: CT scan with contrast of the chest showing small distal right pulmonary embolus.

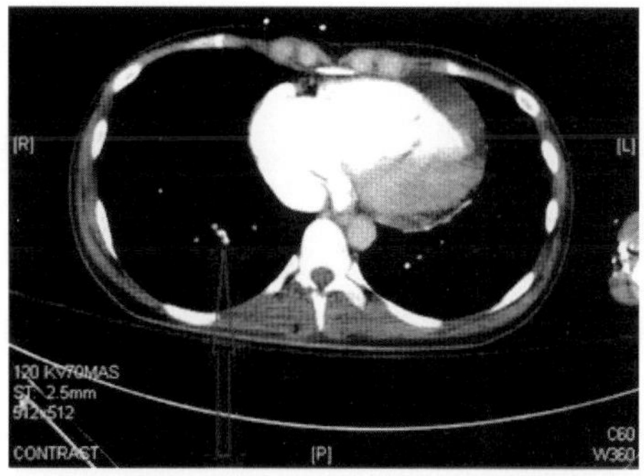

Figure 3: CT scan with contrast of the chest showing small distal right pulmonary embolus.

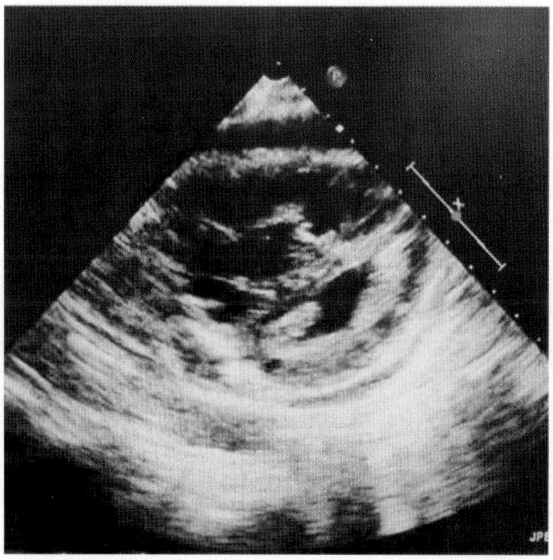

Figure 4: Echocardiogram showing significant dilation of right ventricle along with a slit-like left ventricle.

A Swan-Ganz catheter was placed which showed an initial central venous pressure of 11 millimeters Hg, right ventricular systolic pressure of 40 millimeters Hg/18 millimeters Hg, and a pulmonary artery (PA) pressure of 45 millimeters Hg/24 millimeters Hg with a mean pulmonary artery (PA) pressure of 35 millimeters Hg with wedge pressure of 19

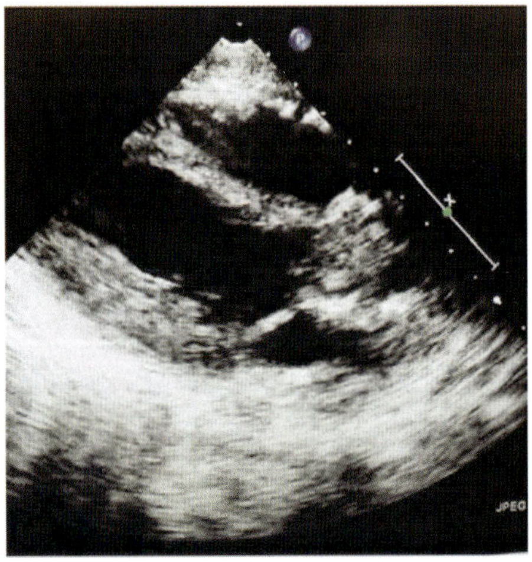

FIGURE 5: Repeat echocardiogram showing larger left ventricle with markedly reduced function, as well as mitigation of previously overloaded right ventricular size and function.

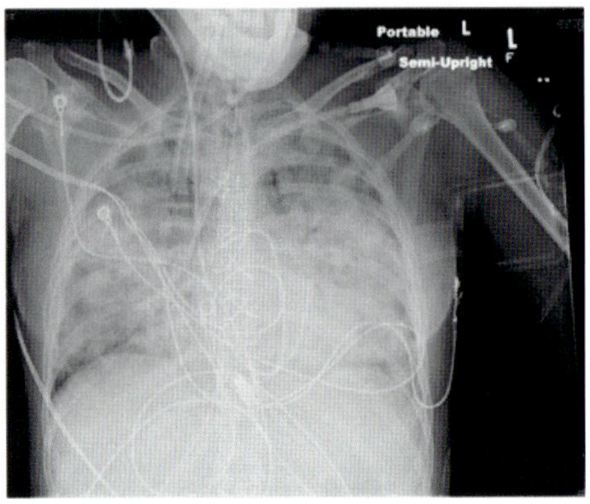

FIGURE 6: Repeat chest X-ray after intubation shows worsening bilateral aeration with developing patchy infiltrates.

millimeters Hg and mixed venous saturation of 60%, cardiac output at 3 liters/minute, and systemic vascular resistance of 500 dynes/second/centimeters^{-5}. Repeat echocardiogram was completed, which in the parasternal long axis showed a larger left ventricle with markedly reduced function, as well as mitigation of the previously overloaded right ventricular size and function (Figure 5). A repeat chest X-ray after intubation showed worsening bilateral aeration with developing patchy infiltrates, not seen on previous imaging (Figure 6). The pulmonary artery catheter measurements showed abnormal right and left sided pressures consistent with the dynamic echocardiographic changes noted on serial imaging.

The patient's laboratory values on current presentation showed an elevated B-type natriuretic peptide of 1,602 nanograms/liter which was thought to be secondary to new onset congestive heart failure and elevated aspartate transaminase and alanine transaminase to 1296 units/liter and 977 units/liter, respectively, possibly secondary to ischemic hepatopathy with acute kidney injury noted with a creatinine of 1.18 milligrams/deciliter. Her troponin level was elevated at 0.06 micrograms/liter prior to the cardiac arrest.

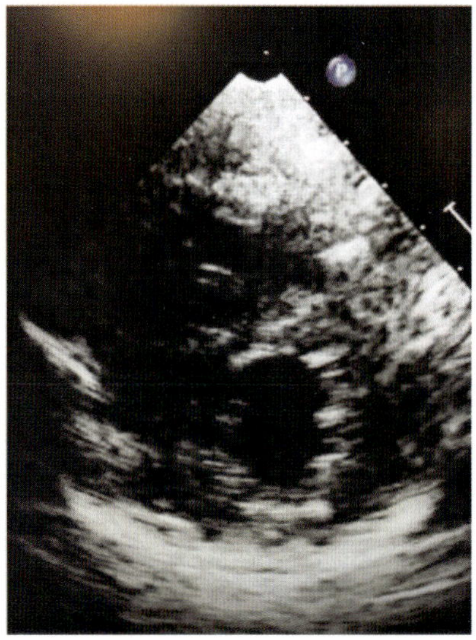

FIGURE 7: Echocardiogram parasternal short axis showing left ventricular chamber back to normal size and function.

With profound hypoxemia and cardiovascular instability after cardiac arrest, the patient was taken to the operating room and placed on central VA-ECMO owing to difficult anatomical peripheral cannulation. She required ECMO support for 14 days prior to decannulation before requiring tracheostomy. Her hospital course was further complicated by compartment syndrome of the left lower extremity requiring emergent bedside fasciotomy as well as arterial thrombus extending from the descending aorta to the superior mesenteric artery for which she underwent open surgical thrombectomy. The patient required continuous renal replacement therapy (CRRT) for oliguric renal failure along with cholecystostomy tube for acalculous cholecystitis.

An extensive workup was performed due to her complicated presentation and severity of illness. Given the patient's poor nutritional status as well as persistent lactic acidosis, a vitamin B1 (thiamine) level was obtained with both plasma and whole blood levels. The plasma level was remarkably low, <2 nanomoles/liter (reference range: 8 to 30 nanomoles/liter), and her vitamin B1 whole blood level was 91 nanomoles/liter (70 to 180 nanomoles/liter). Her vitamin B6 was also low, 15.2 nanomoles/liter (20 to 125 nanomoles/liter).

The patient was initiated on intravenous thiamine prior to laboratory confirmation of low plasma levels. Over the course of her stay, the patient showed significant improvement in her respiratory, cardiovascular, and renal status and was eventually decannulated from VA-ECMO after 14 days with transition to mechanical ventilation and eventual tracheostomy. Her cardiovascular function showed marked improvement both clinically and echocardiographically concurrent with thiamine administration. Three days after initiation of thiamine treatment, her ejection fraction, initially noted at 20 percent while on vasopressors, showed serial increases to 50% and then six days later to 70% (Figure 7). The patient no longer required inotropic support and was weaned off vasopressors. The patient was discharged from the intensive care unit neurologically intact to a telemetry floor and subsequent inpatient rehab after which she was discharged home.

3. Discussion

Beriberi is a rare condition in developed countries [7]. "Shoshin" beriberi is an even less common condition. The diagnosis depends on clinical manifestations of heart failure with the exclusion of other traditional etiologies and prompt response to therapy. With adequate clinical suspicion, the clinical findings can fit a classically pathognomonic picture [8, 9]. Assistance is often needed with additional imaging and lab studies to confirm clinical suspicion.

Transthoracic echocardiography can be used to aid in the diagnosis of this rare condition. Classic echocardiographic findings for cardiac beriberi could include left ventricular enlargement with or without reduced function and can also be accompanied by valvular dysfunction. Empiric therapy with thiamine could be a reasonable option owing to the nonspecific cardiac imaging findings and lack of real-time lab data [10]. In addition, there is virtually no downside to empiric treatment with thiamine in patients with normal renal function as the kidneys can rapidly clear excess thiamine.

Our patient is unique given that she had biventricular failure with dynamic echocardiographic changes necessitating VA-ECMO for profound hemodynamic collapse. Given the stark contrast with recent echocardiographic results, we hypothesize that the eventual cardiac dysfunction initially undetected could have been sequelae of her worsening clinical condition with a nonexistent cardiac reserve secondary to thiamine deficiency. The subsequent hospital course with infection and embolic and thrombotic phenomena were thought to be secondary to mechanical complications of extracorporeal membrane oxygenation as these issues were mitigated with decannulation.

A contrast enhanced chest tomography study done on presentation to the emergency room showed an incidental small distal pulmonary embolus with initial right ventricular strain pattern on echocardiogram. We surmise that the patient had decompensated heart failure on presentation as evidenced by elevated beta natriuretic peptide, transaminitis, and hypoxia. Given her triad of lactic acidosis and hypoxia with confounding pulmonary embolism, her pulmonary vascular resistance increased causing right sided heart failure with subsequent cardiac arrest.

We underscore the importance of serial echocardiography in acutely ill patients. Given her CT evidence of thromboembolic disease with initial echocardiographic images showing severe right ventricular strain, thrombolytic therapy was initially entertained given the clinical picture but repeat echocardiography led to reconsideration of this therapy with VA-ECMO opted for emergently. Given her central cannulation and significant transfusion requirement intraoperatively, thrombolytic therapy for pulmonary embolism quite possibly could have resulted in disastrous consequences.

Beriberi frequently is a diagnosis of exclusion. The patient's initial presentation is unique given her dynamic echocardiographic changes and concurrent pulmonary embolism with initial mixed venous saturation pointing against high output heart failure. We postulate that her venous saturation and cardiac output may have been underestimated given her profound anemia noted previously along with compromised right ventricular output owing to her significant acidosis and hypoxia. Her systemic vascular resistance was noted to be low, a finding unexpected in cardiogenic shock. We attribute this to the direct effects of thiamine deficiency on vasomotor tone similar to previous reports [11].

The patient received thiamine intravenously with rapid improvement in her cardiac hemodynamics on subsequent echocardiographic studies. The patient is currently doing well and has been discharged home after an acute rehabilitation stay of two weeks.

4. Conclusion

Beriberi induced cardiomyopathy is a rare occurrence in developed countries. To our knowledge, there is a paucity of literature supporting VA-ECMO (venoarterial extracorporeal membrane oxygenation) as a bridge while treating cardiac beriberi. We stress the importance in maintaining a high index of suspicion for beriberi with new onset heart failure in a malnourished young patient.

Competing Interests

The authors declare that they have no competing interests.

References

[1] M. Akbarian, N. A. Yankopoulos, and W. H. Abelmann, "Hemodynamic studies in beriberi heart disease," *The American Journal of Medicine*, vol. 41, no. 2, pp. 197–212, 1966.

[2] Pediatric Beriberi Simon S Rabinoqitz, MD, PhD, FAAP; Chief Editor: Jatinder Bhatia, MBBS, FAAP, Medscape online, http://emedicine.medscape.com/article/984721-medication.

[3] M. C. Latham, "Chapter 16. Beriberi and thiamine deficiency," in *Human Nutrition in the Developing World (Food and Nutrition Series-No. 29)*, Rome, Italy, Food and Agriculture Organization of the United Nations (FAO), 1997.

[4] M. Donnino, "Gastrointestinal beriberi: a previously unrecognized syndrome," *Annals of Internal Medicine*, vol. 141, no. 11, pp. 898–899, 2004.

[5] J. Duca, C. J. Lum, and A. M. Lo, "Elevated lactate secondary to gastrointestinal beriberi," *Journal of General Internal Medicine*, vol. 31, no. 1, pp. 133–136, 2016.

[6] G. Dabar, C. Harmouche, B. Habr, M. Riachi, and B. Jaber, "*Shoshin* beriberi in critically-ill patients: case series," *Nutrition Journal*, vol. 14, no. 1, article 51, 2015.

[7] J. D. Yang, K. Acharya, M. Evans, J. D. Marsh, and S. Beland, "Beriberi disease: is it still present in the United States?" *American Journal of Medicine*, vol. 125, no. 10, p. e5, 2012.

[8] S. Narasimha Rao and G. R. Chandak, "Cardiac beriberi: often a missed diagnosis," *Journal of Tropical Pediatrics*, vol. 56, no. 4, Article ID fmp108, pp. 284–285, 2009.

[9] D. P. Naidoo, V. Gathiram, A. Sadhabiriss, and F. Hassen, "Clinical diagnosis of cardiac beriberi," *South African Medical Journal*, vol. 77, no. 3, pp. 125–127, 1990.

[10] H.-S. Lee, S.-A. Lee, H.-S. Shin et al., "A case of cardiac beriberi: a forgotten but memorable disease," *Korean Circulation Journal*, vol. 43, no. 8, pp. 569–572, 2013.

[11] T. Imamura and K. Kinugawa, "Shoshin beriberi with low cardiac output and hemodynamic deterioration treated dramatically by thiamine administration," *International Heart Journal*, vol. 56, no. 5, pp. 568–570, 2015.

19

Heart Failure and Hypothermia in an Infant: Pseudocyanide Syndrome?

J. Scott Baird

Department of Pediatrics, Division of Critical Care Medicine, Columbia University, New York, NY, USA

Correspondence should be addressed to J. Scott Baird; jsb106@cumc.columbia.edu

Academic Editor: Kenneth S. Waxman

Purpose. Mixed or central venous oxygen saturation has not been described during concurrent heart failure and hypothermia in children, both of which may be associated with hyperlactatemia. This report of an infant with heart failure and hypothermia is significant for increased inferior vena cava (IVC) oxygen saturation and hyperlactatemia. *Case Report.* A 36-day-old female was fussy for a day and then developed respiratory distress. In the Pediatric ER, she was tachycardic (260 beats/minute) and hypothermic (32.4 degrees C) with prolonged capillary refill and faint distal pulses. Adenosine was given twice via an intraosseous line for supraventricular tachycardia, with conversion to sinus rhythm. Blood drawn from an IVC catheter was significant for uncorrected (for temperature) oxygen saturation of 94% and lactate 18 mmol/L; corrected and uncorrected IVC oxygen saturation early during rewarming were >90%. During rewarming, declines in uncorrected IVC oxygen saturation and lactate correlated. Hypothermia and hyperlactatemia resolved after 10 and 12 hours. *Conclusions.* Concurrent heart failure and hypothermia in an infant were associated with increased IVC oxygen saturation and hyperlactatemia, similar to lab findings associated with a mitochondrial toxin such as cyanide. Improvement of heart failure and hypothermia were associated with resolution of these lab abnormalities, thus helping to rule out mitochondrial toxins. Additional reports may help better define a pseudocyanide syndrome in this setting.

1. Introduction

Mixed or central venous oxygen saturation (SO_2) is decreased with heart failure and increased with hypothermia; though normal limits for mixed or central venous SO_2 require interpretation within a clinical context, levels below 70% and above 90% are concerns [1]. Hyperlactatemia is common to both heart failure and hypothermia. With concurrent heart failure and hypothermia in children, hyperlactatemia is increased in proportion to heart failure severity [2], but mixed or central venous SO_2 data are lacking. This report of an infant with heart failure and hypothermia is notable for increased inferior vena cava (IVC) SO_2 and hyperlactatemia, similar to the findings associated with a mitochondrial toxin, such as cyanide.

2. Case Report

The Columbia University Medical Center IRB (AAAR0802) exempted this retrospective case report from review.

A 36-day-old female was fussy for a day and then developed respiratory distress. She was born at term, and a New York State newborn screen was negative. In the Pediatric ER, she was tachycardic (260 beats/minute) and hypothermic (32.4 degrees C) with prolonged capillary refill and faint distal pulses. She was placed on continuous positive airway pressure via nasal prongs. Adenosine was given twice via an intraosseous line for supraventricular tachycardia with conversion to sinus rhythm. She was then intubated for worsening respiratory distress and placed on an FiO_2 of 1.0. An echocardiogram was notable for decreased biventricular systolic function and left to right shunting through a patent foramen ovale. A dobutamine infusion was started. Arterial cannulation was unsuccessful; transcutaneous pulse SO_2 was consistently 100% during rewarming. Results from the first blood gas (all blood gas results were reported uncorrected for temperature) drawn from a catheter placed in the IVC (by Seldinger technique; sutured in place after advancing to its full length overlying the L3 vertebral body; Figure 1) were pH 7.01, PCO_2 33 mm Hg, PO_2 101 mm Hg, SO_2 94%,

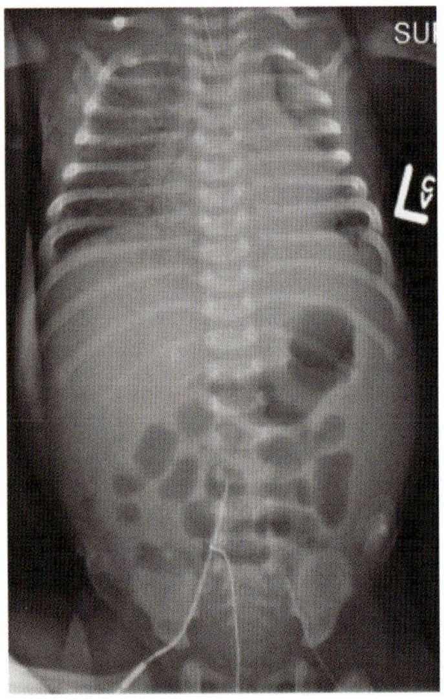

FIGURE 1: Radiograph of infant with heart failure and mild hypothermia showing central venous catheter overlying L3 vertebral body.

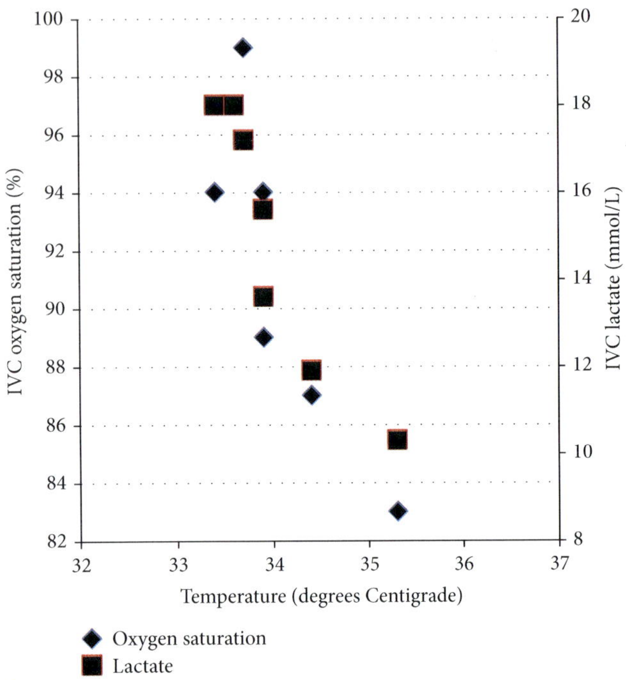

FIGURE 2: Inferior vena cava oxygen saturation (uncorrected for temperature) and lactate during rewarming of infant with heart failure and mild hypothermia.

and lactate 18 mmol/L. Early during rewarming, the IVC SO_2 remained above 90% and was as high as 99% (Figure 2); declines in IVC SO_2 and lactate during the first 3 hours of rewarming correlated (Spearman r: 0.94; $p = 0.002$). An arterial catheter was then placed, and the FiO_2 weaned. B-type natriuretic peptide was increased (4578.5 pg/mL). Capillary refill and distal pulses improved, and dobutamine was discontinued at 8 hours; a repeat echocardiogram the next day showed improved (though still diminished) biventricular systolic function with continued left to right shunting through a patent foramen ovale. Hypothermia and hyperlactatemia resolved over 10 and 12 hours, and IVC SO_2 was 80% on hospital day 2. The patient was diagnosed with supraventricular tachycardia secondary to Wolff-Parkinson-White syndrome. Prior to discharge a week later, serum acylcarnitine profile, lactate, pyruvate, thyroid stimulating hormone, and thyroxine were all normal.

IVC PO_2 values were corrected retrospectively for the patient's temperature [3] (Table 1).

3. Discussion

Concurrent acute heart failure and mild (>32 degrees Centigrade [4]) hypothermia were associated with an increased SO_2, profound metabolic acidosis, and severe hyperlactatemia in blood from the IVC of an infant. Heart failure alone is associated with a decreased mixed venous or central venous SO_2—as well as a decreased IVC SO_2—in neonates [5] as well as infants and children; mild hypothermia alone is associated with an increased—though still normal—mixed venous [6] or central venous [7] SO_2 and is unlikely to be responsible for profound acidosis [4] or severe hyperlactatemia [8, 9]. Resolution of heart failure and mild hypothermia in this infant was associated with resolution of the lab abnormalities: a decrease in cardiac output and tissue metabolic rate, as well as peripheral vasoconstriction and vascular shunting, all improved with resolution of heart failure and hypothermia. Similar lab abnormalities are associated with cyanide toxicity [10, 11], though the pathophysiology is different: as oxidative phosphorylation is disrupted, oxygen extraction and consumption decrease due to the metabolic block, and venous SO_2 increases with hyperlactatemia. Though a metabolic disease or toxin might have been associated with the clinical presentation of this infant, there was ultimately no evidence to support such a diagnosis or its associated pathophysiology.

A clinical controversy regarding blood gas results may have escaped the notice of some pediatric intensivists: correcting blood gas results for the patient's temperature is no longer routine, as recommended [12]. As a result, blood gas specimens are routinely analyzed at 37 degrees Centigrade (normothermia) and so reported. Interestingly, correcting the blood gas results retrospectively in this infant did not alter the findings: early during rewarming (on the first 3 blood gas results), the corrected IVC PO_2 was >80 mm Hg, corresponding generally to SO_2 values on the flat upper part of the oxyhemoglobin dissociation curve. As calculations of SO_2 from PO_2 may be associated with inaccuracies [13], specific SO_2 values were not calculated; however, a leftward shift of the oxyhemoglobin dissociation curve (due both to hypothermia and the presence of fetal hemoglobin in a 5 week old infant) supports IVC SO_2 values > 90% for PO_2 values > 80 mm Hg. It is thus evident that both corrected and uncorrected IVC SO_2 values early during rewarming were increased above normal.

The IVC SO_2 was >90% in 27% (15 of 55) of values from 20 critically ill neonates and infants undergoing cardiopulmonary bypass (mostly with hypothermia), though lactate was only mildly elevated (mean: 2.2 +/− 0.1 mmol/L) [14].

Table 1: Temperature, uncorrected and corrected (for temperature) IVC PO_2, uncorrected IVC SO_2, and IVC lactate in infant with heart failure and mild hypothermia.

Time (minutes)	Temperature (degrees Centigrade)	Uncorrected PO_2 (mm Hg)	Corrected PO_2 (mm Hg)	Uncorrected SO_2 (%)	Lactate (mmol/L)
0	33.4*	101	83	94	18
63	33.6*	100	84	97	18
74	33.7*	174	134	99	17.2
87	33.9*	71	58	94	15.6
106	33.9	59	48	89	13.6
133	34.4	60	50	87	11.9
177	35.3*	49	44	83	10.3

*Interpolated temperatures.

As cardiopulmonary bypass replaces cardiac function, it is possible that heart failure with mild hypothermia in an infant would be associated with more severe hyperlactatemia and an increased IVC SO_2, as noted in this infant. In any case, the trend in lab results from the IVC catheter was consistent during rewarming following cardioversion and suggests that these findings represent an actual association.

Limitations to this report include those related to retrospective case reports generally. Some laboratory data—including arterial blood gas results as well other metabolic testing—were not available due to limited vascular access during acute illness. The FiO_2 was maintained at 1.0 during the first 3 hours of rewarming while the infant's clinical condition stabilized, and this could have contributed to an increased IVC SO_2; however, this effect was not dramatic, as the IVC SO_2 fell to 83% before the FiO_2 was weaned. In any case, pediatric intensivists may benefit from knowing that the SO_2 from a femoral vascular catheter may be as high as 99% in certain clinical conditions, even when the catheter is not arterial. As the IVC catheter was advanced to its full length and sutured in place overlying the L3 vertebral body, proximal catheter migration was not possible, such that the left to right shunt across the patent foramen ovale did not contribute to an increased IVC SO_2.

4. Conclusion

This report offers anecdotal evidence that IVC SO_2 may not always be low in infants with heart failure, while lactic acidosis may be profound in the presence of mild hypothermia: concurrent heart failure and mild hypothermia were likely responsible for the lab abnormalities in this infant, which to some extent mimic the lab abnormalities associated with a mitochondrial toxin such as cyanide. Further study of a pseudocyanide syndrome associated with concurrent heart failure and mild hypothermia in infants may be helpful.

Disclosure

This study was presented in abstract form at the 2017 American Thoracic Society's Annual meeting [15].

References

[1] K. R. Walley, "Use of central venous oxygen saturation to guide therapy," *American Journal of Respiratory and Critical Care Medicine*, vol. 184, no. 5, pp. 514–520, 2011.

[2] S. B. Shinde, K. K. Golam, P. Kumar, and N. D. Patil, "Blood lactate levels during cardiopulmonary bypass for valvular heart surgery," *Annals of Cardiac Anaesthesia*, vol. 8, no. 1, pp. 39–44, 2005.

[3] G. R. Kelman and J. F. Nunn, "Nomograms for correction of blood Po2, Pco2, pH, and base excess for time and temperature," *Journal of Applied Physiology*, vol. 21, no. 5, pp. 1484–1490, 1966.

[4] M. L. Mallet, "Pathophysiology of accidental hypothermia," *QJM: Monthly Journal of the Association of Physicians*, vol. 95, no. 12, pp. 775–785, 2002.

[5] F. B. Plötz, R. A. Van Lingen, and A. P. Bos, "Venous oxygen measurements in the inferior vena cava in neonates with respiratory failure," *Critical Care*, vol. 2, no. 2, pp. 57–60, 1998.

[6] A. Bacher, U. M. Illievich, R. Fitzgerald, G. Ihra, and C. K. Spiss, "Changes in oxygenation variables during progressive hypothermia in anesthetized patients," *Journal of Neurosurgical Anesthesiology*, vol. 9, no. 3, pp. 205–210, 1997.

[7] Z. Hu, L. Xu, Z. Zhu, R. Seal, and P. M. McQuillan, "Effects of hypothermic cardiopulmonary bypass on internal jugular bulb venous oxygen saturation, cerebral oxygen saturation, and bispectral index in pediatric patients undergoing cardiac surgery: A prospective study," *Medicine (United States)*, vol. 95, no. 2, Article ID e2483, 2016.

[8] Q.-J. Zhao, X.-G. Zhang, and L.-X. Wang, "Mild hypothermia therapy reduces blood glucose and lactate and improves neurologic outcomes in patients with severe traumatic brain injury," *Journal of Critical Care*, vol. 26, no. 3, pp. 311–315, 2011.

[9] J. Pirnes and T. Ala-Kokko, "Accidental hypothermia: factors related to long-term hospitalization. A retrospective study from northern Finland," *Internal and Emergency Medicine*, pp. 1–9, 2016.

[10] M. M. Yeh, C. E. Becker, and A. I. Arieff, "Is measurement of venous oxygen saturation useful in the diagnosis of cyanide poisoning?" *American Journal of Medicine*, vol. 93, no. 5, pp. 582-583, 1992.

[11] J. C. Pham, D. T. Huang, F. T. McGeorge, and E. P. Rivers, "Clarification of cyanide's effect on oxygen transport characteristics

in a canine model," *Emergency Medicine Journal*, vol. 24, no. 3, pp. 152–156, 2007.

[12] E. R. Ashwood, G. Kost, and M. Kenny, "Temperature correction of blood-gas and pH measurements," *Clinical Chemistry*, vol. 29, no. 11, pp. 1877–1885, 1983.

[13] P. A. Johnson, D. J. Bihari, R. F. Raper, M. A. Haughton, M. M. Fisher, and R. G. Herkes, "A comparison between direct and calculated oxygen saturation in intensive care," *Anaesthesia and Intensive Care*, vol. 21, no. 1, pp. 72–75, 1993.

[14] M. Redlin, A. Koster, M. Huebler et al., "Regional differences in tissue oxygenation during cardiopulmonary bypass for correction of congenital heart disease in neonates and small infants: Relevance of near-infrared spectroscopy," *The Journal of Thoracic and Cardiovascular Surgery*, vol. 136, no. 4, pp. 962–967, 2008.

[15] J. S. Baird, "Hypothermia and Acute Heart Failure in an Infant: Pseudo-Cyanide Syndrome?" *B67 Interesting and Unusual Pediatric Case Reports*, vol. 195, pp. A4099–A4099, 2017.

Retroperitoneal Paraganglioma-Induced Cardiogenic Shock Rescued by Preoperative Arterial Embolization

N. Houari,[1] S. Touzani,[1] H. Salhi,[2] M.-Y. Alaoui Lamrani,[3] K. Ibnmajdoub,[4] H. El Ouahabi,[2] A. El Bouazzaoui,[1] B. Boukatta,[1] M. Maâroufi,[3] K. Maazaz,[4] and N. Kanjaa[1]

[1]*Anesthesiology & Intensive Care Unit A4, Hassan II University Hospital, Fez, Morocco*
[2]*Endocrinology Department, Hassan II University Hospital, Fez, Morocco*
[3]*Imaging and Interventional Radiology Department, Hassan II University Hospital, Fez, Morocco*
[4]*Visceral Surgery Department, Hassan II University Hospital, Fez, Morocco*

Correspondence should be addressed to N. Houari; nawfal.houari@gmail.com

Academic Editor: Chiara Lazzeri

Background. Catecholamine-induced cardiogenic shock is a rare manifestation of paragangliomas. The high mortality rate of this condition makes the immediate, multidisciplinary approach mandatory. *Case Report.* We report a case of an 18-year-old woman with a retroperitoneal secreting paraganglioma, complicated with a cardiogenic shock and an acute adrenergic myocarditis, requiring hemodynamic support and emergency arterial embolization prior to surgical excision, with a favorable outcome. *Conclusion.* Paraganglioma-induced myocarditis is rare but can be dramatic. Management requires appropriate and immediate hemodynamic support. Embolization may be an alternative to stabilize the patient prior to surgery.

1. Background

Paragangliomas (PG) are rare tumors originating from neural crest cells, arising at various locations along the chain of the sympathetic nervous system as well as the branchiomeric paraganglioma. Complete surgical excision remains the main available treatment and the complexity of the clinical manifestations often makes surgery part of a multidisciplinary approach. Preoperative embolization is still controversial and its role has not been established, especially in cases of paraganglioma-induced adrenergic myocarditis. We report a peculiar case that highlights the importance of preoperative embolization, to stabilize a patient with cardiac manifestations related to a catecholamine-secreting PG.

2. Case Presentation

An 18-year-old female patient was admitted to the endocrinology unit for assessment and preoperative management of a retroperitoneal PG. The patient's past medical history was significant for psoriasis since age 2, for which she has been getting an association of betamethasone and salicylic acid. The patient also reports a history of functional colopathy for the past 3 months. No other significant history of endocrine or tumoral conditions was reported. The patient has been suffering from recurring episodes of excessive perspiration and palpitations over the past 4 years, associated with other symptoms of hypertension such as headaches and tinnitus. The patient also reported multiple episodes of recurrent right-sided abdominal pain worsening over the past year.

Her physical exam upon admission was normal with a BMI (Body Mass Index) = 21.8 kg/m^2, a BP (blood pressure) = 130/90 mmHg bilaterally (no postural hypotension was noted), and a heart rate (HR) =88 beats per minute (bpm). The cutaneous examination showed facial erythrosis and eczematous lesions of the upper and lower extremities. No pigmentation disorders nor cutaneous superficial neurofibromas were noted. EKG analysis showed a sinus rhythm and a left ventricular hypertrophy (LVH). An abdominal computed

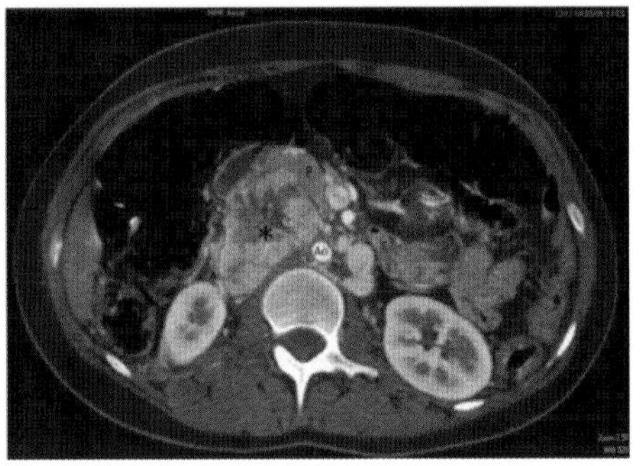

FIGURE 1: A contrast abdominal CT scan showing a 7.0 x 5.0 cm heterogeneous mass (black asterisk) located between the abdominal aorta (Ao) and the inferior vena cava, pushing the head of the pancreas (p).

tomography (CT) scan revealed no adrenal abnormalities but a 7.0 x 5.0 cm tissular-like retroperitoneal mass in contact with the abdominal aorta and the inferior vena cava, intimately related and displacing anteriorly the head of the pancreas (**Figure 1**). Abdominal MRI and elevated urinary methylated metabolites of catecholamines (Metanephrine = 3.2 μmol / 24h (normal range (NR) 0.2 to 1), Normetanephrine = 47.5 μmol / 24 h (NR: 0.4 to 2.1)) confirmed the diagnosis of catecholamine-secreting retroperitoneal PG.

Twenty-four hours after admission, the patient developed a cardiogenic shock. Her initial vital signs were as follows: Glasgow Coma Scale (GCS) = 14 (E4 V4 M6), BP = 82/46 mmHg, HR = 150 bpm, a respiratory rate at 25 cycles per minute with a SpO2 (peripheral oxygen saturation) at 60% with cold distal extremities and cyanosis. Capillary blood glucose was 150 mg/dl. Fluid resuscitation using 500 ml of Ringer Lactate solution and oxygen through high concentration mask were both promptly started and the patient was transferred to the ICU.

On admission, clinical assessment showed signs of heart failure, elevated troponin, and lactates markers and an EKG revealed sinus tachycardia with a frequency of 130 bpm. The patient was hypoxic with a SpO2 at 95% under 9 L/min of oxygen. Two right femoral central lines were placed (venous and arterial) and the patient was started on Noradrenalin (at a rate of 0.5 μg/kg/min). An echocardiography revealed a global hypokinesia with a left ventricular ejection fraction (LVEF) at 15%, requiring the patient to be put on 15 μg/kg/min of Dobutamine as inotropic support.

Seeing how the patient was in no shape to undergo open surgery, we opted for a preoperative radiological percutaneous transarterial embolization (TAE), under local anesthesia. It consisted of coiling of four major feeding vessels, 2 arising from the right renal artery and 2 more from the lumbar arteries (L2 and L3), using hydrogel with Polyzene®-F coating microparticules (**Figure 2**). The patient was gradually weaned off catecholamines during embolization. She was completely weaned off vasoactive drugs in the next 24 hours. 48 hours after embolization, a follow-up echocardiography showed an overall normokinetic left ventricle (LV), an improved FEVG at 50%, and an aortic VTI (velocity time integral) at 20m/s. Lactate levels went back to normal over the next 48 hours. In the postembolization period, the patient experienced several nonsymptomatic hypertension peaks (systolic blood pressure (SBP) = 220mmHg) and received intravenous nicardipine at a rate of 5 mg/H. The extremities warmed up and the daily urine output was maintained.

Three days after embolization, the patient was taken to the operating room for the tumor to be surgically removed through a right subcostal approach. Perioperative exploration found a retroperitoneal soft encapsulated tumor measuring 7.0 cm in diameter, in intimate contact with the abdominal aorta, the right renal vein, and the inferior vena cava (**Figure 3**). Embolization caused no complications. The tumor's adhesions were carefully released from adjacent organs including the right kidney, the duodenum, and the head of the pancreas. There was no need to place a double J ureteral stent preoperatively. Upon manipulation of the mass, there was moderate elevation in the blood pressure that was controlled with intravenous propranolol and nicardipine. A complete resection of the tumor was performed and no adjacent organs were removed or injured during the surgery (**Figure 4**).

The patient experienced episodes of hypotension after the tumor excision and received intravenous noradrenaline at a rate of 0.3 μg/kg/min. The patient was then transferred back to the ICU and extubated in fast track manner. She was weaned off vasoactive drugs in the following 6 hours.

Table 1 sums up the lab work-up of the patient during her stay.

During close ICU monitoring, the patient presented several episodes of hypoglycemia and hypokalemia and was given intravenous supplementation of glucose and potassium. A postoperative echocardiography showed a hyperkinetic myocardium with an enlarged LV, an IVS (interventricular septum) measuring 13 mm, a lateral wall measuring 14 mm, and a much improved LVEF at 70%.

The patient was subsequently discharged after spending 4 days in the ICU and transferred to a general surgery service. Pathological report of the tumor mass confirmed the diagnosis of benign extra-adrenal PG. A one-month echocardiography follow-up noted nothing significant. She now completely recovered and is back to her daily life.

3. Discussion

Paragangliomas (PG) are rare tumors derived from neural crest cells, whose origins may vary along the chain of the autonomic nervous system [1]. Most of PG are located in the head and the neck while deriving from the parasympathetic nervous system and rarely produce catecholamines. On the contrary, most of the PG deriving from the sympathic system are located in the abdomen, produce catecholamines, and are unique, sporadic, benign, and more common in middle-aged women [2].

Patients with functional PG, such as pheochromocytoma, usually present a triad of clinical symptoms (Menard's triad): cephalgia, tachycardia, and diaphoresis, these symptoms being mainly related to high levels of catecholamines in blood. Putting a label on this pathology can sometimes be

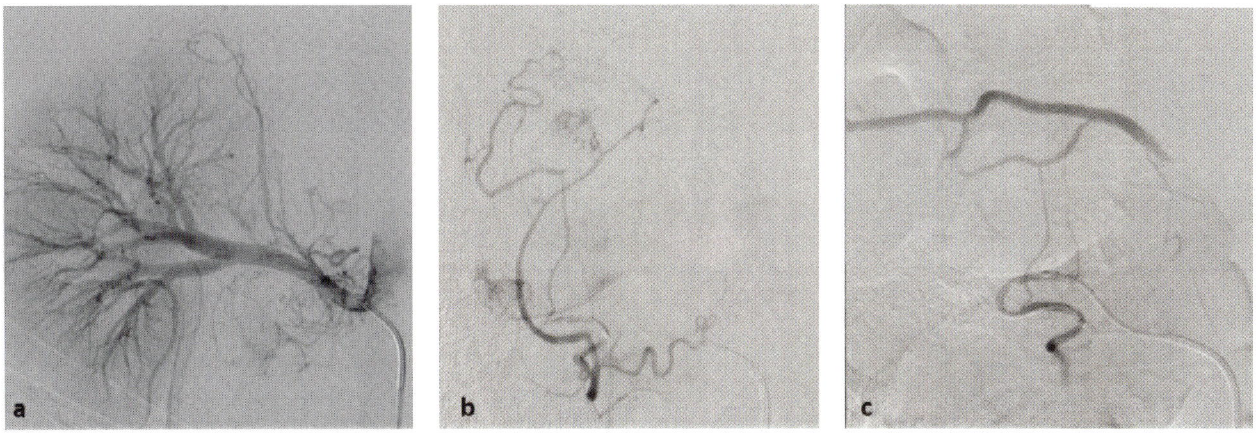

(a) (b) (c)

FIGURE 2: Angiography showing several feeding arteries arising from the right renal artery (a) and the 3rd right lumbar artery (L3) (b). Successful embolization of several arterial arteries: e.g., the 3rd right lumbar artery (c).

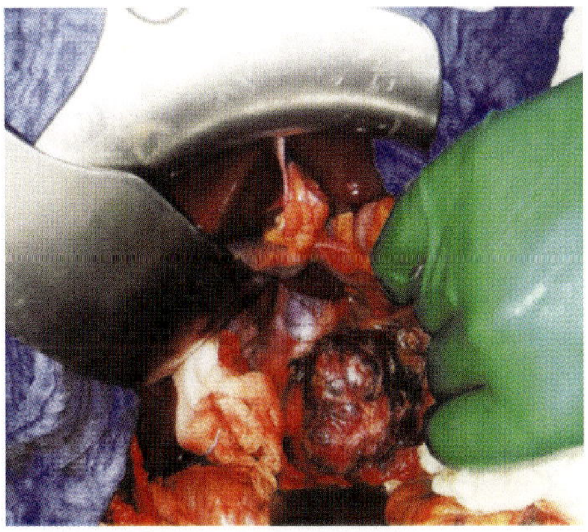

FIGURE 3: Surgical site showing the presence of the paraganglioma with intimate contact with the abdominal aorta and the inferior vena cava after mobilization of the duodenum.

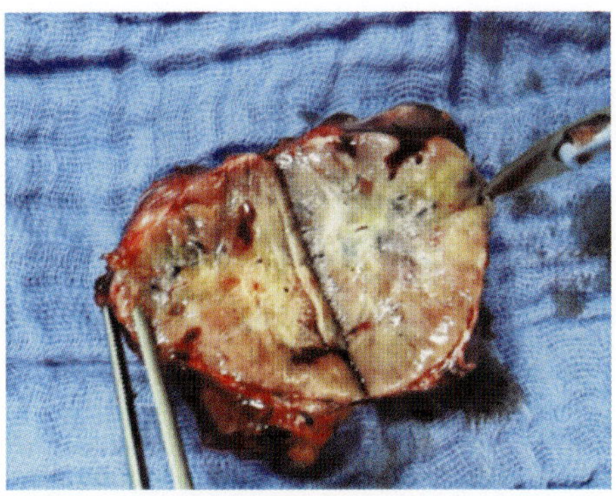

FIGURE 4: Cut gross specimen showing a tan colored mass.

challenging, due to the variability of the clinical presentation, including a variety of life-threatening cardiovascular syndromes, such as hypertensive crisis, acute myocardial infarction (AMI), acute heart failure, shock or profound hypotension, arrhythmia, myocarditis, or cardiomyopathy [3, 4]. The cardiovascular complications seem mainly related to the massive dumping of high levels of catecholamines in blood, especially after the tumor's blood supply has been cut off [5]. Increased catecholamine levels may cause structural and biochemical damage to the myocardium, leading to catecholamine induced cardiomyopathy [6]. This variety of clinical features can explain why the differential diagnosis is often demanding.

There are reports of many cases, as for the case presented herein, of catecholamine-induced shock. Several factors could explain its intricate mechanisms, the main one being the abrupt interruption of catecholamine secretion by the neuroendocrine tumor after a long period of catecholamine-induced hypertension in a patient with a limited circulatory volume and desensitized adrenoceptors [7]. Other factors include the direct toxicity of catecholamines derivatives [8] and the negative inotropic effect of hypocalcemia (as the calcium is sequestrated in the myocytes' sarcoplasm) [9].

AMI cases have also been linked to these tumors. Less than half the patients having had catecholamine-induced myocardial infractions, especially those with preexisting cardiovascular conditions, showed abnormal coronarography [4], which could suggest that myocardial injury in patients with previously healthy hearts is either due to a hemodynamic compromise (an increase in myocardial oxygen demand with a decrease in myocardial oxygen supply) or due to the immediate deleterious effects on cardiac function of catecholamines (accelerated apoptosis and fibrosis) [7]. There were no indications to perform a coronarography in our case given the patient's young age, the absence of preexisting cardiovascular conditions, and the evident, widespread myocardial lesions in the echocardiography findings.

High catecholamine levels lead to faster lipid mobilization, calcium overload, free radical production, and an increased sarcolemmal permeability [10], thus causing either myocarditis through direct myocardial damage or hypertrophic/dilated cardiomyopathy. The latter, far more frequent, can occur at any age, even during childhood [6].

Table 1: The patient's lab work-up evolution during the hospital stay.

	Admission Day -1 (Endocrinology Unit)	Day 0 (Cardiogenic Shock)	H+6 (After Embolization)	Day 2	Day 4 (Tumor Resection)	Postop Day 1
Hemoglobin (G/DL)	16	16.9	12	10.4	11	10.2
Leukocytes (E/MM^3)	8750	22210	9950	9220	8980	8020
Platelets (G/L)	687	512	373	316	270	294
PT	70	64	81	97	-	95
PTT	31.5	30/30	30	31	-	38.5
Glucose (G/L)	1.33		1.85			
Albumin	49	41	38	32	31	29
Protein	82	67	63	60	52	53
Urea	0.35	0.59	0.25	0.16	0.08	0.07
Creatinine (MG/L)	7	9	7	5	5	5
CRP (MG/L)	1	3	18	45	78	125
Sodium (MMOL/L)	140	137	132	131	134	133
Potassium (MMOL/L)	4.4	5.5	4.6	3.3	2.9	4.5
Chloride	101	97	99	102	101	105
Calcium (MG/L)	106	89	96	-	79	85
Magnesium		24	21			
Phosphorus	43					16
Alkaline Reserve	26	20	25	21	21	21
AST	63	174	180	78	53	49
ALT	54	362	502	351	177	138
CK		204				
CK-MB		201				
Troponin	-	1.96	1.1	0.73	0.46	0.18
PH		7.5				
PACO2		30.2				
HCO3-		23.6				
PAO2		150				
Arterial Lactate		1.25	0.43			

In most cases, myocardial damage caused by catecholamine-induced cardiomyopathy is reversible through proper treatment and/or surgical excision. Treatment consists of continuous inotropic support, and in some cases (during the acute phase of the cardiogenic shock) even the use of circulatory assistance such as Extracorporeal Membrane Oxygenation (ECMO) and Intra-Aortic Balloon Pump (IABP) [9, 11, 12]. Some patients improved right after medication onset, and others required up to several months for their symptoms to resolve [7].

Preoperative arterial embolization of pheochromocytomas or paragangliomas is not routinely performed because of the theoretical risk of catecholamine release in circulation resulting in hypertensive crisis. However, it can be performed under strict monitoring to reduce vascular supply in large, hypervascularized tumors, thus facilitating surgical excision [13–16]. However, there are no indications that this procedure significantly reduces perioperative blood loss, surgical time, or hospital stay [17, 18].

To the best of our knowledge, arterial embolization has only been described once in cases of catecholamine-induced refractory cardiogenic shock. It aimed to wean a patient in cardiogenic shock from emergency extracorporeal life support (ECLS) as a bridge to final surgery [11]. After the procedure, the patient improved, and ECLS was weaned in 48h without complications, and adrenalectomy was performed after 10 weeks.

Considering the severity of the clinical manifestations and the fact that the patient's condition was already labeled, we decided to carry out an emergency arterial embolization under strict monitoring right after the first signs of cardiogenic shock. This procedure allowed our team to wean the patient off inotropic and vasoactive drugs in a matter of hours.

There is no consensus for the exact delay of surgery after an episode of catecholamine-induced cardiomyopathy. It can range from a few days to several weeks [9, 11]. Some authors report carrying out surgery during the acute phase, with no significant perioperative complications and an improved postoperative cardiac function [12, 19]. In our case, surgery was scheduled right after stabilization to avoid a full-blown relapse.

4. Conclusion

Our case is a good example of how challenging the diagnosis of PG can be, especially when it lacks the typical clinical presentation, and is manifested by cardiovascular events, as it is the case with pheochromocytoma/paraganglioma-induced adrenergic myocarditis. Management requires appropriate and immediate hemodynamic support and circulatory assistance may prove mandatory when it comes to refractory cardiogenic shock. Surgical resection after adequate medical preparation is still the main treatment and it is necessary for histological assessment, but preoperative endovascular embolization can prove to be a great, less risky, alternative to stabilize patients prior to surgery.

Acknowledgments

The authors would like to thank Dr. Hajar Laamarti for her invaluable help in translating this article.

References

[1] A. S. Tischler, "Pheochromocytoma and extra-adrenal paraganglioma: Updates," *Archives of Pathology & Laboratory Medicine*, vol. 132, pp. 1272–1284, 2008.

[2] D. Erickson, Y. C. Kudva, M. J. Ebersold et al., "Benign paragangliomas: clinical presentation and treatment outcomes in 236 patients," *The Journal of Clinical Endocrinology & Metabolism*, vol. 86, no. 11, pp. 5210–5216, 2001.

[3] N. Kanjaa, M. Khatouf, A. Elhijri et al., "Phéochromocytomes. Formes graves et inhabituelles," *Annales Françaises d'Anesthésie et de Réanimation*, vol. 18, no. 4, pp. 458–464, 1999.

[4] A. E. Bouazzaoui, N. Hammas, N. Houari et al., "Syndrome coronaire aigu: un mode de révélation peu fréquent du phéochromocytome," *Pan African Medical Journal*, vol. 22, 2015.

[5] P. Charon, A Hamwi, P. Laigneau, and P. Beroud, "Forme pseudo-coronarienne de rupture hémorragique d'un pheochromocytome. A propos d'une observation," *Annales De Cardiologie Et D'Angeiologie*, vol. 40, pp. 193–197, 1991.

[6] J. R. Kizer, L. S. Koniaris, J. D. Edelman, and M. G. S. J. Sutton, "Pheochromocytoma crisis, cardiomyopathy, and hemodynamic collapse," *CHEST*, vol. 118, no. 4, pp. 1221–1223, 2000.

[7] A. Prejbisz, J. W. Lenders, G. Eisenhofer, and A. Januszewicz, "Cardiovascular manifestations of phaeochromocytoma," *Journal of Hypertension*, vol. 29, no. 11, pp. 2049–2060, 2011.

[8] P. K. Ganguly, R. E. Beamish, and N. S. Dhalla, "Catecholamine cardiotoxicity in pheochromocytoma," *American Heart Journal*, vol. 117, no. 6, pp. 1399-1400, 1989.

[9] G. Sojod, M. Diana, J. Wall, J. D'Agostino, D. Mutter, and J. Marescaux, "Successful extracorporeal membrane oxygenation treatment for pheochromocytoma-induced acute cardiac failure.," *The American Journal of Emergency Medicine*, vol. 30, no. 6, pp. 1017–e1, 2012.

[10] A. Adameova, Y. Abdellatif, and N. S. Dhalla, "Role of the excessive amounts of circulating catecholamines and glucocorticoids in stress-induced heart disease," *Canadian Journal of Physiology and Pharmacology*, vol. 87, no. 7, pp. 493–514, 2009.

[11] H. Vagner, T. M. Hey, B. Elle, and M. K. Jensen, "Embolisation of pheochromocytoma to stabilise and wean a patient in cardiogenic shock from emergency extracorporeal life support," *BMJ Case Reports*, 2015.

[12] S. Ritter, T. Guertler, C. A. Meier, and M. Genoni, "Cardiogenic shock due to pheochromocytoma rescued by extracorporeal membrane oxygenation," *Interactive CardioVascular and Thoracic Surgery*, vol. 13, no. 1, pp. 112-113, 2011.

[13] J. H. Rosing, R. Brooke Jeffrey, T. A. Longacre, and R. S. Greco, "Massive extra-adrenal retroperitoneal paraganglioma: Pre-operative embolization and resection," *Digestive Diseases and Sciences*, vol. 54, no. 8, pp. 1621–1624, 2009.

[14] S. Morita, Y. Furuta, A. Honma, F. Suzuki, K. Fujita, and S. Fukuda, "Preoperative Embolization and Postoperative Complications of Carotid Body Tumors," *Nippon Jibiinkoka Gakkai Kaiho*, vol. 111, no. 3, pp. 96–101, 2008.

[15] F. Nakamura, R. A. Silva, V. P. Santos, Á. Razuk Filho, and R. A. Caffaro, "Embolização pré operatória no tratamento de paraganglioma abdominal: relato de caso," *Revista do Colégio Brasileiro de Cirurgiões*, vol. 37, no. 2, pp. 159–161, 2010.

[16] M. Shakir, G. Blossom, and J. Lippert, "Anterior mediastinal paraganglioma: A case for preoperative embolization," *World Journal of Surgical Oncology*, vol. 10, article no. 134, 2012.

[17] C. C. Boedeker, G. J. Ridder, and J. Schipper, "Paragangliomas of the head and neck: Diagnosis and treatment," *Familial Cancer*, vol. 4, no. 1, pp. 55–59, 2005.

[18] E. D. P. Miranda, R. I. Lopes, G. P. Padovani et al., "Malignant paraganglioma in children treated with embolization prior to surgical excision," *World Journal of Surgical Oncology*, vol. 14, no. 1, article no. 26, 2016.

[19] J. Vandwalle, R. Spie, G. Jarry, V. Agaesse, J. Petit, and F. Saint, "Phéochromocytome et défaillance cardiaque : une indication exceptionnelle de surrénalectomie en urgence ou semi-urgence," *Progrès en Urologie*, vol. 20, no. 7, pp. 498–502, 2010.

21

Euglycemic Diabetic Ketoacidosis in a Patient with Cocaine Intoxication

Asma Abu-Abed Abdin,[1] Muhammad Hamza,[2] Muhammad S. Khan,[3] and Awab Ahmed[3]

[1]*Jordan University for Science and Technology, P.O. Box 3030, Irbid 22110, Jordan*
[2]*Department of Medicine, Dow Medical College, Baba-E-Urdu Road, Karachi 74200, Pakistan*
[3]*Section of Pulmonary & Critical Care Medicine, University of Oklahoma Health Sciences Center, 920 Stanton L Young Boulevard, Oklahoma City, OK 73104, USA*

Correspondence should be addressed to Muhammad S. Khan; muhammad-khan@ouhsc.edu

Academic Editor: Moritoki Egi

Diabetic ketoacidosis (DKA) is characterized by elevated anion gap metabolic acidosis, hyperglycemia, and elevated ketones in urine and blood. Hyperglycemia is a key component of DKA; however, a subset of DKA patients can present with near-normal blood glucose, an entity described as "euglycemic DKA." This rare phenomenon is thought to be due to starvation and food restriction in insulin dependent diabetic patients. Cocaine abuse is considered a trigger for development of DKA. Cocaine also has anorexic effects. We describe an interesting case of euglycemic DKA in a middle-aged diabetic female presenting with elevated anion gap metabolic acidosis, with near-normal blood glucose, in the settings of noncompliance to insulin and cocaine abuse. We have postulated that cocaine abuse was implicated in the pathophysiology of euglycemic DKA in this case. This case highlights complex physiological interplay between type-1 diabetes, noncompliance to insulin, and cocaine abuse leading to DKA, with starvation physiology causing development of euglycemic DKA.

1. Introduction

The hallmark of diabetic ketoacidosis (DKA) is hyperglycemia, metabolic acidosis, and increased ketones [1]. The absence of hyperglycemia, defined as serum glucose concentration greater than 250 mg/dL [1], makes the diagnosis of DKA less obvious in a patient with elevated serum anion gap metabolic acidosis and positive serum and urine ketones. However, euglycemic DKA has been well described in the literature mainly in type-1 diabetic patients, starvation, gestational diabetes, and more recently the settings SGLT inhibitor use. We describe a case of middle-aged women, who presented with severe metabolic acidosis, ketonemia, and near-normal blood glucose in the settings of noncompliance to insulin and cocaine use leading to poor oral intake. This case report also reviews possible physiologic interplay between lack of insulin and cocaine use leading to DKA.

2. Case

A fifty-seven-year-old female presented to emergency room with altered mental status, nausea, vomiting, and abdominal pain. The patient was in usual state of health 2 days before presentation, when she developed intermittent dull epigastric pain. The patient was able to tolerate the pain initially, but on day of presentation the pain became severe and persistent and she started having nonbilious vomiting. She also became somnolent and tachypneic and therefore the decision was made to bring her to the emergency room. Her past medical history was significant for diabetes mellitus and she was on insulin monotherapy. The family reported that for the last few weeks the patient was noncompliant with using insulin. On initial evaluation her vital signs were remarkable for temperature of 37 degree Celsius, pulse of 120/minutes, blood pressure (BP) of 134/78 mmHg, respiratory rate of 24 breath/minute, and oxygen saturation of

95% on 2-liter nasal cannula. Pertinent examination findings included obtunded patient who did not wake up to deep sternal rub, dry oral mucosa, and a weak gag reflex. Her pulmonary and cardiovascular examination was unremarkable. Admission labs indicated severe uncompensated metabolic acidosis with arterial blood gas showing pH of 7.02, $PaCO_2$ of 14, PaO_2 of 134, calculated bicarbonate of 4, and oxygen saturation of 97%. Serum chemistries indicated sodium 137 mEq/L (136–145 mEq/L), potassium 4.4 mEq/L (3.5–5.1 mEq/L), chloride 82 mEq/L (97–109 mEq/L), bicarbonate < 10 mEq/L (23–32 mEq/L), blood urea nitrogen (BUN) 32 mg/dL (7–17 mg/dL), serum creatinine 2.84 mg/dL (0.7–1.1 mg/dL), serum glucose 172 mg/dL (66–111 mg/dL), measured serum anion gap 46 (4–14), and measured serum osmolality 324 mOsm/kg (280–300 mOsm/kg). Her urine analysis was positive for ketones. Urine and serum drug screen was positive for cocaine. Other labs including complete blood count, lactic acid, serum Tylenol levels, and liver function tests were within normal limits. Admission chest roentgenogram was unremarkable (Figure 1).

Given concern for severe uncompensated metabolic acidosis and decreased sensorium, the patient was intubated for airway protection. Initial differential diagnosis included toxic alcohol ingestion, euglycemic diabetic ketoacidosis, alcoholic ketoacidosis, and starvation ketoacidosis. The serum ethanol, methanol, ethylene glycol, and propylene glycol were undetectable on admission labs and serum beta-hydroxybutyrate (BHB) levels were significantly elevated 15.95 mmol/L (0.02–0.27 mmol/L) confirming the diagnosis of euglycemic diabetic ketoacidosis. As the patient's blood glucose was 172 mg/dL on admission, we initially administered 1 liter bolus of intravenous (IV) 5% Dextrose and 0.45% normal saline (D5-1/2 NS), followed by a maintenance rate of 250 cc/hour, supplemented with 20 mEq of potassium chloride IV per liter of D5-1/2 NS. Insulin drip was initiated at a rate of 0.1 units/kg/hour. Finger stick blood glucose was checked hourly to maintain blood glucose between 150 and 200 mg/dL. Basic metabolic panel and BHB levels were checked at four-hour interval. After initial 4 liters of volume resuscitation, the patient's anion gap started to close and in 18 hours period her gap closed completely as shown in Table 1.

The patient was subsequently transitioned to subcutaneous insulin. Her mentation improved and she was extubated. After extubation patient confirmed that she was on a cocaine binge for 2 days and missed her insulin doses during that time. The patient was transferred out of medical intensive care unit and was discharged from hospital subsequently.

3. Discussion

Diabetic ketoacidosis (DKA) is defined by the American Diabetes Association as having a combination of hyperglycemia (glucose > 250 mg/dL), acidosis (arterial pH < 7.3 and bicarbonate < 15 mEq/L), and ketosis (moderate ketonuria or ketonemia) [1]. Normally, human bodies have balance between insulin levels and their counter regulatory hormones which include glucagon, epinephrine, cortisol, and growth hormone. Any factor that causes decrease in insulin levels or increase in its counter regulatory hormones or both will lead to development of DKA [1].

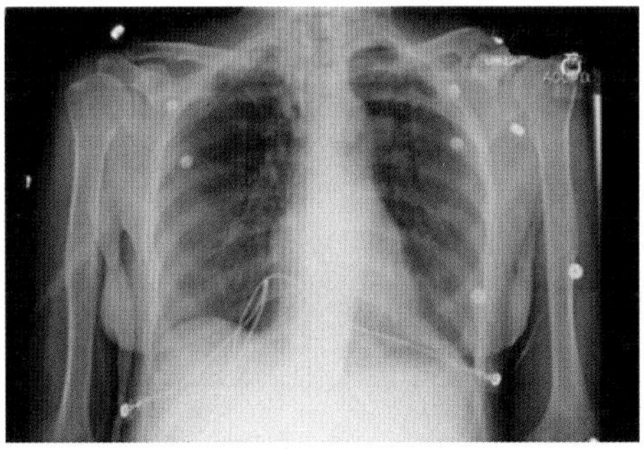

FIGURE 1: Chest X-ray on admission.

Rare cases of DKA have been found to occur in the absence of true hyperglycemia; such cases are called euglycemic DKA. This phenomenon was first reported by Munro et al., when 37 out of 211 studied DKA cases were found to be normoglycemic (defined as a serum glucose level of 300 mg/dL (16.7 mmol/L) or lower and a plasma bicarbonate level of 10 mmol/L or lower at presentation) [2]. Thereafter, these criteria have been adjusted to consider serum glucose level of 200 mg/dL as a threshold for the diagnosis of euglycemic DKA. The underlying mechanism of this rare entity is either decreased hepatic production of glucose during fasting states or enhanced urinary excretion of glucose induced by increase in counter regulatory hormones, with the former being the more important; that is, when a diabetic patient is exposed to any triggering factor for DKA and is fasting for any cause while continuing his insulin treatment regularly, the liver will be in a state of glycogen depletion, which in turn leads to decreased hepatic glucose production and increased lipolysis and fatty acid production, and this finally will lead to decreased glucose production while ketone bodies formation is continuous, ending in a state of euglycemic DKA [3]. Some of the causes that have been reported to induce euglycemic DKA include low caloric intake and starvation or prolonged vomiting, pregnancy, pancreatitis, insulin pump use, and SGLT2 inhibitors [4–9]. Table 2 gives major differentiating points between hyperglycemia DKA and euglycemic DKA.

Euglycemic DKA can be distinguished from other forms of ketoacidosis including starvation ketoacidosis, and alcoholic ketoacidosis, by clinical history and serum bicarbonate levels. The serum bicarbonate concentration in starvation ketoacidosis is usually more than 18 mEq/L [10]. The absence of other causes of elevated anion gap metabolic acidosis such as lactic acidosis, elevated toxic serum alcohols (methanol, ethylene glycol, etc.), drug toxicity, paraldehyde ingestion, and renal failure can distinguish DKA.

In the current case, the patient presented with severe uncompensated metabolic acidosis, ketonuria, and ketonemia in the absence of true hyperglycemia. After excluding other possibilities of wide anion gap metabolic acidosis including ethanol, methanol, or ethylene glycol ingestion, the diagnosis of euglycemic DKA was made and it was treated accordingly by IV 5% Dextrose, 0.45% normal saline, and

Table 1: Basic metabolic panel, beta-hydroxybutyrate, and serum pH from time of admission to closure of anion gap.

	Admission	Six hours apart	Four hours apart	Four hours apart	Four hours apart	Four hours apart
Sodium	137 mEq/L	139 mEq/L	139 mEq/L	138 mEq/L	138 mEq/L	137 mEq/L
Potassium	4.4 mEq/L	4.8 mEq/L	4.3 mEq/L	4.1 mEq/L	3.9 mEq/L	4.2 mEq/L
Chloride	82 mEq/L	102 mEq/L	103 mEq/L	105 mEq/L	107 mEq/L	107 mEq/L
Bicarbonate	<10 mEq/L	<10 mEq/L	10 mEq/L	15 mEq/L	21 mEq/L	22 mEq/L
Blood urea nitrogen	32 mg/dL	25 mg/dL	22 mg/dL	19 mg/dL	15 mg/dL	14 mg/dL
Creatinine	2.84 mg/dL	1.82 mg/dL	1.69 mg/dL	1.66 mg/dL	1.20 mg/dL	1.06 mg/dL
Glucose	172 mg/dL	251 mg/dL	180 mg/dL	198 mg/dL	166 mg/dL	95 mg/dL
Anion gap	46	28	26	18	10	8
B-Hydroxybutyrate	—	15.95 mmol/L	—	4.51 mmol/L	—	0.05 mmol/L
pH	7.02	7.13	7.26	7.34	7.36	7.38

Table 2: Major differences between hyperglycemic DKA and euglycemic DKA.

Hyperglycemic DKA	Euglycemic DKA
Blood glucose > 250 mg/dL, arterial pH < 7.3, and serum bicarbonate < 18 mEq/L	Blood glucose < 200 mg/dL, arterial pH < 7.3, and serum bicarbonate < 18 mEq/L
Insulin deficiency and increased counter regulatory hormones causing hyperglycemia	Insulin deficiency and increased counter regulatory hormones causing hyperglycemia and starvation from any cause euglycemia
Triggered by infections, concurrent illnesses, and dehydration	As a result of decreased circulating glucose in starvation, cirrhosis, exogenous insulin use, SGLT-2 inhibitors, pancreatitis, depression, and so forth

insulin drip. The patient was screened positive for cocaine in serum and urine drug screen, and thereafter she admitted that she had been on binge cocaine intake for two days before presentation. Interestingly, cocaine has been reported to be a trigger for DKA in many diabetic patients. This is attributed to cocaine's stimulatory effect on cortisol, epinephrine, and norepinephrine release from the adrenal gland [11, 12]. This increase in counter regulatory hormones is the underlying cause for having DKA with hyperglycemia in such patients.

In this patient, two counter regulatory factors played a role culminating in development of euglycemic DKA. We hypothesize that, with history of noncompliance to insulin and while being on cocaine binge, the patient developed hyperglycemic DKA for two reasons: firstly, from lack of exogenous insulin and secondly from hyperglycemic effect of cocaine via adrenocortical hormones as described above. Conversely, as cocaine has been shown to cause anorexic effect via suppression of feeding centers in central nervous system [13, 14] and while being on cocaine binge, the patient developed poor oral intake. This starvation effect led to drop in her blood sugar to normal range. Interestingly, the anorexic, thus, hypoglycemic effects of cocaine were more pronounced in our patient, hence overshadowing the initial hyperglycemia resulting in euglycemic DKA.

In conclusion, euglycemic DKA should be included in differential diagnosis in patients presenting with elevated anion gap metabolic acidosis and near-normal blood glucose, especially in the setting of cocaine abuse. Volume resuscitation and insulin drip initiation remain the cornerstone of treatment and early diagnosis through high index of suspicion is paramount in order to start the right treatment.

Competing Interests

The authors declare that they have no competing interests.

References

[1] E. A. Nyenwe and A. E. Kitabchi, "The evolution of diabetic ketoacidosis: an update of its etiology, pathogenesis and management," *Metabolism*, vol. 65, no. 4, pp. 507–521, 2016.

[2] J. F. Munro, I. W. Campbell, A. C. McCuish, and L. J. Duncan, "Euglycaemic diabetic ketoacidosis," *British Medical Journal*, vol. 2, no. 5866, pp. 578–580, 1973.

[3] M. S. Rauf, "Euglycemic ketoacidosis," *Pakistan Journal of Medical Sciences*, vol. 24, no. 1, pp. 161–162, 2008.

[4] F. Joseph, L. Anderson, N. Goenka, and J. Vora, "Starvation-induced true diabetic euglycemic ketoacidosis in severe depression," *Journal of General Internal Medicine*, vol. 24, no. 1, pp. 129–131, 2009.

[5] A. Gelaye, A. Haidar, C. Kassab, S. Kazmi, and P. Sinha, "Severe Ketoacidosis Associated with Canagliflozin (Invokana): a safety concern," *Case Reports in Critical Care*, vol. 2016, Article ID 1656182, 3 pages, 2016.

[6] M. Chico, S. N. Levine, and D. F. Lewis, "Normoglycemic diabetic ketoacidosis in pregnancy," *Journal of Perinatology*, vol. 28, no. 4, pp. 310–312, 2008.

[7] J. Rosenstock and E. Ferrannini, "Euglycemic diabetic ketoacidosis: a predictable, detectable, and preventable safety concern with SGLT2 inhibitors," *Diabetes Care*, vol. 38, no. 9, pp. 1638–1642, 2015.

[8] J. Prater and J. Chaiban, "Euglycemic diabetic ketoacidosis with acute pancreatitis in a patient not known to have diabetes," *Endocrine Practice*, vol. 1, no. 2, pp. e88–e91, 2015.

[9] E. A. Warner, G. S. Greene, M. S. Buchsbaum, D. S. Cooper, and B. E. Robinson, "Diabetic ketoacidosis associated with cocaine use," *Archives of Internal Medicine*, vol. 158, no. 16, pp. 1799–1802, 1998.

[10] A. E. Kitabchi, G. E. Umpierrez, J. M. Miles, and J. N. Fisher, "Hyperglycemic crises in adult patients with diabetes," *Diabetes Care*, vol. 32, no. 7, pp. 1335–1343, 2009.

[11] E. A. Nyenwe, R. S. Loganathan, S. Blum et al., "Active use of cocaine: an independent risk factor for recurrent diabetic ketoacidosis in a city hospital," *Endocrine Practice*, vol. 13, no. 1, pp. 22–29, 2007.

[12] A. S. Kashyap, K. P. Anand, and S. Kashyap, "Cocaine use a risk factor for DKA," *Endocrine Abstracts*, vol. 7, abstract P249, 2004.

[13] D. C. Balopole, C. D. Hansult, and D. Dorph, "Effect of cocaine on food intake in rats," *Psychopharmacology*, vol. 64, no. 1, pp. 121–122, 1979.

[14] S. J. Cooper and G. A. van der Hoek, "Cocaine: a microstructural analysis of its effects on feeding and associated behaviour in the rat," *Brain Research*, vol. 608, no. 1, pp. 45–51, 1993.

22

Starvation Ketoacidosis: A Cause of Severe Anion Gap Metabolic Acidosis in Pregnancy

Nupur Sinha, Sindhaghatta Venkatram, and Gilda Diaz-Fuentes

Division of Pulmonary and Critical Care Medicine, Bronx Lebanon Hospital Center and Albert Einstein College of Medicine, Bronx, NY 10457, USA

Correspondence should be addressed to Nupur Sinha; nsinha@bronxleb.org

Academic Editor: Won S. Park

Pregnancy is a diabetogenic state characterized by relative insulin resistance, enhanced lipolysis, elevated free fatty acids and increased ketogenesis. In this setting, short period of starvation can precipitate ketoacidosis. This sequence of events is recognized as "accelerated starvation." Metabolic acidosis during pregnancy may have adverse impact on fetal neural development including impaired intelligence and fetal demise. Short periods of starvation during pregnancy may present as severe anion gap metabolic acidosis (AGMA). We present a 41-year-old female in her 32nd week of pregnancy, admitted with severe AGMA with pH 7.16, anion gap 31, and bicarbonate of 5 mg/dL with normal lactate levels. She was intubated and accepted to medical intensive care unit. Urine and serum acetone were positive. Evaluation for all causes of AGMA was negative. The diagnosis of starvation ketoacidosis was established in absence of other causes of AGMA. Intravenous fluids, dextrose, thiamine, and folic acid were administered with resolution of acidosis, early extubation, and subsequent normal delivery of a healthy baby at full term. Rapid reversal of acidosis and favorable outcome are achieved with early administration of dextrose containing fluids.

1. Introduction

A relative insulin deficient state has been well described in pregnancy. This is due to placentally derived hormones including glucagon, cortisol, and human placental lactogen which are increased in periods of stress [1]. The insulin resistance increases with gestational age and confers susceptibility to ketosis. Superimposed fasting and stress due to any cause may predispose to severe ketoacidosis. The exaggerated response to fasting with increased ketone formation in second trimester of pregnancy was first described by Felig and Lynch in 1970 [2].

Several studies suggest that the development of acidosis has an adverse maternal and fetal impact including fetal neurological impairment and fetal loss. Severe acidosis occurs rarely in pregnancy and is usually a result of diabetic ketoacidosis in women with type 1 diabetes mellitus, lactic acidosis secondary to sepsis, or rare conditions with metabolic consequences such as acute fatty liver of pregnancy. Similar metabolic changes are seen with poor dietary intake or prolonged fasting and resulting acidosis is referred to as "starvation ketoacidosis" [3]. Starvation ketoacidosis is encountered in many settings like prolonged fasting, malnutrition, gastric banding eating disorder, Atkins diet, and alcoholism, but seldom recognized, and is rarely a severe acidosis outside pregnancy [1, 4–7].

We report a very rare case of a pregnant patient presenting with acute severe starvation ketoacidosis after a period of vomiting, with favorable outcome after timely identification and intervention, stressing the importance of early recognition of this life-threatening entity as a cause of acute severe anion gap metabolic acidosis (AGMA).

2. Case Report

A 41-year-old female in her sixth pregnancy at 32nd week of gestation was admitted to the intensive care unit with history of recurrent vomiting for four days. Vomiting had worsened for 48 hours, last two episodes being bloody, prompting her to seek medical attention. She denied any fever, chills,

TABLE 1: Laboratory parameters.

	At admission	12 hours	24 hours	48 hours
pH	7.158	7.199	7.248	7.403
pCO_2 (mmHg)	19.0	8.8	20.6	24.1
pO_2 (mmHg)	29.4 (venous)	135	246	187
HCO_3^- (mg/dL)	5	4	10	16
Anion gap (mmoles/L)	31	29	16	12
Acetone	Moderate	Moderate	Negative	Negative
Lactate (mmoles/L)	1.4	1.0	1.0	1.0
Glucose (mg/dL)	83	80	110	155
Creatinine (mg/dL)	1.4	1.4	1.1	1.2
Potassium (mEq/L)	5.5	3.7	3.1	3.0
Hemoglobin (g/dL)	14.2	12.7	10.1	9.2
Albumin (g/dL)	4.1	—	3.1	3.1
AST (U/L)	37	—	29	34
ALT (U/L)	41	—	34	35
Alkaline phosphatase (U/L)	152	—	116	115
Bilirubin (mg/dL)	0.2	—	0.3	0.3
Serum osmolality (mOsm/Kg)	309	—	—	283
Urine osmolality (mOsm/Kg)	632	—	—	—
Urine analysis	Ketones 2+	—	—	—

abdominal pain, diarrhea, or urinary symptoms. She denied any past, personal, or family medical history and had no surgery in the past. Social history included occasional alcohol use which was continued during pregnancy. Urine toxicology screen was positive for cannabinoids. Patient was afebrile at the time of admission, appeared dehydrated, and was tachycardic and tachypneic, but normotensive. Initial laboratory (Table 1) revealed mild leukocytosis at 16,000 per cubic mm; severe AGMA with pH—7.162, PCO_2—13, bicarbonate—5, and anion gap—31; and acute renal failure with creatinine—1.4 and normal lactate—1.4. Urine was positive for proteins and acetone. Acetone was present in moderate quantities in serum. Serum alcohol levels, acetylsalicylic acid, and acetaminophen levels were undetectable. Serum glucose level was 83 mg/dL and ammonia level 49 mcg/dL. Mild transaminitis was noted, with normal creatinine kinase (CK) levels. Patient required intubation and mechanical ventilation for worsening respiratory distress with Kussmaul's breathing and mild hematemesis. Esophagogastroduodenoscopy (EGD) revealed nonbleeding esophageal ulcerations. All septic work-up including blood, urine cultures, and chest roentgenogram were negative for infection. Initially, patient received normal saline, which was soon switched to 5% dextrose in lactated ringer mainly to avoid hyperchloremic acidosis. Thiamine and folic acid were given in view of prior alcohol use. Viability of fetus was confirmed by cardiotocographic tracings. Bicarbonate administration was considered but not given as acidosis resolved by 36 hrs and patient was successfully extubated on day 4 of hospital admission. Hydroxyproline levels, iron levels, ferritin levels, serum, and urine osmolarity were normal. Patient denied any use of antifreeze or any other toxic ingestion. A final diagnosis of starvation ketoacidosis due to recurrent vomiting with resulting poor oral intake, leading to severe AGMA and persistent hypokalemia, was made. Electrolytes were replaced and patient was monitored for refeeding syndrome. Patient was discharged with adequate follow-ups and delivered a healthy female baby by normal vaginal delivery at full term. The toxicology screen on the newborn was negative for cannabinoids. Her neurodevelopment is appropriate for age as noted in her most recent 18-month clinic visit.

3. Discussion

Metabolic acidosis of any etiology during pregnancy is concerning as it may lead to fetal lactic acidosis and hypoxemia [8]. Several studies have reported varying degree of adverse impact of maternal acidosis on neural development [8], including impaired intelligence [8–10] and fetal demise [11]. Identification of the underlying cause and timely intervention are of utmost importance in improving the fetal outcome.

In a patient presenting with increased AGMA, differential includes lactic acidosis, ketoacidosis (diabetic, starvation, or alcohol-associated), or toxic ingestions (methanol, ethylene glycol, and aspirin) [12].

Under normal circumstances with optimal glucose availability and normal insulin secretion, glycolysis generates pyruvate which enters the citric acid cycle for energy generation by the production of ATP. In any situation of low glucose availability, due to either starvation or insulin deficiency, there is deficiency of pyruvate entering the citric acid cycle due to depletion of glycogen stores. Alternative sources of energy in such circumstances are provided by generation of acetyl CoA from beta oxidation of fatty acids. The amount of acetyl CoA produced may exceed the capacity of the citric acid cycle, resulting in the generation of beta-hydroxybutyrate, acetoacetate, and acetone. The latter does not participate in energy generation and is either exhaled or excreted. Beta-hydroxybutyrate and acetoacetate are used as an alternative energy supply but their accumulation results in metabolic acidosis [1]. In an otherwise healthy individual, starvation requires at least 14 days to reach maximum severity, with mildly elevated ketoacids and pH usually being above 7.3 [1, 13]. Sufficient endogenous insulin secretion continues and prevents significant free fatty acid formation. Ketoacidosis is more severe in states of glycogen depletion, as seen in individuals with history of excess alcohol intake, and is augmented by lower insulin levels and perhaps higher levels of counterregulatory hormones as a result of volume depletion [1].

Normal pregnancy is characterized by relative insulin resistance, enhanced lipolysis, elevated levels of free fatty acids, and increased ketogenesis and even a short period of starvation may precipitate ketoacidosis [8]. Felig and Lynch first described the increased tendency to ketosis in pregnant women and demonstrated an exaggerated response to fasting during the second trimester, with increased ketone formation compared to nonpregnant women [2]. This concept was further clarified by Metzger et al., who demonstrated significantly higher levels of free fatty acids and beta-hydroxybutyrate after 12 hours of fasting in pregnant patients in their third trimester compared to the nonpregnant group [14]. This exaggerated response in late pregnancy is described as "accelerated starvation" and is possibly a mechanism for rapidly adapting the mother to the metabolism of fat so that less expendable fuels such as glucose and amino acids can be spared for the growth of the fetus. It is postulated that the predisposition to ketosis is the result of a relative lack of insulin, augmented by the presence of placentally derived counterregulatory hormones such as glucagon, cortisol, and human placental lactogen. These hormones are increased during periods of stress such as vomiting [1].

Predisposition to acidosis is further augmented in late pregnancy by state of respiratory alkalosis due to central respiratory stimulation by progesterone, lung volume changes, and altered compliance leading to hyperventilation and a reduction in PCO_2 [15, 16]. The chronic respiratory alkalosis is compensated by renal bicarbonate excretion, resulting in lower plasma bicarbonate concentration and reduced buffering capacity [15, 17], thus contributing to increased ketotic tendency in third trimester pregnancy [15, 18].

In our case, bicarbonate level of 5 was remarkable as vomiting leads to metabolic alkalosis secondary to loss of hydrochloride. Serum lactate levels were normal which made the diagnosis of lactic acidosis unlikely. Diabetic ketoacidosis was ruled out by normal glucose levels, absence of prior history of diabetes, and normal HbA1C. Additionally, she has remained nondiabetic during future follow-ups with us, thus ruling out the possibility of euglycemic diabetic ketoacidosis. She denied any history of eating disorders, including anorexia, or being on any specific diet. Patient denied any toxic ingestion or recent alcohol intake. Serum salicylate, alcohol, and acetaminophen levels were negative. Extensive search of literature did not reveal association of cannabinoids with severe ketoacidosis [19–21]. The rare differential of transient oxoprolinuria [22] was considered but hydroxyproline levels and ammonia levels were normal. In view of mild transaminitis and low platelets, HELLP syndrome was considered but discarded in absence of hemolysis and thrombocytopenia. Her normotensive status, absence of history of hypertension, and only mild proteinuria ruled out the diagnosis of preeclampsia. Starvation ketoacidosis was the most plausible diagnosis. We hypothesize that accumulation of ketones in this woman with recurrent vomiting and poor intake of 4-day duration in her third trimester pregnancy, augmented by underlying state of depleted glycogen stores in the setting of history of alcohol intake, may have resulted in profound starvation and resulting acidosis. The rapid resolution of the AGMA following administration of dextrose containing intravenous fluids supports our diagnosis.

Starvation ketosis in pregnancy has been described in the literature [1, 3, 11, 15, 18, 23–25], but the few cases presenting with such severe acidosis have been associated with diabetes mellitus. Recently a single case of a pregnant patient with severe acidosis was reported in association with muscular dystrophy [26]. Almost all reported cases required emergent Caesarian section in addition to dextrose administration. Only one reported case [3] resolved with administration of 10% dextrose.

This case is unique on account of the extreme severity of ketoacidosis in the setting of acute starvation, absence of comorbidity, and the favorable fetal and maternal outcome with early administration of dextrose containing fluids.

4. Conclusion

Starvation ketoacidosis in pregnancy may present as severe anion gap metabolic acidosis after short period of acute starvation. Third trimester pregnancies are prone to ketosis and starvation ketoacidosis may develop rapidly in the presence of inadequate caloric intake. The mother may appear well despite the severity of metabolic derangement, which can help differentiate this from other causes of raised anion gap metabolic acidosis.

Early recognition of the pregnant patient at risk for starvation ketoacidosis is essential for fetal outcome. Late recognition and thereby delay in treatment are associated with a greater risk for impaired neurodevelopment.

Intensivist and obstetricians should be aware of this entity especially in a pregnant patient with concurrent history of alcohol use. We recommend timely provision of carbohydrates in cases of suspected starvation in pregnancy; this allows endogenous insulin secretion and inhibits further ketone production. In patients with marginal insulin reserves, glucose levels should be monitored closely and introduction of insulin along with dextrose may be considered as part of the treatment.

Abbreviations

AGMA: Anion gap metabolic acidosis
CK: Creatinine kinase
EGD: Esophagogastroduodenoscopy
HELLP: Hemolysis, elevated liver enzymes, and low platelets.

Disclosure

None of the authors has a financial relationship with a commercial entity that has an interest in the subject of the paper. No financial support was used for the study.

References

[1] C. J. Frise, L. Mackillop, K. Joash, and C. Williamson, "Starvation ketoacidosis in pregnancy," *European Journal of Obstetrics & Gynecology and Reproductive Biology*, vol. 167, no. 1, pp. 1–7, 2013.

[2] P. Felig and V. Lynch, "Starvation in human pregnancy: hypoglycemia, hypoinsulinemia, and hyperketonemia," *Science*, vol. 170, no. 3961, pp. 990–992, 1970.

[3] N. Burbos, A. M. Shiner, and E. Morris, "Severe metabolic acidosis as a consequence of acute starvation in pregnancy," *Archives of Gynecology and Obstetrics*, vol. 279, no. 3, pp. 399–400, 2009.

[4] P. J. Hilton, W. McKinnon, G. A. Lord, J.-M. R. Peron, and L. G. Forni, "Unexplained acidosis of malnutrition: a study by ion-exchange chromatography/mass spectrometry," *Biomedical Chromatography*, vol. 20, no. 12, pp. 1386–1389, 2006.

[5] D. Bruegger, M. Rehm, L. da Silva, F. Christ, and U. Finsterer, "Severe metabolic acidosis resulting from a dislocated gastric band," *Obesity Surgery*, vol. 14, no. 4, pp. 555–558, 2004.

[6] A. Napoli, M. Framarino, A. Colatrella et al., "Eating disorders and diabetic ketoacidosis in a pregnant woman with type 1 diabetes: a case report," *Eating and Weight Disorders*, vol. 16, no. 2, pp. e146–e149, 2011.

[7] T.-Y. Chen, W. Smith, J. L. Rosenstock, and K.-D. Lessnau, "A life-threatening complication of Atkins diet," *The Lancet*, vol. 367, no. 9514, p. 958, 2006.

[8] J. A. Parker and D. L. Conway, "Diabetic ketoacidosis in pregnancy," *Obstetrics and Gynecology Clinics of North America*, vol. 34, no. 3, pp. 533–543, 2007.

[9] J. A. Churcill, H. W. Berendes, and J. Nemore, "Neuropsychological deficits in children of diabetic mothers," *The American Journal of Obstetrics & Gynecology*, vol. 105, no. 2, pp. 257–268, 1969.

[10] T. Rizzo, B. E. Metzger, W. J. Burns, and K. Burns, "Correlations between antepartum maternal metabolism and child intelligence," *The New England Journal of Medicine*, vol. 325, no. 13, pp. 911–916, 1991.

[11] J. M. Land, C. H. D. A'Court, M. D. G. Gillmer, and J. G. G. Ledingham, "Severe non-diabetic keto-acidosis causing intrauterine death," *British Journal of Obstetrics and Gynaecology*, vol. 99, no. 1, pp. 77–79, 1992.

[12] P. A. Gabow, "Disorders associated with an altered anion gap," *Kidney International*, vol. 27, no. 2, pp. 472–483, 1985.

[13] O. E. Owen, S. Caprio, G. A. Reichard Jr., M. A. Mozzoli, G. Boden, and R. S. Owen, "Ketosis of starvation: a revisit and new perspectives," *Clinics in Endocrinology and Metabolism*, vol. 12, no. 2, pp. 359–379, 1983.

[14] B. E. Metzger, V. Ravnikar, R. A. Vileisis, and N. Freinkel, "'Accelerated starvation' and the skipped breakfast in late normal pregnancy," *The Lancet*, vol. 1, no. 8272, pp. 588–592, 1982.

[15] A. Patel, D. Felstead, M. Doraiswami, G. M. Stocks, and U. Waheed, "Acute starvation in pregnancy: a cause of severe metabolic acidosis," *International Journal of Obstetric Anesthesia*, vol. 20, no. 3, pp. 253–256, 2011.

[16] D. W. Cugell, N. R. Frank, E. A. Gaensler, and T. L. Badger, "Pulmonary function in pregnancy. I. Serial observations in normal women," *The American Review of Tuberculosis*, vol. 67, no. 5, pp. 568–597, 1953.

[17] V. S. Lim, A. I. Katz, and M. D. Lindheimer, "Acid-base regulation in pregnancy," *The American Journal of Physiology*, vol. 231, no. 6, pp. 1764–1769, 1976.

[18] C. A. Mahoney, "Extreme gestational starvation ketoacidosis: case report and review of pathophysiology," *The American Journal of Kidney Diseases*, vol. 20, no. 3, pp. 276–280, 1992.

[19] B. Tofighi and J. D. Lee, "Internet highs—seizures after consumption of synthetic cannabinoids purchased online," *Journal of Addiction Medicine*, vol. 6, no. 3, pp. 240–241, 2012.

[20] CDC report, "Severe illness associated with synthetic cannabinoid use—Brunswick, Georgia," *Morbidity and Mortality Weekly Report*, vol. 62, no. 46, p. 939, 2013.

[21] O. A. Abodunde, J. Nakda, N. Nweke, and R. L. Veera, "Cannabinoid hyperemesis syndrome presenting with acute renal failure," *Journal of Medical Cases*, vol. 4, no. 3, pp. 173–175, 2013.

[22] T. Kuhara, Y. Inoue, M. Ohse, B. F. Krasnikov, and A. J. L. Cooper, "Urinary 2-hydroxy-5-oxoproline, the lactam form of α-ketoglutaramate, is markedly increased in urea cycle disorders," *Analytical and Bioanalytical Chemistry*, vol. 400, no. 7, pp. 1843–1851, 2011.

[23] S. Keay and R. Fox, "Maternal ketoacidosis complicating acute starvation in pregnancy," *Journal of Obstetrics and Gynaecology*, vol. 20, no. 5, p. 539, 2000.

[24] B. Franke, D. Carr, and M. H. Hatem, "A case of euglycaemic diabetic ketoacidosis in pregnancy," *Diabetic Medicine*, vol. 18, no. 10, pp. 858–859, 2001.

[25] M. Chico, S. N. Levine, and D. F. Lewis, "Normoglycemic diabetic ketoacidosis in pregnancy," *Journal of Perinatology*, vol. 28, no. 4, pp. 310–312, 2008.

[26] N. Cecere, C. Hubinont, A. K. Kadingi et al., "Extreme maternal metabolic acidosis leading to fetal distress and emergency caesarean section," *Case Reports in Obstetrics and Gynecology*, vol. 2013, Article ID 847942, 3 pages, 2013.

23

A Case of Leptospirosis-Associated Severe Pulmonary Hemorrhagic Syndrome Successfully Treated with Venovenous Extracorporeal Membrane Oxygenation

Nao Umei and Shingo Ichiba

Department of Surgical Intensive Care Medicine, Nippon Medical School Hospital, Tokyo, Japan

Correspondence should be addressed to Shingo Ichiba; ecmoshingo@gmail.com

Academic Editor: Chiara Lazzeri

Background. In patients with leptospirosis-associated severe pulmonary hemorrhagic syndrome (SPHS), hypoxemia is the most common cause of death despite maximal mechanical ventilation. *Case.* A 50-year-old male sushi chef who had never traveled outside Japan presented with a 2-day history of fever and muscle pain. On admission, the patient had thrombocytopenia, renal insufficiency, and jaundice. His condition continued to deteriorate, with decreasing platelet count, worsening renal function, hyperbilirubinemia, hypotension, and respiratory distress. On day 5 after onset of symptoms, he required intubation and mechanical ventilation. Bronchoscopy showed diffuse endobronchial bleeding. His respiratory status worsened rapidly with a partial pressure of arterial oxygen to fraction of inspired oxygen ratio of 70, necessitating venovenous extracorporeal membrane oxygenation (V-V ECMO) and treatment with an inotrope, renal replacement therapy, and broad-spectrum antibiotics including benzylpenicillin. Anticoagulation was maintained at the minimum level. His condition improved, and he was weaned off ECMO on day 15 and discharged on day 19 after onset of symptoms. The leptospirosis diagnosis was confirmed by leptospiral DNA detection in urine samples by polymerase chain reaction and the results of paired serum antibody titer testing. *Conclusions.* V-V ECMO may prevent mortality in patients with leptospirosis-induced SPHS that does not respond to conventional therapy.

1. Introduction

Leptospirosis presents with acute influenza-like symptoms such as headache, chills, fever, vomiting, and muscle pain. Although leptospirosis can present with mild nonspecific flu-like symptoms, in its severe form, called Weil disease, it causes symptoms such as jaundice, bleeding, and renal failure [1, 2]. Rapid hemorrhagic tendency, jaundice, renal dysfunction, rhabdomyolysis, and myocardial pericarditis appear 4-5 days after disease onset. Jaundice, bleeding, and impaired renal function usually diminish after several weeks. However, pulmonary involvement occurs in 20–70% of leptospirosis cases, with pulmonary hemorrhage constituting a major cause of death [3–6]. The mortality rate in leptospirosis cases with severe pulmonary hemorrhagic syndrome (SPHS) is 30–60% even with adequate treatment [4, 7]. In this report, we describe a case of life-threatening leptospirosis with SPHS that occurred in urban Tokyo and that was successfully managed with venovenous extracorporeal membrane oxygenation (V-V ECMO).

2. Case Presentation

A 50-year-old male sushi chef who had never traveled outside Japan presented with a 2-day history of fever and muscle pain. Laboratory investigation yielded the following results: white blood cells (WBC): 7780/μL; platelets: 89000/μL; C-reactive protein (CRP): 36.4 mg/dL; blood urea nitrogen (BUN): 47 mg/dL; creatinine: 2.41 mg/dL; and total bilirubin (T-Bil): 2.0 mg/dL. The day after he was admitted to the hospital, the patient's condition worsened, as indicated by the laboratory data: WBC: 6700/μL; platelets: 50000/μL; CRP: 32.49 mg/dL; BUN: 66 mg/dL; creatinine: 2.81 mg/dL; and T-Bil: 5.6 mg/dL. He was presumptively diagnosed with bacterial pneumonia, atypical pneumonia, and miliary tuberculosis. He was also diagnosed with leptospirosis on the basis

TABLE 1: Extracorporeal membrane oxygenation settings.

ECMO day	1	2	3	4	5	6	7	8	9	10	11
Flow (L/min)	4.2	3.5	3	2	2	1.5	1.5	1.5	1.5	1.5	1.5
Gas flow (L/min)	4	4	4	4	4	4	4	4	4	4	4
F_DO_2	1	1	1	1	1	1	1	1	1	1	1
Motor RPM	2865	2500	2300	1800	1800	1500	1500	1500	1500	1500	1500

F_DO_2: fraction of delivered oxygen to the oxygenator; RPM: revolutions per minute.

of jaundice, renal failure, and thrombocytopenia. He was administered the broad-spectrum antibiotics ceftriaxone, levofloxacin, and minocycline on the first day of admission to the referral hospital. Vancomycin and meropenem were administered on the second day. He was also given the antitubercular agents—isoniazid, rifampicin, pyrazinamide, and ethambutol—even though the results of a tuberculosis screening test were negative. Despite these treatments, his systolic blood pressure dropped to 70 mmHg, and his respiratory condition deteriorated; he was intubated 5 days after the onset of symptoms, which is three days after admission to the previous hospital. An X-ray showed bilateral alveolar infiltrates, and blood gas analysis revealed the following: pH: 7.390; partial pressure of arterial carbon dioxide ($PaCO_2$): 28.3 mmHg; and partial pressure of arterial oxygen (PaO_2): 70.4 mmHg HCO_3^- 16.8 mmol/L with fraction of inspired oxygen (F_IO_2) of 1.0 as well as positive end-expiratory pressure (PEEP) of 10 cm H_2O. The patient developed a life-threatening condition with septic shock and severe acute respiratory failure, despite optimal medical treatment. He was referred to our center for ECMO. Our ECMO team decided to initiate V-V ECMO at the previous hospital and transport the patient on V-V ECMO because the patient was severely hypoxic and needed maximal doses of norepinephrine, epinephrine, and vasopressin to stabilize his cardiac condition. Cannulation was performed via the right femoral vein with 25-French drainage cannulae (HLS Cannulae Maquet Cardiopulmonary, Hirrlingen, Germany) for access and via the right internal jugular vein with 23-French cannulae for return. The ECMO circuit was an adult ECMO bypass custom tubing pack consisting of a Rotaflow® centrifugal pump (Maquet Cardiopulmonary GmbH, Hirrlingen, Germany) and gas exchanger (MERA NHP Excelung NSH-R HPO-23WH-C®, Senko Medical Inc., Tokyo, Japan). V-V ECMO was initiated at a blood flow rate of 4.0 L/min, with sweep gas flow through the oxygenator at 4.0 L/min of 100% oxygen. After the procedure, the patient's SpO_2 was 94%, heart rate was 131 beats/min, and blood pressure was 142/74 mmHg on 0.1 μg/kg/min of epinephrine and 0.3 μg/kg/min of norepinephrine. He was transported to our center via ground ambulance.

After he was transported to our ICU, we maintained the ECMO blood flow at >3.0 L/min during the first 3 days of ECMO because his activated partial thromboplastin time was maintained at around 40–50 s, which was lower than normal because of bleeding (Table 1). After bleeding was controlled, we decreased the ECMO blood flow gradually to 1.5 L/min when peripheral capillary oxygen saturation (SpO_2) was over 90%. During V-V ECMO the mechanical ventilation was set at the lung rest setting, which consisted of a driving pressure of 5 cm of water, PEEP of 12 cm of water, and F_IO_2 of 0.4. Fiber-optic bronchoscopy showed diffuse endobronchial bleeding. The patient was systemically heparinized to maintain an activated partial thromboplastin time of 40–50 seconds, which was lower than the normal value for V-V ECMO. Dobutamine was initiated at 3 μg/kg/min because transthoracic echocardiography showed that the ejection fraction was 30%, mitral regurgitation was moderate, and tricuspid regurgitation was severe. After initiation of dobutamine, his cardiac function improved, epinephrine was stopped the next day, and norepinephrine was stopped the day after that. He remained oliguric and needed renal replacement therapy for 7 days. At the time of presentation to our center, his WBC count was 18,000/μL, CRP level was 24.52 mg/dL, and procalcitonin level was > 100 ng/mL. Although we thought of a wide variety of infections as differential diagnoses, we strongly suspected leptospirosis on the basis of severe acute respiratory failure, myocardial pericarditis, renal failure, jaundice, and thrombocytopenia, which made us continue the broad-spectrum antibiotics, levofloxacin, vancomycin, meropenem, antitubercular agents, and add benzylpenicillin. Because of pulmonary hemorrhage, he was given a platelet transfusion (20 units) for the first 3 days of V-V ECMO therapy. Even though his pulmonary hemorrhage improved on day 8 of V-V ECMO, computed tomography scans showed bilateral ground-glass opacities, bilateral pleural effusion, and atelectasis. Rehabilitation, including sitting on the edge of the bed and standing, was initiated. On day 6 of ECMO therapy, polymerase chain reaction analysis of urine samples collected at the previous hospital confirmed the presence of leptospiral DNA. The tests for tuberculosis, *Legionella* urinary antigen, pneumococcal antigen, serum *Mycoplasma* antibody, and *Chlamydia pneumoniae* antibody all yielded negative results. We switched the intravenous antibiotics from broad-spectrum antibiotics to benzylpenicillin (12 million units/day).

On day 11 of ECMO therapy, blood tests showed improvements in platelet count and serum CRP, creatinine, and T-Bil levels (Figure 1). In addition, the amount of sputum decreased, and improvements were observed in his chest X-ray (Figure 2), compliance, and oxygenation (Figure 3); therefore, we performed a 2-hour trial off-test. The patient tolerated the trial without O_2 flow to the oxygenator; therefore, we decided to wean him off ECMO. He was extubated 2 days after being taken off ECMO and transferred back to the previous hospital 2 days after extubation. His last blood gas analysis

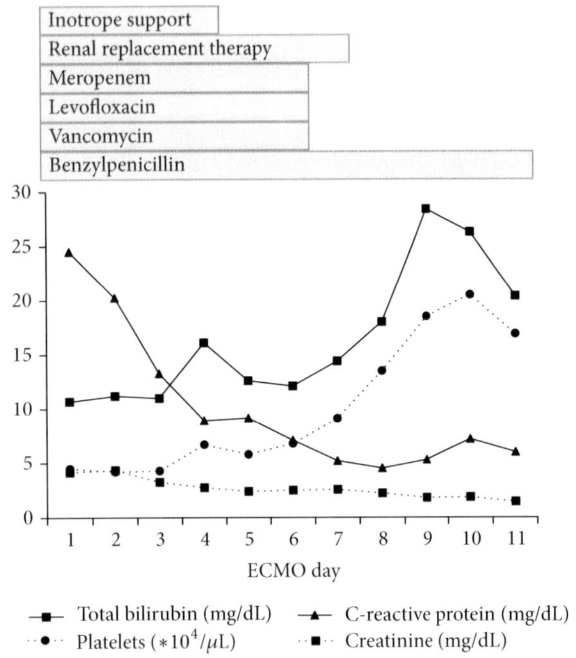

FIGURE 1: Summary of laboratory data and therapeutic course.

revealed the following results: pH: 7.468; $PaCO_2$: 36.6 mmHg; PaO_2: 67.2 mmHg; and HCO_3^-: 26.2 mmol/L on room air. Laboratory investigation revealed the following results: WBC: 7400/μL; platelets: 256000/μL; CRP: 1.13 mg/dL; BUN: 29.1 mg/dL; creatinine: 1.36 mg/dL; and T-Bil: 7.9 mg/dL. Finally, paired serum antibody titer testing (on days 5 and 19 after the onset of symptoms) showed a fourfold or higher increase in antibody titers for *Leptospira interrogans* serovar Copenhageni and *Leptospira interrogans* serovar Icterohaemorrhagiae, confirming the diagnosis of leptospirosis.

3. Discussion

In the present report, we describe the case of a patient with leptospirosis-associated SPHS combined with jaundice, acute renal failure, and cardiomyopathy. The present case report is important because our findings suggest the possibility of improving patient survival by using V-V ECMO in patients with leptospirosis-associated SPHS.

In most leptospirosis cases, the pulmonary symptoms usually appear 4–6 days after disease onset. The disease may progress rapidly and result in death in less than 72 hours [8]. SPHS, also described as the severe pulmonary form of leptospirosis (SPFL), is believed to be the major form of death in leptospirosis infection [8]. SPFL also manifests as pulmonary hemorrhage, which is usually massive and leads to respiratory insufficiency and death by asphyxiation. It is also similar to the pathological expression of diffuse alveolar hemorrhage [9]. To our knowledge, there are no reports comparing leptospirosis-associated SPHS with non-leptospirosis SPHS. We believe that the fundamental strategy for the treatment of pulmonary insufficiency due to the clinicopathological features mentioned above would be identical for both conditions, including mechanical ventilation with higher PEEP and management of coagulopathy. In some catastrophic cases with severe hypoxemia unresponsive to conventional medical treatment, ECMO is required, under cautious anticoagulation therapy.

The pathophysiology of pulmonary injury in leptospirosis is poorly understood. The pulmonary injury may be caused by an undefined leptospiral toxin that induces endothelial damage in pulmonary capillaries, or by host immune responses [6, 10, 11]. Methylprednisolone has been used for treatment of SPHS on the basis of the pathogenetic mechanism of lung injury; however, no significant mortality benefit has been observed in patients already on mechanical ventilation [12]. Trivedi et al. evaluated the efficacy of cyclophosphamide and plasma exchange in patients with leptospiral pulmonary hemorrhage. However, patients with severe disease may not tolerate the transient hypoxemia associated with plasma exchange [13]. High-frequency oscillatory ventilation may be effective for pulmonary hemorrhage treatment; however, it may result in significant hemodynamic instability [14]. Alternatively, V-V ECMO, which supports pulmonary function and minimizes the damage induced by mechanical ventilation, could be useful until the lungs recover. Liao et al. have reported the successful use of V-V ECMO for the treatment of severe respiratory failure due to alveolar bleeding and acute respiratory distress syndrome [15]. They initiated ECMO on day 4 because the PaO_2/F_IO_2 ratio was 162; ECMO was maintained for 6 days, and extubation was performed 4 days after ECMO discontinuation. Arokianathan et al. reported that, after transportation to the ECMO center, the patient was maintained on ECMO for 8 days and extubated 2 days after ECMO discontinuation [16]. In the present case, ECMO was initiated on day 5 after onset of symptoms, when SPHS developed, and continued for 11 days; the patient was extubated 2 days after ECMO discontinuation.

Liao et al. used 4 units of platelets, 12 units of red cell concentrate, and 24 units of fresh frozen plasma during ECMO management [15]. The transfusion of 60 units of platelets was required to maintain the platelet count at >50,000/μL, which is the limit specified in our ECMO management protocol for patients with bleeding complications. We also administered 8 units of red cell concentrate and 4 units of fresh frozen plasma because of massive pulmonary alveolar bleeding. Although blood transfusions are inevitable for the management of alveolar bleeding, ECMO is useful as an adjunct therapy until alveolar bleeding stops and respiratory condition improves in patients with leptospirosis.

Our patient's WBC count was 7780/μL on the day of his admission to the previous hospital, which was not very high. De Silva et al. reported in their large prospective study that total white cell counts showed a decline over the first 5 days of illness and then rose until the end of second week [17]. It is supposed that the delayed increase in the WBC count may have coincided with the initiation of lung injury, which was also seen in our patient's clinical course.

The cause of severe respiratory failure in the present case was massive alveolar bleeding and pulmonary edema. Marked alveolar bleeding was observed during bronchoscopy. In addition, cardiogenic pulmonary edema secondary

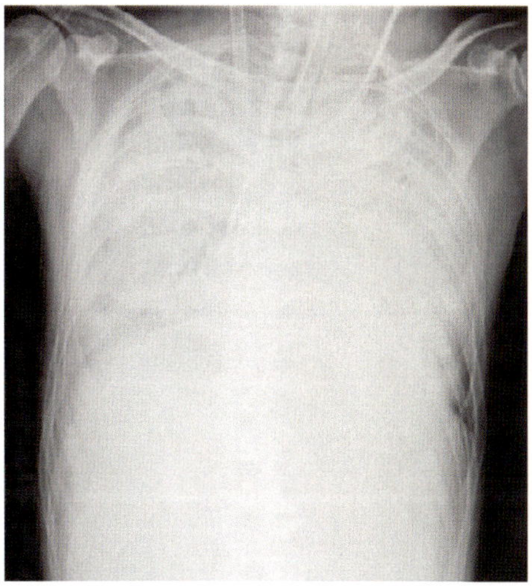

(a) Chest X-ray of patient on day 1 of extracorporeal membrane oxygenation

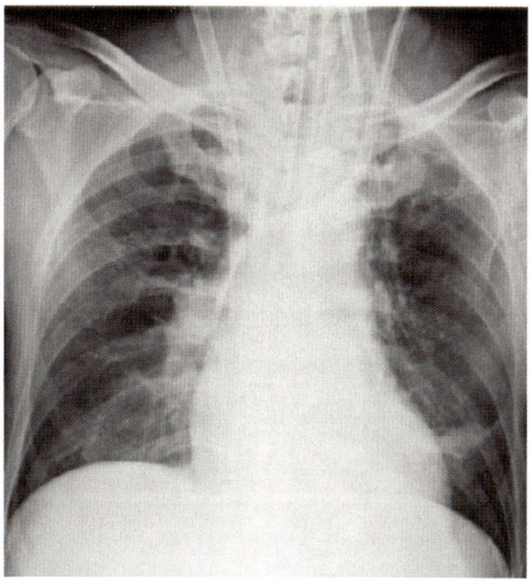

(b) Chest X-ray of patient on day 11 of extracorporeal membrane oxygenation

FIGURE 2

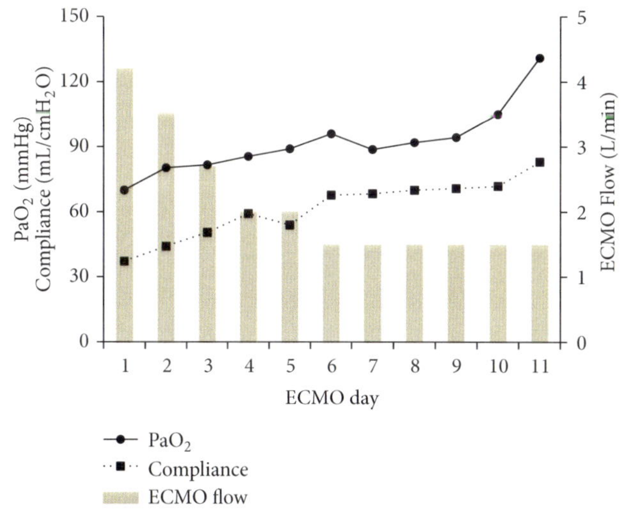

FIGURE 3: Partial pressure of arterial oxygen (PaO_2) and compliance during extracorporeal membrane oxygenation therapy.

to myocarditis may make respiratory failure worse. Moreover, the Jarisch-Herxheimer reaction may be associated with deterioration of respiratory status [18].

Leptospirosis is endemic in tropical regions and extremely rare in urban areas. However, patients without a history of traveling to tropical regions such as Southeast Asia and Latin America can develop leptospirosis in urban areas. If a patient has flu-like symptoms and multiple organ failure, it is important to rule out leptospirosis as a differential diagnosis. The course of the disease should be carefully monitored in the intensive care unit as respiratory distress may progress rapidly. In addition, V-V ECMO therapy should be considered early in case of difficulty in maintaining adequate oxygenation by conventional mechanical ventilation because respiratory distress is the most common cause of death in these cases.

In conclusion, we successfully treated a patient with leptospirosis-associated SPHS by using V-V ECMO with careful anticoagulation therapy. Our findings indicate that the survival of patients with leptospirosis could be improved by using V-V ECMO.

References

[1] D. A. Haake and P. N. Levett, "Leptospirosis in humans," *Current Topics in Microbiology and Immunology*, vol. 387, pp. 65–97, 2015.

[2] P. N. Levett, "Leptospirosis," *Clinical Microbiology Reviews*, vol. 14, no. 2, pp. 296–326, 2001.

[3] V. Leung, M.-L. Luong, and M. Libman, "Leptospirosis: Pulmonary hemorrhage in a returned traveller," *Canadian Medical Association Journal*, vol. 183, no. 7, pp. E423–E427, 2011.

[4] M. Dolhnikoff, T. Mauad, E. P. Bethlem, and C. R. R. Carvalho, "Leptospiral pneumonias," *Current Opinion in Pulmonary Medicine*, vol. 13, no. 3, pp. 230–235, 2007.

[5] T. Panaphut, S. Domrongkitchaiporn, A. Vibhagool, B. Thinkamrop, and W. Susaengrat, "Ceftriaxone compared with sodium penicillin G for treatment of severe leptospirosis," *Clinical Infectious Diseases*, vol. 36, no. 12, pp. 1507–1513, 2003.

[6] M. A. Martinez Garcia, A. de Diego, R. Damia, and J. L. Lopez Hontagas, "Pulmonary involvement in leptospirosis," *European journal of clinical microbiology & infectious diseases*, vol. 19, no. 6, pp. 471–474, 2000.

[7] S. R. R. Vieira and J. S. Brauner, "Leptospirosis as a cause of acute respiratory failure: clinical features and outcome in 35 critical care patients.," *The Brazilian journal of infectious diseases : an official publication of the Brazilian Society of Infectious Diseases*, vol. 6, no. 3, pp. 135–139, 2002.

[8] J. J. Pereira Da Silva, M. O. Dalston, J. E. M. De Carvalho, S. Setúbal, J. M. C. De Oliveira, and M. M. Pereira, "Clinicopathological and immunohistochemical features of the severe

pulmonary form of leptospirosis," *Journal of the Brazilian Society of Tropical Medicine*, vol. 35, no. 4, pp. 395–399, 2002.

[9] M. S. Park, "Diffuse alveolar hemorrhage," *Tuberculosis and Respiratory Diseases*, vol. 74, no. 4, pp. 151–162, 2013.

[10] E. P. Bethlem and C. R. R. Carvalho, "Pulmonary leptospirosis," *Current Opinion in Pulmonary Medicine*, vol. 6, no. 5, pp. 436–441, 2000.

[11] M. Dolhnikoff, T. Mauad, E. P. Bethlem, and C. R. R. Carvalho, "Pathology and pathophysiology of pulmonary manifestations in leptospirosis," *The Brazilian Journal of Infectious Diseases*, vol. 11, no. 1, pp. 142–148, 2007.

[12] V. V. Shenoy, V. S. Nagar, A. A. Chowdhury, P. S. Bhalgat, and N. I. Juvale, "Pulmonary leptospirosis: An excellent response to bolus methylprednisolone," *Postgraduate Medical Journal*, vol. 82, no. 971, pp. 602–606, 2006.

[13] S. V. Trivedi, A. H. Vasava, L. C. Bhatia, T. C. Patel, N. K. Patel, and N. T. Patel, "Plasma exchange with immunosuppression in pulmonary alveolar haemorrhage due to leptospirosis," *Indian Journal of Medical Research*, vol. 131, no. 3, pp. 429–433, 2010.

[14] M. B. M. Nor, A. Md Ralib, N. A. Ibrahim, and M. R. Abdul-Ghani, "High frequency oscillatory ventilation in leptospirosis pulmonary hemorrhage syndrome: A case series study," *Indian Journal of Critical Care Medicine*, vol. 20, no. 6, pp. 342–348, 2016.

[15] C.-Y. Liao, R.-J. Ben, H.-M. Wu et al., "Acute respiratory distress syndrome manifested by leptospirosis successfully teated by extracorporeal membrane oxygenation (ECMO)," *Internal Medicine*, vol. 54, no. 22, pp. 2943–2946, 2015.

[16] D. Arokianathan, K. Trower, S. Pooboni, A. Sosnowski, P. Moss, and H. Thaker, "Leptospirosis: A case report of a patient with pulmonary haemorrhage successfully managed with extra corporeal membrane oxygenation," *The Journal of infection*, vol. 50, no. 2, pp. 158–162, 2005.

[17] N. L. De Silva, M. Niloofa, N. Fernando et al., "Changes in full blood count parameters in leptospirosis: A prospective study," *International Archives of Medicine*, vol. 7, no. 1, article no. 31, 2014.

[18] G. Guerrier and E. D'Ortenzio, "The Jarisch-Herxheimer Reaction in Leptospirosis: A Systematic Review," *PLoS ONE*, vol. 8, no. 3, Article ID e59266, 2013.

Spontaneous Tumor Lysis Syndrome due to Uterine Leiomyosarcoma with Lung Metastases

Vivek Alaigh[1] and Debapriya Datta[2]

[1]*Department of Medicine, University of CT Health Center, 263 Farmington Avenue, Farmington, CT 06030, USA*
[2]*Division of Pulmonary-Critical Care Medicine, University of CT Health Center, Farmington, CT 06030, USA*

Correspondence should be addressed to Debapriya Datta; ddatta@uchc.edu

Academic Editor: Ricardo Oliveira

Tumor lysis syndrome (TLS) is an oncologic emergency characterized by a combination of metabolic derangements (hyperuricemia, hyperkalemia, hyperphosphatemia, and hypocalcemia) caused by rapid turnover from cell destruction in certain cancers. These metabolic derangements can lead to seizures, cardiac arrhythmias, renal failure, and death. TLS is usually seen after the initiation of chemotherapy for hematologic malignancies. TLS occurring spontaneously, without initiation of chemotherapy, is rare and its occurrence in solid tumors is rarer still. We report a case of spontaneous TLS in a patient with leiomyosarcoma of the uterus, with metastasis to lung. Such a case has never been reported before.

1. Introduction

Tumor lysis syndrome (TLS) is an oncologic emergency resulting from lysis of tumor cells with release of intracellular contents into the circulation [1]. It consists of hyperuricemia, hyperkalemia, hyperphosphatemia, and hypocalcemia caused by rapid breakdown of tumor cells [2]. These derangements can lead to seizures, cardiac arrhythmias, renal failure, and death.

TLS is most commonly seen during the initiation of chemotherapy in aggressive hematologic malignancies, such as acute myeloid leukemia, acute lymphoblastic leukemia, and non-Hodgkin's lymphoma [3]. Less often, it has been seen in the treatment of solid bulky tumors that are sensitive to chemotherapy, such as breast cancer and small cell lung cancer [3]. Of note, there is not a systemic relationship between the size of a solid tumor and the occurrence of TLS. TLS occurring spontaneously without prior treatment is rare, though reported in hematologic malignancies. Even rarer is spontaneous TLS in solid tumors. Rarely does TLS occur spontaneously with solid tumors. There has not been any previously documented case of spontaneous TLS occurring in a uterine malignancy with lung metastases.

2. Case Description

A 58-year-old Caucasian female with no significant past medical history presented from a community hospital with a 3-week history of abdominal distension and constipation. She also complained of nausea, fatigue, shortness of breath with exertion, and decreased appetite. On examination, the patient had an extremely firm and distended lower abdomen with tenderness in the right lower quadrant. The rest of her examination was otherwise unremarkable. A computed tomogram (CT) scan of the abdomen showed a large heterogeneous, partially necrotic abdominal-pelvic mass, 16.3 cm by 20.2 cm in size (Figure 1), and peritoneal carcinomatosis with small ascites. Chest CT scan (Figure 2) showed a moderate right-sided pleural effusion, as well as bilateral pulmonary nodules with mediastinal lymphadenopathy. Pertinent laboratory values on admission included potassium of 3.2 mg/dL, bicarbonate of 28.2 mg/dL, creatinine of 1 mg/dL, and phosphorus of 3.6 mg/dL.

Because of the size of her tumor, she was subsequently transferred to a tertiary health center for further evaluation and possible surgery. As seen in Table 1, the patient on admission was found to have hyperkalemia (potassium 6.2 mg/dL),

Table 1: Progression of the patient's electrolyte derangements.

Patient disposition	Potassium (mg/dL)	Phosphorus (mg/dL)	Ionized calcium (mmol/L)	Uric acid (mg/dL)	Creatinine (mg/dL)	Bicarbonate (mg/dL)	LDH (mg/dL)	Lactate (mmol/L)
Admission to community hospital	3.2	3.6	N/A	N/A	1	28.2	774	3.8
Prior to transfer to tertiary care center	6.2	9.8	N/A	15.1	2.3	19.4	N/A	2.3
Admission to tertiary care center	6.2	9.8	1	15.1	3	9	N/A	11.1
On ICU admission	6.5	11.5	1.07	16.1	2.8	14	1243	5.5
Prior to death	4.3	6.5	1.14	7	2.3	17	1066	5

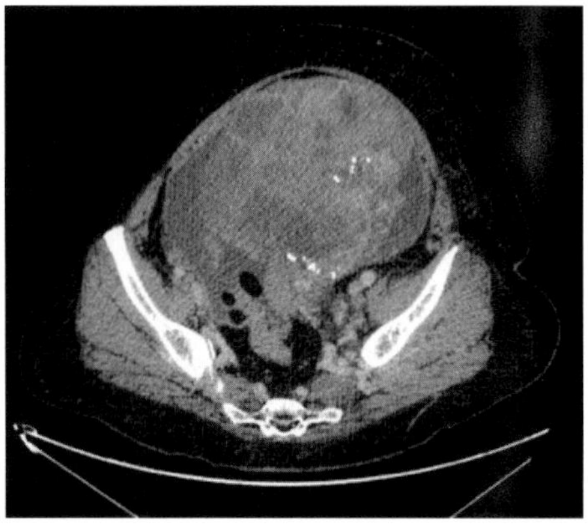

Figure 1: CT scan of the abdomen showing a large heterogeneous, partially necrotic abdominal-pelvic mass, 16.3 cm by 20.2 cm in size.

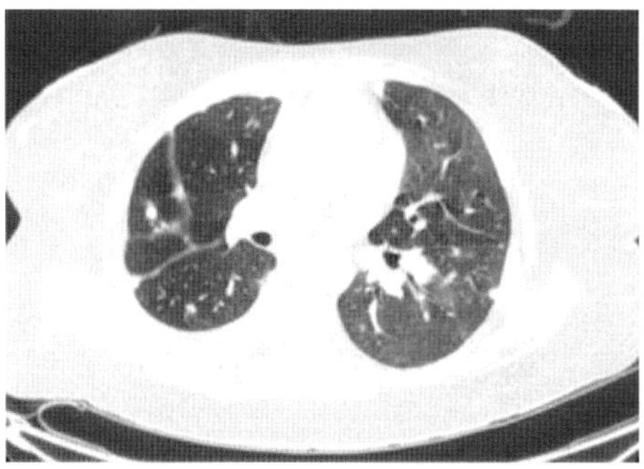

Figure 2: CT scan of chest showing a moderate right-sided pleural effusion, as well as bilateral pulmonary nodules with hilar adenopathy.

hyperphosphatemia (phosphate 9.8 mg/dL), hyperuricemia (uric acid 15.1 mg/dL), and hypocalcemia (ionized calcium of 1 mmol/L), without having received any chemotherapy for her malignancy. She additionally went into renal failure (creatinine of 3 mg/dL) and severe metabolic acidosis (bicarbonate of 9 mg/dL with an arterial pH of 7.259). She also had a lactate of 11.1 mg/dL. LDH was also elevated at 1263 U/L, roughly six times the upper limit of normal. Based on these abnormalities, laboratory TLS was diagnosed; given her renal failure, she also had evidence of clinical TLS.

The patient's electrolytes worsened, with potassium of 6.5 mg/dL, phosphorus of 11.1 mg/dL, and a uric acid of 16.1 mg/dL. She also had a lactic acid level of 11.1 mg/dL. She was transferred to the ICU due to hypotension (blood pressure of 62/49 mm Hg), requiring vasopressor support, and increased work of breathing due to her profound acidosis (for which she was placed on rescue noninvasive bilevel positive airway pressure). Her renal failure was treated with intravenous normal saline (her creatinine eventually trended down to 2.3 mg/dL) while her hyperuricemia was treated with rasburicase 6 mg (uric acid trended down to 7 mg/dL). She was additionally started on a sodium bicarbonate infusion for severe metabolic acidosis (bicarbonate improved to 17 mg/dL). She was given kayexalate, D50, insulin, and calcium gluconate for her hyperkalemia, which eventually corrected to 4.3 mg/dL. LDH and lactic acid trended down to 1066 mg/dL and 5.6 mg/dL, respectively.

Final pathology from the biopsies of the abdominal mass and lung nodules taken at the community hospital was consistent with leiomyosarcoma with metastases to the lungs. The patient however was deemed a poor surgical candidate for debulking as well as a poor candidate for dialysis. She was additionally unable to be weaned off of vasopressor support. Given the patient's poor prognosis, the patient opted for comfort care. She was placed on hospice and expired subsequently.

3. Discussion

The Cairo-Bishop laboratory criteria of TLS, established in 2004, define laboratory TLS as meeting two of the following: uric acid > 8 mg/dL, potassium > 6.5 mg/dL, phosphorus > 4.5 mg/dL in adults (or a 25% increase from baseline in all), and calcium < 7 mg/dL (or a 25% decrease from baseline) [4]. These criteria were created in the setting of chemotherapy use (three days before chemotherapy or seven days after chemotherapy) as well as adequate hydration and use of a uric acid lowering agent. In addition, clinical TLS was defined as laboratory TLS as mentioned above plus creatinine > 1.5 times the upper limit of normal, oliguria cardiac arrhythmias, neuromuscular irritability, seizures, and sudden death [4].

TLS primarily occurs after initiating chemotherapy in hematologic malignancies. Aggressive non-Hodgkin's lymphoma (such as Burkitt's lymphoma), acute myeloid leukemia, and acute lymphoblastic leukemia have the highest risk of TLS [3, 4]. TLS develops because of rapid cell breakdown with chemotherapy [5]. TLS is rare in solid tumors unless they are large bulky tumors and/or they are highly chemosensitive.

According to a risk-stratification system, for TLS, high-risk group was defined as >5% risk for developing TLS [5]. This group consisted of hematologic malignancies such as Burkitt's lymphoma, diffuse B-celll lymphoma; ALL with WBC > 100,000/microL. Intermediate risk group (risk 1–5% for developing TLS) includes hematologic malignancies such as ALL with WBC < 100,000/microL, early lymphoblastic lymphoma, chronic lymphocytic leukemia, and bulky chemosensitive tumors such as germ cell tumors and small cell lung cancer. Most solid tumors are considered low risk (risk of TLS < 1%). Other malignancies at low risk for TLS include multiple myeloma, chronic myeloid leukemia, and acute myeloid leukemia with WBC < 25,000/microL [5].

Prophylactic uric acid lowering therapy is important in the prevention of TLS in malignancies that have the potential to develop it. Intravenous hydration promotes the excretion of uric acid; additionally, allopurinol blocks the production of uric acid by inhibiting xanthine oxidase. In malignancies with a high risk of developing TLS, aggressive intravenous hydration as well as rasburicase (although controversial for prophylactic use), which converts uric acid to a readily excreted metabolite, should be given prophylactically [5]. For intermediate risk patients, allopurinol should be used. For patients at low risk for TLS, IV hydration should be administered for prevention of TLS; administration of prophylactic uric acid lowering therapy is not recommended [5, 6].

Intravenous hydration and correction of other electrolyte derangements such as hyperkalemia are crucial in the management for TLS. Correction of hyperkalemia can be achieved via kayexalate as well as dialysis [3]. IV calcium should not be administered, however, to patients with hyperphosphatemia, because it promotes calcium phosphate precipitates [5]. A patient who does not respond to these measures may need renal replacement therapy to manage electrolyte abnormalities and renal failure [3, 5]. The mechanism behind renal failure can be attributed to calcium phosphate precipitation as well as to uric acid crystallization that occurs at the level of the renal tubules. Rasburicase is often recommended if there is evidence of renal failure and/or if there is a persistently rising uric acid level (typically if greater than 10 mg/dL). Often, when prognosis is poor, a palliative approach is suggested [7, 8].

Spontaneous tumor lysis syndrome makes up for only 15% of TLS cases and is typically seen in highly aggressive hematologic malignancies [8, 9]. There have been previous case reports of spontaneous TLS in solid tumors such as in lung cancers [10, 11], breast cancers [12, 13], germ cell tumors [14, 15], and prostate cancer [16]. However the prevalence is difficult to determine [16].

Additionally, TLS occurring in vaginal, vulvar, and ovarian cancers has been previously reported [7, 17]. However, those cases were related to the initiation of chemotherapy. Based on review of the literature, this is the only case of uterine leiomyosarcoma, where tumor lysis occurred spontaneously without the patient receiving chemotherapy.

The mechanism of occurrence of spontaneous TLS is hypothesized to be the consequence of necrosis developing in a large tumor as vascular supply is compromised by tumor growth and necrosis of tumor cells progress to tumor lysis from necrotic tumor cell contents being released into circulation [8]. The existing cases in literature including the current case indicate that, in solid tumors, tumor burden, especially with tumors that are highly proliferative and/or have areas of necrosis, may be a risk factor for the development of spontaneous TLS [10]. In the case of the patient mentioned above, it is likely her tumor burden with areas of necrosis that predisposed her to develop spontaneous TLS. This case highlights recognition of tumor lysis syndrome even with ordinary abdominal symptoms in the setting of metabolic derangements.

4. Conclusion

This case illustrates a presentation of spontaneous TLS in a gynecologic solid tumor which has not been previously reported. This case demonstrates that TLS may occur in large solid tumors even without the initiation of chemotherapy. Patients with large tumors should be closely monitored for metabolic derangements that may indicate the development of spontaneous TLS.

Disclosure

An earlier version of this work was presented as an abstract at CHEST 2016 Annual Meeting Abstracts.

References

[1] K. R. Hande and G. C. Garrow, "Acute tumor lysis syndrome in patients with high-grade non-Hodgkin's lymphoma," *The American Journal of Medicine*, vol. 94, no. 2, pp. 133–139, 1993.

[2] M. S. Cairo and M. Bishop, "Tumour lysis syndrome: new therapeutic strategies and classification," *British Journal of Haematology*, vol. 127, no. 1, pp. 3–11, 2004.

[3] S. C. Howard, D. P. Jones, and C.-H. Pui, "The tumor lysis syndrome," *New England Journal of Medicine*, vol. 364, no. 19, pp. 1844–1854, 2011.

[4] M. S. Cairo, B. Coiffier, A. Reiter, and A. Younes, "Recommendations for the evaluation of risk and prophylaxis of tumour lysis syndrome (TLS) in adults and children with malignant diseases: an expert TLS panel consensus," *British Journal of Haematology*, vol. 149, no. 4, pp. 578–586, 2010.

[5] B. Coiffier, A. Altman, C.-H. Pui, A. Younes, and M. S. Cairo, "Guidelines for the management of pediatric and adult tumor lysis syndrome: An evidence-based review," *Journal of Clinical Oncology*, vol. 26, no. 16, pp. 2767–2778, 2008.

[6] X. Gbaguidi, L. Goodrich, F. Roca, P. Suel, and P. Chassagne, "Bulky solid tumors in elderly adults: beware of spontaneous

tumor lysis syndrome," *Journal of the American Geriatrics Society*, vol. 64, no. 1, pp. 235–237, 2016.

[7] A. E. Mirrakhimov, P. Voore, M. Khan, and A. M. Ali, "Tumor lysis syndrome: a clinical review," *World Journal of Critical Care Medicine*, vol. 4, no. 2, pp. 130–138, 2015.

[8] A. Will and E. Tholouli, "The clinical management of tumour lysis syndrome in haematological malignancies," *British Journal of Haematology*, vol. 154, no. 1, pp. 3–13, 2011.

[9] A. E. Mirrakhimov, A. M. Ali, M. Khan, and A. Barbaryan, "Tumor lysis syndrome in solid tumors: an up to date review of the literature," *Rare Tumors*, vol. 6, article 5389, no. 2, 2014.

[10] C. Shenoy, "Acute spontaneous tumor lysis syndrome in a patient with squamous cell carcinoma of the lung," *Quarterly Journal of Medicine*, vol. 102, no. 1, pp. 71–73, 2009.

[11] J. Feld, H. Mehta, and R. L. Burkes, "Acute spontaneous tumor lysis syndrome in adenocarcinoma of the lung: a case report," *American Journal of Clinical Oncology: Cancer Clinical Trials*, vol. 23, no. 5, pp. 491–493, 2000.

[12] A. Elfar, M. Teleb, C. E. Rodriguez-Castro, and Z. Nahleh, "Spontaneous tumor lysis syndrome in breast cancer: a case report and discussion," *journal of Cancer Therapeutics and Research*, vol. 2, no. 1, p. 9, 2013.

[13] N. T. Sklarin and M. Markham, "Spontaneous recurrent tumor lysis syndrome in breast cancer," *American Journal of Clinical Oncology: Cancer Clinical Trials*, vol. 18, no. 1, pp. 71–73, 1995.

[14] G. Pentheroudakis, V. O'Neill, P. Vasey, and S. Kaye, "Spontaneous acute tumour lysis syndrome in patients with metastatic germ cell tumours: Report of two cases," *Supportive Care in Cancer*, vol. 9, no. 7, pp. 554–557, 2001.

[15] V. D'Alessandro, A. Greco, C. Clemente et al., "Severe spontaneous acute tumor lysis syndrome and hypoglycemia in patient with germ cell tumor," *Tumori*, vol. 96, no. 6, pp. 1040–1043, 2010.

[16] C.-J. Lin, R.-K. Hsieh, K.-H. Lim, H.-H. Chen, Y.-C. Cheng, and C.-J. Wu, "Fatal spontaneous tumor lysis syndrome in a patient with metastatic, androgen-independent prostate cancer," *Southern Medical Journal*, vol. 100, no. 9, pp. 916-917, 2007.

[17] Y. Hiraizumi, S. Kamoi, Y. Inde, K. Kurose, Y. Ohaki, and T. Takeshita, "A case of tumor lysis syndrome following chemotherapy for a uterine epithelioid leiomyosarcoma with focal rhabdomyosarcomatous differentiation," *Journal of Obstetrics and Gynaecology Research*, vol. 37, no. 7, pp. 947–952, 2011.

25

Uncommon Occurrences of Air Embolism: Description of Cases and Review of the Literature

Giorgio Berlot, Adriano Rinaldi, Marco Moscheni, Massimo Ferluga, and Perla Rossini

Anesthesia and Intensive Care Department, Cattinara Hospital, Azienda Sanitaria Universitaria Integrata di Trieste, University of Trieste, Strada di Fiume 447, 34149 Trieste, Italy

Correspondence should be addressed to Giorgio Berlot; berlot@inwind.it

Academic Editor: Zsolt Molnár

Many different risk factors have been associated with the occurrence of gas embolism making this potentially lethal complication easily avoidable. However, this condition can occur in circumstances not commonly reported. Three different and extremely uncommon cases of gas embolism are presented and discussed: the first was caused by the voluntary ingestion of hydrogen peroxide, the second occurred during a retrograde cholangiopancreatography, and the last followed the intrapleural injection of Urokinase. Whereas in the first patient the gas embolism was associated with only relatively mild digestive symptoms, in the remaining two it caused a massive cerebral ischemia and an extended myocardial infarction, respectively. Despite a hyperbaric oxygen therapy performed timely in each case, only the first patient survived. The classical risk factors associated with gas embolism like indwelling central venous catheters, diving accidents, etc. are rather well known and thus somewhat preventable; however, a number of less common and difficult-to-recognize causes can determine this condition, making the correct diagnosis elusive and delaying the hyperbaric oxygen therapy, whose window of opportunity is rather narrow. Thus, a gas embolism should be suspected in the presence of not otherwise explainable sudden neurologic and/or cardiovascular symptoms also in circumstances not typically considered at risk.

1. Introduction

The term gas embolism (GE) indicates an array of clinical conditions determined by the entry of gases like air, oxygen (O_2), carbon dioxide (CO_2), or nitrogen (N), and so on, into the bloodstream driven by the pressure gradient existing between the atmosphere and the venous system [1]. The severity of the clinical picture basically depends on some gas-related factors, including the body's position, the blood solubility, the patient's overall health, the volume, and the rate of accumulation [2, 3]; indeed, even small amounts can determine severe clinical consequences if located in critical locations: in humans, the injection of as few as 1 to 2 ml of air in the arterial circulation has been associated with neurologic damage and extremely severe consequences, even cardiac arrest, have been described after the injection of 2 ml only of air into the cerebral circulation [4–8]. In the past few decades, a better knowledge of the pathophysiology of GE determined an increased awareness of the underlying risk factors and clinical manifestations and prompted the publication of a number of clinical and experimental studies [7, 9–13].

Here we report and discuss three cases of GE determined by unusual causes, including the voluntary ingestion of hydrogen peroxide (HP), an endoscopic procedure, and the Urokinase instillation adjunctive to the chest tube drainage in a case of pleural empyema.

2. Cases Report

2.1. Case Number 1. A 60-year-old woman was transferred from another hospital after the voluntary ingestion of 400 ml of 5% hydrogen peroxide (HP). At the admission, she was awake and complained of mild diffuse abdominal pain; on examination, the abdomen appeared slightly distended and the bowel sounds were increased. Once in our ICU, the HBOT started 7 hours after the ingestion and was performed according to the US Navy Table 6 (Figure 1). A pre-HBOT abdominal CT scan demonstrated multiple gas

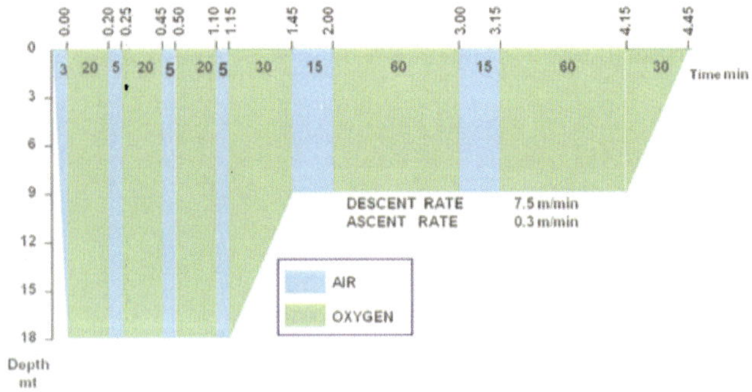

Figure 1: US Navy decompression Table 6.

bubbles distributed in the peripheral branches of the portal system and in the lumen of the upper mesenteric, ileocolic, and colic veins (Figure 2(a)), which appeared reduced after the treatment (Figure 2(b)). On the following day, a TEE demonstrated a PFO. Three days later she was discharged home free of symptoms.

2.2. Case Number 2. A 62-year-old woman underwent an endoscopic retrograde cholangiography (ERCP) using air to dilate the duodenum in another hospital. During the procedure, performed under light iv. sedation, the patient suddenly presented seizures, spontaneous decerebrate posture, bilateral mydriasis, associated with atrial fibrillation, and arterial desaturation; at this point she was tracheally intubated and mechanically ventilated. A CT scan of the head demonstrated many small gas bubbles within the subarachnoid spaces, the intrasellar space, and the basal nuclei (Figures 3(a) and 3(b)). The patient was taken immediately to our HBOT facility; the treatment started 4 hours and 45 minutes after the onset of symptoms and followed the US Navy Table 6 (Figure 1). A CT scan obtained immediately thereafter showed the reduction of the subarachnoid air and a single right frontal bubble; there was an effacement of the right hemispheric sulci and a 4 mm-left bound deviation of the midline (Figure 3(c)). Mannitol and hypertonic saline were given to decrease the intracranial pressure (ICP) and the sedation was maintained with iv. Thiopentone. On the next morning, at the CT scan of the brain the midline shift was increased up to 11 mm and the basal cisternae were not visible (Figure 3(d)). At the suspension of the sedation, the patient presented right myoclonus, bilateral left deviation of the eyes and left hyperextension at the painful stimulation. A wide right craniotomy was then performed to reduce the ICP but the brain herniated through the cranial breach (Figure 3(e)). The patient returned to the initial hospital three days later and died in vegetative state seven months after the described episode.

2.3. Case Number 3. A 72-year-old male patient underwent a left thoracostomy for the positioning of a chest tube to treat an empyema complicating a mesothelioma. On the day after, Urokinase was injected through the chest tube, which was clamped immediately thereafter. Approximately 10 minutes later, the patient suddenly became unconscious and cyanotic. At the arrival of the medical emergency team, the patient was comatose, anisocoric, bradycardic, and hypotensive. The patient was intubated and mechanically ventilated at FIO_2 100%; at the same time, fluids, dobutamine, and norepinephrine were started. The CT scan of the chest and of the brain demonstrated a massive GE with evidence of multiple air bubbles inside the thoracic aorta, the left cardiac ventricle, the coronary arteries, and the cortical vessels (Figure 4). The HBOT started three hours after the onset of symptoms and followed the US Navy Table 6 (Figure 1). During the treatment the patient underwent repeated episodes of ventricular tachycardia and fibrillation treated according to the BLS guidelines and for this reason it has not been possible to follow the US Navy Table 6A, which was our first choice; thirty minutes before the end of the procedure an asystole appeared and the CPR was stopped 20 minutes after its occurrence. The autopsy failed to demonstrate any laceration of the lung, whose surface presented multiple wide hemorrhagic areas; the cause of the cardiogenic shock was ascribed to a hyper acute extensive myocardial infarction; a wide ischemic area was present also in the right frontal lobe (Figure 5).

3. Discussion

Several different pathologic and nonpathologic conditions have been associated with the occurrence of GE, including thoracic penetrating injuries, mechanical ventilation with elevated pressures of insufflations, surgical procedures performed in the sitting position, endoscopic maneuvers, air aspiration from central venous catheters (CVC), or their subcutaneous tracks, sexual intercourses, diving accidents, etc. [14]. Whatever the cause, after the penetration in the venous system the gas bubbles can travel along different routes (Figure 6): first, they can join the venae cavae and move upward into the internal jugular vein (IJV) due to both its continuity with the upper vena cava and its shorter length; GE in this location impede the cerebral venous drainage. Second, they can reach the lung circulation and obstruct the right ventricular outflow. Finally, they can migrate towards the systemic circulation via physiologic intrapulmonary shunts, the pulmonary capillaries, or a patent foramen ovale (PFO). Once in the aorta, the GE can move and plug the microvascular network everywhere, determining a multisystem disorder whose features are primarily related to either the ischemia or the subsequent inflammatory reaction of the involved organs [15]. Then, it appears that the GE-related symptoms vary according to their location, those determined by arterial GE (AGE) being more severe and sudden than those caused by venous GE (VGE), provided that the latter do not exert cardiovascular or neurologic effects.

The incidence of GE in different studies ranges from 1 in 772 to 2,65 per 100.000 hospitalizations [1]; this extremely wide difference is probably due to the lack of specificity of symptoms and/or the diagnostic tools used. Actually, as more and more invasive diagnostic and therapeutic procedures requiring the cannulation of large veins and/or the insufflation of gas inside the body cavities are performed, it is hypothesizable that an elevated number of GE do not cause

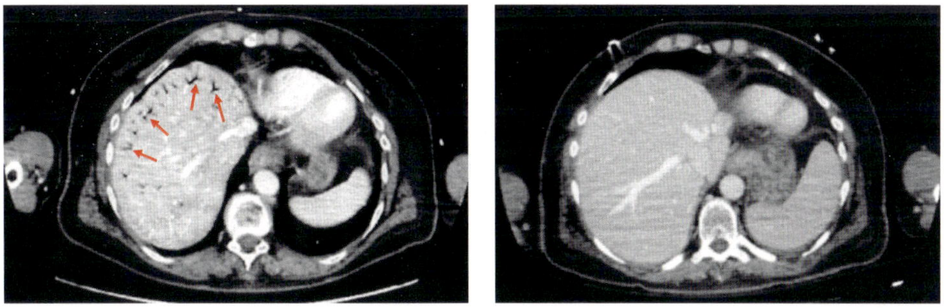

(a) (b)

FIGURE 2: Abdominal CT scan: (a) GE in the peripheral branch of the portal system after HP ingestion; (b) reduction of the GE after HBOT.

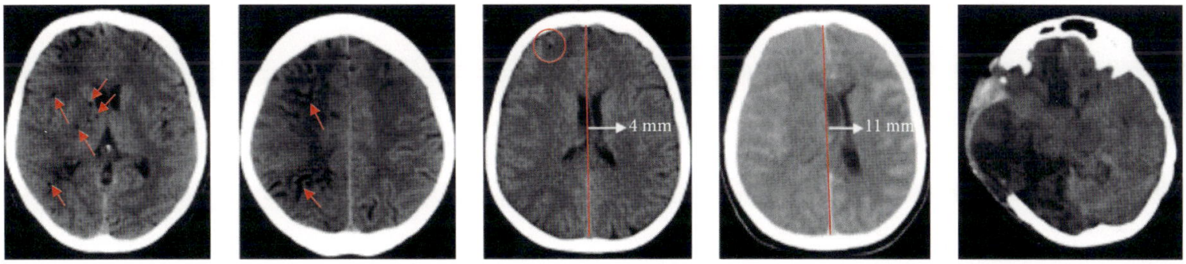

(a) (b) (c) (d) (e)

FIGURE 3: Head CT scan: (a) before HBOT: gas bubbles in the basal nuclei and (b) within the subarachnoid spaces (arrows); (c) immediately after HBOT: single right frontal bubble (circle) and 4 mm: leftward deviation of the midline (arrow); (d) 14 hours after HBOT 4 mm: leftward deviation of the midline; (e) 5 days after right decompressive craniectomy: massive brain herniation with right hemispheric and left frontal ischemia.

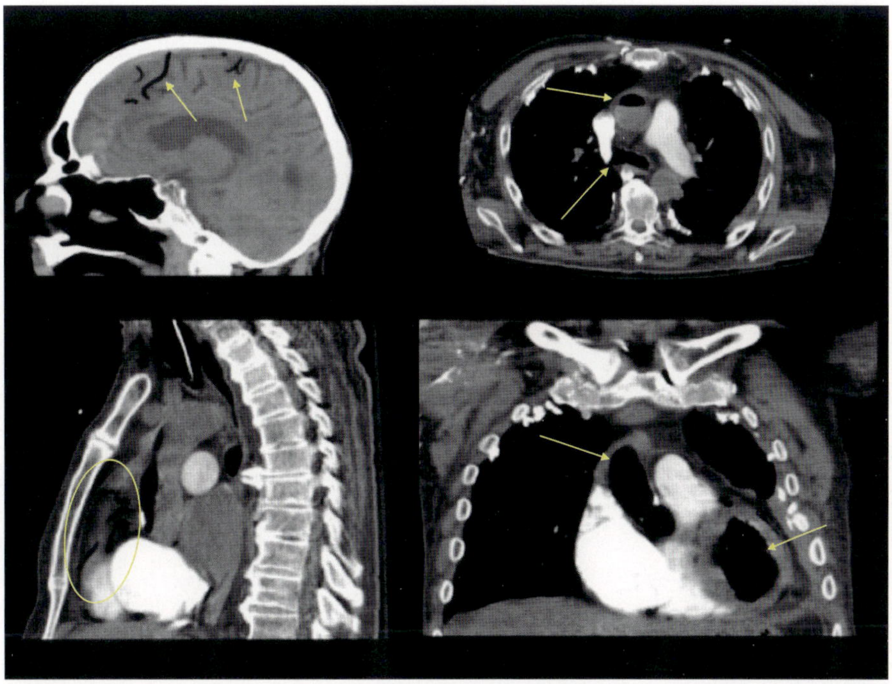

FIGURE 4: (a): Air within the cortical vessels (arrows); (b) air within the ascending and thoracic descending aorta (arrows); (c) air within the coronary arteries (circle); (d) air within the aortic arch and the left ventricle.

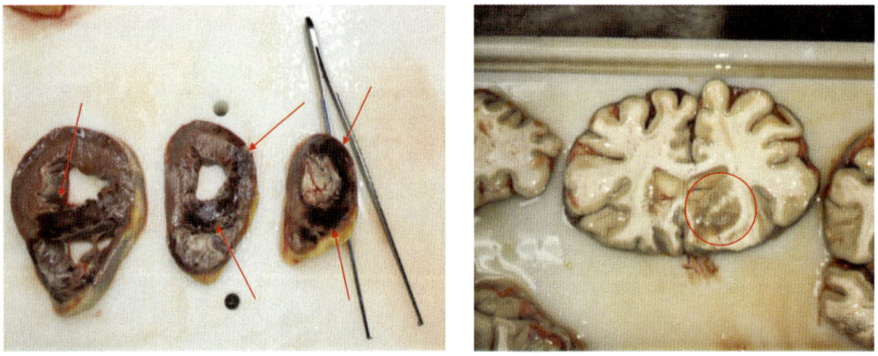

(a) (b)

Figure 5: (a) Acute myocardial infarction involving extensively the right ventricle and the septum; (b) acute cerebral infarction downstream the arteries obstructed by the GE.

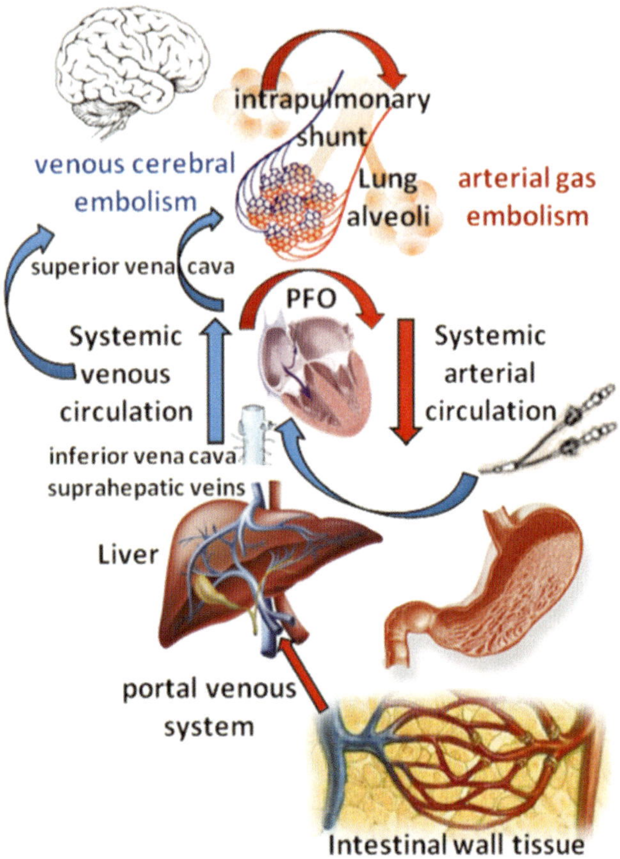

Figure 6: Routes of dissemination of GE.

symptoms or go unnoticed [1]. Hence, the diagnosis of GE is based primarily on the clinical suspicion, on presence of risk factors, and on the use of monitoring techniques that are able to detect air bubbles floating into the bloodstream, including the precordial Doppler ultrasound probe and the transesophageal echocardiography (TEE); the final diagnosis and the severity of the involvement of the target organs are established with the CT scan [1, 2].

The treatment of serious forms of GE warrants an aggressive approach, consisting in (a) the endotracheal intubation and mechanical ventilation with 100% O_2; (b) the positioning of the patient in the Trendelenburg and left lateral decubitus to reduce the amount of GE floating to the brain and facilitate the egress of air from the right ventricle; (c) the aspiration of bubble from the right ventricle via a CVC; and (d), most importantly, the Hyperbaric Oxygen Therapy (HBOT), to be performed on an emergency basis to reduce the volume of the GE. Its rationale is based on sound chemicophysical principles, including the reduction of the volume of the bubbles (Boyle's law) and the increased solubility of the culprit gas (Henry's law) leading to a better oxygenation of the ischemic tissues; moreover, HBOT has been associated with the reduction of the inflammatory reaction in the ischemic areas by limiting the activation and the adhesion of the leukocytes upon the endothelium [16–18]. The window of opportunity of HBOT is relatively narrow, as demonstrated by Blanc [19] who reported a better outcome in patients with cerebral GE treated < 6 hours after the event as compared with those treated after this interval; however, patients with GE can gain advantage from a HBOT even after a significant delay [20–22]. Even if quite often the source of GE is immediately clear or easily detectable, there are many variables, including the rarity of reported cases, the presence of confounding factors, and the failed recognition of triggering events which can make the diagnosis extremely elusive and delay if not impede the appropriate treatment.

In ICU patients, the diagnosis of GE can be relatively straightforward as a limited number of causes can prompt its occurrence; conversely, far more difficulties are present in non-ICU patients due to uncommon triggering events like those exposed above.

This is well represented by the first patient, who ingested a consistent amount of HP. This substance, which has multiple uses including antisepsis, is hydrolyzed by the enzyme catalase via the reaction: $2H_2O_2 \longrightarrow 2\ H_2O + O_2 + \text{heat}$; the amount of released O_2 is related to both the amount and the concentration of HP: as an example, one milliliter of 6% HP releases approximately 10 mL of O_2 [23]. The ingestion of HP can exert deleterious effects via different mechanisms, including (a) the direct cytotoxic action on the gastric mucosa possibly leading to erosions and perforations; (b) the increase of the intragastric volume and pressure determined by the high amounts of O_2 derived by its hydrolysis; and (c) the absorption of O_2 bubbles through the gastroduodenal wall and its passage into the portal system where it can determine portal hypertension; moreover, the gas bubbles can migrate from the liver sinusoids or preexisting portocaval shunts into the inferior vena thus reducing the venous return [24, 25]. Our patient did not present these major complications despite the relevant volume of highly concentrated HP ingested, making the choice of treatment uncertain. Actually, the role of HBOT in asymptomatic patients is not clear, as some patients treated conservatively were discharged without consequences [23, 26], probably due to a more rapid scavenging of O_2 bubbles as compared with those containing N only as it occurs in diving accidents [23]; thus, the HBOT was performed more to prevent a systemic embolization (a PFO which was demonstrated in the following days) than to reduce the volume of gas bubbles located in the portal circulation, which often dissolve spontaneously [27]. An immediate treatment is not warranted in case of a VGA confined to the portal system; actually, the patient improved and her abdominal symptoms resolved completely even if the HBOT was initiated after as long as 7 hours from the ingestion of HP.

The second patient suffered from the most uncommon complication of ERCP, consisting in the penetration of gas into the portal vein [28]. Different risk factors have been identified, including preexisting conditions, such as inflammation, previous surgeries, or a stone-induced decubitus of the biliary tract, and procedure-related factors, such as the irritation caused by the contrast medium, the sphincterotomy, the placement of a metal stent, and elevated volumes of air insufflated at pressure to distend the gastroduodenal tract [29, 30]. In our patient, this latter mechanism likely determined the intramural dissection of small veins and the subsequent passage of air bubbles into the suprahepatic veins through the hepatic sinusoids or via preexisting shunts between the portal and inferior cava vein [31]. The severe neurologic symptoms and their abrupt onset must be ascribed either to the concurrent presence of a retrograde VGE in the right IJV, and/or to air bubbles escaping into the systemic circulation through a intrapulmonary shunt or the transcapillary route that determined a massive ischemic injury in the territory of the right middle cerebral artery [30, 32, 33]. The diagnosis of cerebral GE was particularly difficult due to a number of circumstances, including the sedation, the lack of preliminary symptoms, and, most importantly, the extremely uncommon occurrence of this complication [29, 34, 35]. Despite the aggressive and multimodal treatment of this patient, which included also a decompressive craniotomy besides HBOT, the ischemic damage was so relevant that the neurologic conditions failed to improve in the following months.

The third case is somewhat puzzling, as the patient died in refractory cardiogenic shock likely due to the intracoronary AGE in the absence of any port of entry for air discovered at the autopsy. Actually, other authors have described the occurrence of GE in patients undergoing one or even repeated pleural lavages with fibrinolytic agents, sometimes after several days from the positioning of the chest tube. In our patient, we hypothesized that the injected Urokinase lysed one or more clots on the surface of the hemorrhagic areas demonstrated at the autopsy thus permitting the gas contained into the empyema to penetrate the pulmonary vessels and to cause a GE involving multiple vascular beds.

In all our patients the HBOT was performed according US Navy Table 6 which is currently used to treat patients involved in diving accident.

When discussing GE the key question is if it could have been somewhat prevented or recognized in an early phase as the treatment is time-dependent and the HBOT facilities can be difficult to reach due to technical factors, including weather or altitude limitations for helicopters and traffic jam for surface transportation. In the described cases, the prevention of GE clearly was not feasible in case number 1 but it could have been avoided using CO_2 to inflate the duodenum in the second case. In patient number 3, this issue is difficult to establish, as other cases have been described in patients undergoing lung or pleural biopsies under thoracoscopy [36, 37]. In these circumstances, a high index of suspicion is warranted to detect as soon as possible neurologic and/or cardiovascular abnormalities possibly caused by a GE and to shorten the treatment-free interval.

4. Conclusions

Gas embolism can occur in circumstances other than those classically considered at risk thus making the diagnosis elusive. Any sudden change in mental status and/or hemodynamic alterations not otherwise explainable should raise the suspicion of GE during even minimally invasive procedures that can create a communication between air or other gases and the vascular system. If the suspicion of AGE is confirmed and there are no contraindications—like untreated pneumothorax—it is of primary importance to start the HBOT, which is a very safe medical procedure if it is done properly, as soon as possible in order to improve the correction of ischemia and the outcome of the patient.

You should also consider the possibility of HBOT treatments once a day for 90 minutes with a FiO_2 100% at 2 ATA if there are sequels after the main treatment.

Authors' Contributions

Each author was involved in the treatment of the described case and contributed to the preparation of the manuscript.

References

[1] C. McCarthy, S. Behravesh, S. Naidu, and R. Oklu, "Air Embolism: Practical Tips for Prevention and Treatment," *Journal of Clinical Medicine*, vol. 5, no. 11, p. 93, 2016.

[2] M. A. Mirski, A. V. Lele, L. Fitzsimmons, and T. J. K. Toung, "Diagnosis and treatment of vascular air embolism," *Anesthesiology*, vol. 106, no. 1, pp. 164–177, 2007.

[3] S. Gordy and S. Rowell, "Vascular air embolism," *International Journal of Critical Illness & Injury Science*, vol. 3, no. 1, pp. 73–76, 2013.

[4] B. Goldfarb and H. T. Bahnson, "Early and late effects on the heart of small amounts of air in the coronary circulation," *The Journal of Thoracic and Cardiovascular Surgery*, vol. 46, pp. 368–378, 1963.

[5] L. Michel, D. C. Poskanzer, K. A. McKusick, G. L. Nardi, and R. A. Malt, "Fatal Paradoxical Air Embolism to the Brain: Complication of Central Venous Catherization," *Journal of Parenteral and Enteral Nutrition*, vol. 6, no. 1, pp. 68–70, 1982.

[6] P. Halpern, A. Greenstein, Y. Melamed, U. Taitelman, I. Sznajder, and F. Zveibil, "Arterial air embolism after penetrating lung injury," *Critical Care Medicine*, vol. 11, no. 5, pp. 392-393, 1983.

[7] A. N. Thomas and B. G. Stephens, "Air embolism: A cause of morbidity and death after penetrating chest trauma," *Journal of Trauma - Injury Infection and Critical Care*, vol. 14, no. 8, pp. 633–638, 1974.

[8] A. Nozari, E. Dilekoz, I. Sukhotinsky et al., "Microemboli may link spreading depression, migraine aura, and patent foramen ovale," *Annals of Neurology*, vol. 67, no. 2, pp. 221–229, 2010.

[9] W. J. Waldo, N. N. Harlaftis, and P. N. Symbas, "Systemic air embolism: Does it occur after experimental penetrating lung injury?" *The Journal of Thoracic and Cardiovascular Surgery*, vol. 71, pp. 96–101, 1976.

[10] J. M. Graham, A. C. Beall Jr., K. L. Mattox, and G. D. Vaughan, "Systemic air embolism following penetrating trauma to the lung," *CHEST*, vol. 72, no. 4, pp. 449–454, 1977.

[11] G. H. Meier, W. J. Wood, and P. N. Symbas, "Systemic air embolism from penetrating lung injury," *The Annals of Thoracic Surgery*, vol. 27, pp. 161–168, 1979.

[12] R. B. Ponn, "Systemic air embolism in experimental penetrating lung injury," *The Journal of Thoracic and Cardiovascular Surgery*, vol. 74, pp. 296–298, 1976.

[13] W. H. Van Mason, E. G. Damon, A. R. Dickinson, and T. O. Nevison, "Arterial Gas Emboli After Blast Injury," *Proceedings of the Society for Experimental Biology and Medicine*, vol. 136, no. 4, pp. 1253–1255, 1971.

[14] D. Mathieu, S. Tissier, and M. Boulo, "Gas embolism," in *Handbook on Hyperbaric Medicine*, pp. 221–225, Springer, Berlin, Germany, 2006.

[15] M. Barak and Y. Katz, "Microbubbles: pathophysiology and clinical implications," *CHEST*, vol. 128, no. 4, pp. 2918–2932, 2005.

[16] C. E. Hammarlund, "The physiologic effects of hyperbaric oxygenation," in *Hyperbaric medicine practice*, pp. 41–43, Best Publishing, Flagstaff, AZ, 3rd edition, 2008.

[17] G. Oriani, A. Marroni, and F. Wattel, *Handbook on Hyperbaric Medicine*, Springer Milan, Milano, 1996.

[18] S. Van Poucke, P. Jorens, and L. Beaucourt, "Phisiologic effects of hyperbaric oxygen om ischemia-reperfusion phenomenon," in *Handbook on Hyperbaric Medicine*, vol. 126, pp. 18–22, Springer, 2006.

[19] P. Blanc, A. Boussuges, K. Henriette, J. Sainty, and M. Deleflie, "Iatrogenic cerebral air embolism: importance of an early hyperbaric oxygenation," *Intensive Care Medicine*, vol. 28, no. 5, pp. 559–563, 2002.

[20] C. G. Wherrett, R. J. Mehran, and M.-A. Beaulieu, "Cerebral arterial gas embolism following diagnostic bronchoscopy: Delayed treatment with hyperbaric oxygen," *Canadian Journal of Anesthesia*, vol. 49, no. 1, pp. 96–99, 2002.

[21] E. M. Dunbar, R. Fox, B. Watson, and P. Akrill, "Successful late treatment of venous air embolism with hyperbaric oxygen," *Postgraduate Medical Journal*, vol. 66, no. 776, pp. 469-470, 1990.

[22] J. T. Mader and W. H. Hulet, "Delayed Hyperbaric Treatment of Cerebral Air Embolism: Report of a Case," *JAMA Neurology*, vol. 36, no. 8, pp. 504-505, 1979.

[23] L. K. French, B. Z. Horowitz, and N. J. McKeown, "Hydrogen peroxide ingestion associated with portal venousgas and treatment with hyperbaric oxygen: A case seriesand review of the literature," *Clinical Toxicology*, vol. 48, no. 6, pp. 533–538, 2010.

[24] J. M. Moon, B. J. Chun, and Y. I. Min, "Hemorrhagic gastritis and gas emboli after ingesting 3% hydrogen peroxide," *The Journal of Emergency Medicine*, vol. 30, no. 4, pp. 403–406, 2006.

[25] B. E. Watt, A. T. Proudfoot, and J. A. Vale, "Hydrogen peroxide poisoning," *Toxicological Reviews*, vol. 23, no. 1, pp. 51–57, 2004.

[26] T. A. Luu, M. T. Kelley, J. A. Strauch, and K. Avradopoulos, "Portal vein gas embolism from hydrogen peroxide ingestion," *Annals of Emergency Medicine*, vol. 21, no. 11, pp. 1391–1393, 1992.

[27] S. M. Hendriksen, N. L. Menth, B. C. Westgard et al., "Hyperbaric oxygen therapy for the prevention of arterial gas embolism in food grade hydrogen peroxide ingestion," *The American Journal of Emergency Medicine*, vol. 35, no. 5, pp. 809–809.e8, 2017.

[28] V. Chandrasekhara, M. A. Khashab, V. R. Muthusamy et al., "Adverse events associated with ERCP," *Gastrointestinal Endoscopy*, vol. 85, no. 1, pp. 32–47, 2017.

[29] S. Donepudi, D. Chavalitdhamrong, L. Pu, and P. V. Draganov, "Air embolism complicating gastrointestinal endoscopy: a systematic review," *World Journal of Gastrointestinal Endoscopy*, vol. 5, no. 8, pp. 359–365, 2013.

[30] M. Bisceglia, A. Simeone, R. Forlano, A. Andriulli, and A. Pilotto, "Fatal systemic venous air embolism during endoscopic retrograde cholangiopancreatography," *Advances in Anatomic Pathology*, vol. 16, no. 4, pp. 255–262, 2009.

[31] C. Nern, D. Bellut, N. Husain, A. Pangalu, U. Schwarz, and A. Valavanis, "Fatal Cerebral Venous Air Embolism during Endoscopic Retrograde Cholangiopancreatography - Case Report and Review of the Literature," *Clinical Neuroradiology*, vol. 22, no. 4, pp. 371–374, 2012.

[32] J. G. Heckmann, C. J. G. Lang, K. Kindler, W. Huk, F. J. Erbguth, and B. Neundörfer, "Neurologic manifestations of cerebral air embolism as a complication of central venous catheterization," *Critical Care Medicine*, vol. 28, no. 5, pp. 1621–1625, 2000.

[33] B. P. Murphy, F. J. Harford, and F. S. Cramer, "Cerebral air embolism resulting from invasive medical procedures. Treatment with hyberbaric oxygen," *Annals of Surgery*, vol. 201, no. 2, pp. 242–245, 1985.

[34] B. Wills-Sanin, Y. R. Cárdenas, L. Polanco, O. Rivero, S. Suarez, and A. F. Buitrago, "Air Embolism after Endoscopic Retrograde Cholangiopancreatography in a Patient with Budd Chiari Syndrome," *Case Reports in Critical Care*, vol. 2014, pp. 1–4, 2014.

[35] J. Fernandez-Fernandez, H. Real-Noval, and E. Rodriguez-Rodriguez, "Massive cerebral air embolism following endoscopic retrograde cholangiopancreatography. A case report and review of the literature," *Revue Neurologique*, vol. 63, no. 11, pp. 497–500, 2016.

[36] M. Menéndez-González, P. Oliva-Nacarino, and A. Álvarez-Cofiño, "Cerebral gas embolism caused by pleural fibrinolytic treatment," *Stroke*, vol. 38, no. 9, pp. 2602–2604, 2007.

[37] J. M. Galvis, D. R. Nunley, T. Zheyi, and L. A. V. Dinglasan, "Left ventricle and systemic air embolism after percutaneous lung biopsy," *Respiratory Medicine Case Reports*, vol. 22, pp. 206–208, 2017.

Central Venous Line Insertion Revealing Partial Anomalous Pulmonary Venous Return: Diagnosis and Management

Bashar Alzghoul,[1] Ayoub Innabi,[1] Aditya Chada,[2] Ahmad R. Tarawneh,[2] Krishna Kakkera,[2] and Khaled Khasawneh[2]

[1]*Department of Internal Medicine, University of Arkansas for Medical Sciences, Little Rock, AR, USA*
[2]*Division of Pulmonary and Critical Care Medicine, University of Arkansas for Medical Sciences, Little Rock, AR, USA*

Correspondence should be addressed to Bashar Alzghoul; bnalzghoul@uams.edu

Academic Editor: Gil Klinger

Central venous line malposition is a well-known complication of line insertion. Rarely, it can be mal-positioned in an anomalous pulmonary vein. We present an unusual case of a 56-year-old woman that was found to have partial anomalous pulmonary venous return on central venous line insertion. In this report, we describe a systematic approach to diagnosis and management of this unusual situation.

1. Introduction

Partial anomalous pulmonary venous return (PAPVR) is a rare congenital anomaly that occurs during embryologic development when at least one pulmonary vein fails to communicate with the left atrium; instead, it drains directly or indirectly in the right atrium. It remains asymptomatic most of the time and is discovered incidentally or postmortem [1]. There have been few reports in literature of PAPVR discovered after central venous line (CVL) insertion. We report a 56-year-old woman that was found to have left upper PAPVR on CVL insertion. In addition, we conducted literature review of similar cases reported before and suggested a systematic approach to diagnosis and management.

2. Case Presentation

A 56-year-old woman with a medical history of multiple sclerosis, quadriplegia, sacral decubitus ulcer, chronic osteomyelitis, chronic deep vein thrombosis (DVT), chronic steroids use, and chronic Foley catheter use presented to the emergency department with severe sepsis due to multiple potential sources including urinary tract infection, soft tissue infection, or osteomyelitis. Vital signs were significant for blood pressure of 85/59 mmHg, heart rate of 63 beats per minute, respiratory rate of 33 breaths per minute, and oxygen saturation of 83% on room air. At the beginning, patient declined intubation so she was placed on 100% oxygen via nonrebreather mask. Arterial blood gas (ABG) on 100% oxygen was 7.29/49/55. Initial chest X-ray (CXR) showed small bilateral pleural effusions with suspected left lower lobe infiltrate. Despite intravenous (IV) fluid resuscitation, broad spectrum IV antibiotics, and stress dose steroids, patient became more hypotensive and IV norepinephrine was started through a right femoral CVL that was placed in the emergency department. Patient was started on heparin drip for suspected pulmonary embolism that was stopped later due to large bleeding from femoral line site and consideration of pneumonia as the cause of hypoxemia. Patient agreed later to be intubated and decision was made to remove femoral line and place a 7.0 Fr triple-lumen CVL through the left internal jugular vein (IJ) over a guidewire and under full ultrasound (U/S) guidance, which was placed easily with no complications. A CXR was obtained to confirm placement which showed that the catheter tip did not cross the midline; instead, it was extending towards the left of the aortic arch probably into an anomalous vein as read by the radiologists (Figure 1). Ultrasound examination of the neck showed

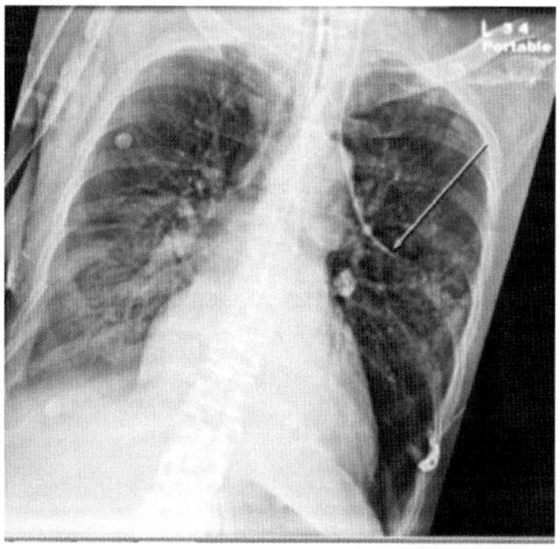

FIGURE 1: Single frontal view CXR showing the tip of the left IJ CVL extending left of the aortic arch towards the left lung field.

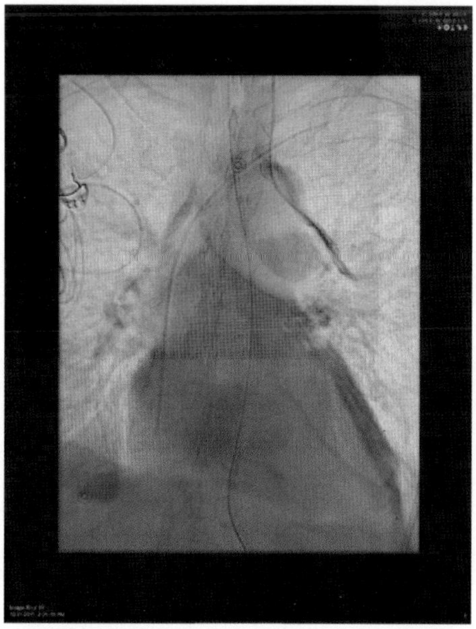

FIGURE 2: Fluoroscopy study showing left IJ CVL extending through the anomalous pulmonary vein.

proper catheter placement in the left IJ. A pressure transducer was connected which showed a venous wave form with a pressure of 10 mmHg. ABG obtained from the catheter on continuous mechanical ventilation (FiO_2 = 50%, positive end expiratory pressure = 5 CM H_2O) showed PaO_2 of 102 mmHg compared to 79 mmHg from radial arterial site. A transthoracic echocardiography, which was done to evaluate cardiac function, did not show evidence of atrial septal defect or any other cardiac malformation. Fluoroscopy study was used to place a left peripherally inserted central catheter (PICC) and to confirm the location of the left IJ CVL which demonstrated contrast injection in an anomalous pulmonary vein (Figure 2). We concluded that the patient has partial anomalous pulmonary venous return (PAPVR) and the left IJ CVL was removed. The PICC line was used instead for central access.

3. Discussion

Central venous lines (CVLs) insertion is a very common procedure that is performed by practitioners of different specialties for varied indications. Among these indications are drug administration, parenteral nutrition, renal replacement therapy, cardiac catheterization, and trans-venous pacing of the heart [2]. Malposition of CVL insertion is relatively common due to operator and technical factors in part. However, it can be due to congenital and acquired abnormalities of the venous system that leads to abnormal positioning of the line. In some cases, CVL malposition can lead to catastrophic complications [3, 4]. Thus, it is critically important for practitioners to identify malposition of CVLs and take evidence based appropriate actions depending on the situation.

CXR is routinely used to confirm the location of the CVL, which ideally should be at the junction between the

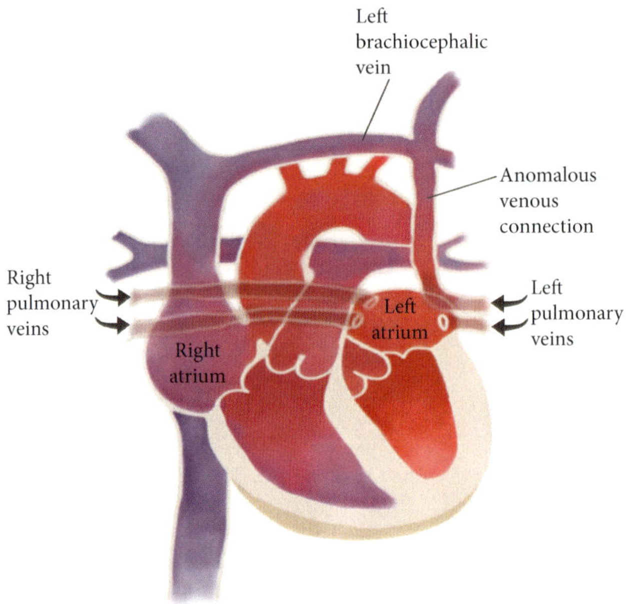

FIGURE 3: Schematic illustration of the anatomy of the CVL inserted accidentally in an anomalous pulmonary vein connected to the right atrium via the brachiocephalic vein.

superior vena cava (SVC) and the right atrium. There are multiple radiographic landmarks that can be utilized on CXR to confirm that the CVL is in the right location [5]. In our case, we encountered an unusual location of the CVL on the CXR where the catheter tip did not cross the midline; instead, it was extending laterally towards the left lung field, left of the aortic arch. The CVL was clearly mal-positioned, but the question that we had was where exactly was the line inserted: Was it inserted in the carotid artery? Does the patient have a persistent left SVC?

We decided to follow a systematic approach that showed the CVL was inserted in an anomalous pulmonary vein. This finding might be encountered by other practitioners in critical situations where someone needs to make fast decisions, so it is important to be familiar with the anatomy.

The pulmonary veins originally arise from a common pulmonary vein that buds from the left atrium during the embryologic development. It then joins the splanchnic venous plexus in the lung buds. If any or all of the pulmonary veins fail to connect to the left atrium, it will eventually divert the blood directly or indirectly to the right atrium [1, 6]. Figure 3 shows a schematic view of left upper partial anomalous pulmonary venous return (PAPVR). On cadaveric studies, PAPVR was reported in up to 0.7% of the cases [1]. It was first described by Winslow in 1739 [7, 8]. There are scarce cases in literature of accidental diagnosis of PAPVR in adults after CVL insertion. We did a literature review using PubMed and Google scholar search engines using the key words (Central Venous) and (partial anomalous). We included cases of adult patients who were diagnosed to have PAPVR after CVL insertion and ended up with 10 cases. As illustrated in Table 1, we managed to summarize the approach that was followed in these cases. We tried in this article to highlight the diagnostic and management approach followed in other reported cases and suggest a systematic approach to follow when encountering similar situation.

First we used the U/S to examine the course of the CVL in the neck to confirm whether the CVL was inserted in the IJ vein or in the carotid artery. Of note, U/S examination of the chest can be used sometimes to localize the tip of CVL; however, it needs an experienced operator and may not detect the final intrathoracic placement of the CVL all the time [9]. Second, we connected the CVL to a pressure transducer which showed a venous wave form. Among the cases reported in literature, Wylam and Schmidt [6] were the only to describe pulsating arterial wave form. They attributed that to wedging of the tip of the catheter in a pulmonary venous branch, which would subsequently reflect the pressure tracing from that of the upstream pulmonary artery. However, in their case, the patient had moderate pulmonary hypertension diagnosed by heart catheterization. Third, we obtained ABG from the CVL and from arterial site. In our case, the PaO2 was paradoxically higher from the CVL compared to arterial sample. This paradoxical finding was reported in four of the 10 cases [6, 10–12]. In addition, PO_2 was reported to be high in four other cases, but no arterial sample was obtained to compare [13–16]. The high PO_2 can be explained by the fact that the catheter tip is collecting blood directly from the pulmonary venous blood flow before intermixing with systemic venous blood [15]. The fourth step would be to confirm placement via definitive radiologic method. In our case, since we decided to substitute the CVL with a PICC, we used fluoroscopy studies to define the anatomy. From this, it might be unnecessary to use CT/CTA only to establish the diagnosis of CVL insertion in an aberrant pulmonary vein unless it was indicated for some other reason.

Table 1: Summary of the approach followed in 10 cases reported in literature of adult patients found to have PAPVR on CVL insertion.

Article	Year	Side	Indication	Pulmonary systemic connection site	Paradoxical paO_2	Wave form	Fluoroscopy	CTA/CT chest	U/S confirmation	Pulmonary HTN	Management
Wylam and Schmidt [6]	1990	Left IJ	Sepsis	Left upper pulmonary vein to left brachiocephalic	√	Pulsatile	√	No	n/a	√	Repositioned
Cheng et al. [10]	2002	Left IJ	Sepsis	Left upper pulmonary vein to left brachiocephalic	√	Venous	√	No	√	n/a	Removed
Townley [13]	2003	Left IJ	Venous access	Left lung	High PO_2 but no arterial sample to compare	Venous	No	No	n/a	n/a	Removed
Chintu et al. [18]	2008	Left IJ	Hemodialysis	Left upper pulmonary vein to left brachiocephalic	n/a	n/a	√	No	n/a	n/a	Removed
Javangula et al. [14]	2010	Left IJ	Sepsis	Left upper pulmonary vein to left brachiocephalic	High PO_2 but no arterial sample to compare	Venous	√	CTA	√	No	Repositioned
Habito and Kalva [17]	2011	Left IJ	Chemotherapy	Right upper pulmonary vein to SVC	n/a	n/a	√	CTA	n/a	n/a	Repositioned
Brandt and Artmeier-Brandt [15]	2015	Left subclavian	Venous access in the setting of trauma	Left upper pulmonary vein to left brachiocephalic vein	High PO_2 but no arterial sample to compare	Venous	No	CTA	n/a	n/a	n/a

Table 1: Continued.

Article	Year	Side	Indication	Pulmonary systemic connection site	Paradoxical paO_2	Wave form	Fluoroscopy	CTA/CT chest	U/S confirmation	Pulmonary HTN	Management
Khanna et al. [11]	2014	Left IJ	Intraoperative venous access	Left upper pulmonary vein to left brachiocephalic	√	Venous	No	Regular CT without contrast	n/a	n/a	Used for 2 days
Chirinos et al. [16]	2014	Left IJ	Hemodialysis	Left upper pulmonary vein to left brachiocephalic	High PO_2 but no arterial sample to compare	Venous	Yes	CTA	n/a	n/a	Removed
Grillot et al. [12]	2016	Left IJ	Hemodialysis	Left upper pulmonary vein to left brachiocephalic	√	Venous	No	CTA	√	n/a	Used for 7 days

n/a: not available.

Instead, one can use the constellation of findings described above and confirm the diagnosis using simple fluoroscopy studies.

There are no enough cases in literature to examine the safety of using the CVL inserted in an anomalous pulmonary vein. In our case, we opted to remove the catheter since we had alternative options. Other authors opted for reposition of the catheter under fluoroscopy guidance [6, 14, 17]. However, Khanna and colleagues [11] reported using the CVL safely for two days as venous access. In addition, Grillot and colleagues [12] reported using it for seven days for hemodialysis.

4. Conclusion

It is important to be familiar with PAPVR as a cause of CVL malposition. When encountered, the systematic approach can help establish the diagnosis. This includes ultrasound confirmation of venous access, checking blood gases from the CVL and concurrently from an arterial site which is expected to show high PO_2 that might be paradoxically higher than the arterial side, checking the pressure wave, and using fluoroscopy to confirm radiologically.

Acknowledgments

The authors express great gratitude for Maya Amer, BAR, for graphic design and assistance.

References

[1] J. E. J. Healy, "An anatomic survey of anomalous pulmonary veins: their clinical significance," *The Journal of Thoracic Surgery*, vol. 23, pp. 433–444, 1952.

[2] P. L. Tan and M. Gibson, "Central venous catheters: the role of radiology," *Clin. Radiol*, vol. 61, pp. 13–22, 2006.

[3] F. Gibson and A. Bodenham, "Misplaced central venous catheters: applied anatomy and practical management," *British Journal of Anesthesia*, vol. 110, 2013.

[4] L. Wang, Z.-S. Liu, and C.-A. Wang, "Malposition of central venous catheter: presentation and management," *Chinese Medical Journal*, vol. 129, no. 2, pp. 227–234, 2016.

[5] M. Wirsing, C. Schummer, R. Neumann, J. Steenbeck, P. Schmidt, and W. Schummer, "Is traditional reading of the bedside chest radiograph appropriate to detect intraatrial central venous catheter position?" *Chest*, vol. 134, no. 3, pp. 527–533, 2008.

[6] M. E. Wylam and G. A. Schmidt, "Serendipitous discovery during jugular catheterization. Partial anomalous pulmonary venous connection," *Chest*, vol. 98, no. 2, pp. 493–495, 1990.

[7] Winslow. No Title. J. Mem Acad Roy Sci. 113 (1739).

[8] N. M. Ammash, J. B. Seward, C. A. Warnes, H. M. Connolly, P. W. O'Leary, and G. K. Danielson, "Partial anomalous pulmonary venous connection: Diagnosis by transesophageal echocardiography," *Journal of the American College of Cardiology*, vol. 29, no. 6, pp. 1351–1358, 1997.

[9] H. Kamalipour, S. Ahmadi, K. Kamali, A. Moaref, M. Shafa, and P. Kamalipour, "Ultrasound for localization of central venous catheter: a good alternative to chest X-ray?" *Anesthesiology and Pain Medicine*, vol. 6, no. 5, Article ID e38834, 2016.

[10] C. J. C. Cheng, B. L. Lim, and B. S. Tan, "Inadvertent catheterisation of a partial anomalous pulmonary venous channel during central venous cannulation," *Anaesthesia*, vol. 57, no. 2, pp. 198–200, 2002.

[11] A. K. Khanna, A. Maheshwari, M. J. Popovich, and P. Mathur, "Incidental discovery of a partial anomalous pulmonary venous connection in the surgical critical care unit," *Journal of Clinical Anesthesia*, vol. 26, 2014.

[12] N. Grillot, S. Figueiredo, A. Aubry, P.-E. Leblanc, and J. Duranteau, "Unusual dialysis catheter position due to partial anomalous pulmonary venous return: diagnosis and management," *Anaesthesia Critical Care and Pain Medicine*, vol. 35, no. 3, pp. 233–235, 2016.

[13] S. A. Townley, "Central venous catheter malposition in an anomalous pulmonary vein," *European Journal of Anaesthesiology*, vol. 20, no. 12, pp. 985-986, 2003.

[14] K. Javangula, J. Cole, M. Cross, and P. H. Kay, "An unusual manifestation of left partial anomalous pulmonary venous connection," *Interactive Cardiovascular and Thoracic Surgery*, vol. 11, no. 6, pp. 846-847, 2010.

[15] L. Brandt and U. Artmeier-Brandt, "Partial anomalous pulmonary venous connection as incidental finding: explanation for apparently paradoxical central venous blood gas analysis results," *Anaesthesist*, vol. 64, no. 10, pp. 754–757, 2015.

[16] J. C. Chirinos, J. A. Neyra, J. Patel, and A. R. Rodan, "Hemodialysis catheter insertion: is increased PO_2 a sign of arterial cannulation? A case report," *BMC Nephrology*, vol. 15, article 127, 2014.

[17] C. M. R. Habito and S. P. Kalva, "Partial Anomalous Pulmonary Venous Return Detected Incidentally during Port Placement," *J. Vasc. Interv. Radiol*, vol. 23, 2012.

[18] M. R. Chintu, S. Chinnappa, and S. Bhandari, "Aberrant positioning of a central venous dialysis catheter to reveal a left-sided partial anomalous pulmonary venous connection," *Vascular Health and Risk Management*, vol. 4, no. 5, pp. 1141–1143, 2008.

Mechanical Ventilation Weaning in Inclusion Body Myositis: Feasibility of Isokinetic Inspiratory Muscle Training as an Adjunct Therapy

Leonardo Cordeiro de Souza,[1,2] Josué Felipe Campos,[2] Leandro Possidente Daher,[2] Priscila Furtado da Silva,[2] Alex Ventura,[2] Pollyana Zamborlini do Prado,[2] Daniele Brasil,[2] Debora Mendonça,[2] and Jocemir Ronaldo Lugon[3]

[1] *Medical Science Post-Graduation Program, Universidade Federal Fluminense, Niterói, RJ, Brazil*
[2] *Intensive Care Division, Hospital e Clínica São Gonçalo, São Gonçalo, RJ, Brazil*
[3] *Nephrology Division, Department of Medicine, Medical School, Universidade Federal Fluminense, Niterói, RJ, Brazil*

Correspondence should be addressed to Leonardo Cordeiro de Souza; leonardo.uti@gmail.com

Academic Editor: Nicolas Nin

Inclusion body myositis is a rare myopathy associated with a high rate of respiratory complications. This condition usually requires prolonged mechanical ventilation and prolonged intensive care stay. The unsuccessful weaning is mainly related to respiratory muscle weakness that does not promptly respond to immunosuppressive therapy. We are reporting a case of a patient in whom the use of an inspiratory muscle-training program which started after a two-week period of mechanical ventilation was associated with a successful weaning in one week and hospital discharge after 2 subsequent weeks.

1. Introduction

In 1971, the term "inclusion body myositis" (IBM) was coined to describe a subset of patients with chronic myositis, whose muscle biopsy showed besides inflammation, muscle fibres containing vacuoles and abnormal filaments, and characteristic inclusions in cytoplasm and nucleus [1]. The inclusion body myositis is grouped with dermatomyositis and polymyositis as idiopathic inflammatory myopathies [2]. The disease is characterized by a proximal myopathy, which progressively leads to functional disability. It is more common in adults in their fifties [1, 2]. Respiratory complications can reach a prevalence of 45%. Weakness/fatigue of respiratory muscles with interstitial pneumonia and dysphagia are the main causes of death [2–4]. The use of mechanical ventilation is required in most cases, but weaning is hardly achieved [4, 5]. We are reporting a case in whom an inspiratory muscle training program (IMT) using an isokinetic electronic load device which started after a two-week period of mechanical ventilation was associated with a successful weaning in one week.

2. Case Report

A 43-year-old male was admitted to the intensive care of the hospital with symmetrical muscle weakness in the pelvic and scapular girdles. He reported a history of Guillain-Barré syndrome in 2005 without motor sequelae. His initial laboratory exams were haemoglobin of 16.1 g/dL; leukocytes of 13,030/mm^3 with 3% young forms and 13% of lymphocytes; urea of 23 mg/dL; creatinine of 0.34 mg/dL; Na of 131 mEq/L; K of 5.5 mEq/L; Cl of 97 mEq/L; AST of 51 U/L; ALT of 49 U/L; lactate of 1.1 mEq/L; LDL of 926 U/L; CK of 145 U/L; and CRP of 4.6 mg/dL.

He evolved with acute respiratory failure type II (PaO_2 < 60 mmHg and $PaCO_2$ > 45 mmHg) requiring orotracheal intubation and mechanical ventilation that was set on a pressure controlled mode. His cerebrospinal fluid showed

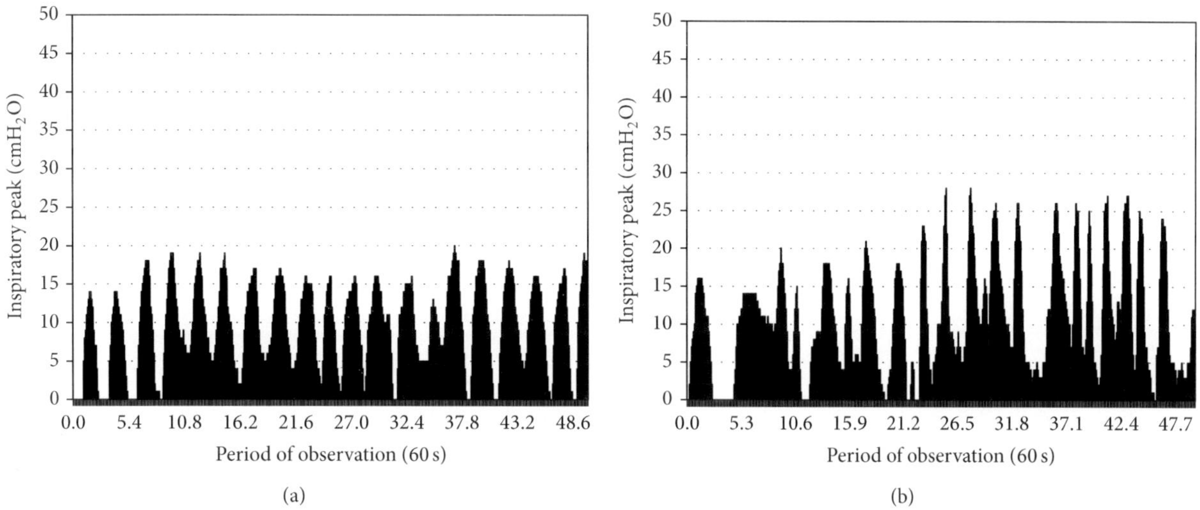

FIGURE 1: Graphics of inspiratory peaks by TIE index method. (a) At start of program on mechanical ventilation dependence; (b) 14 days after treatment associated with successful weaning.

the presence of lymphocytes, monocytes, neutrophils, and macrophages, blood cultures were negative for bacterial or fungal agents, and serological tests for toxoplasmosis, herpes, varicella, and HIV were all negative. A deltoid muscle biopsy showed a mononuclear interstitial inflammatory infiltrate with fibres exhibiting rimmed vacuoles, findings that were thought to be compatible with the diagnosis of inclusion body myositis.

During his stay in the ICU, he received a course of intravenous immunoglobulin (0.4 g/kg per day for 5 days) and oral prednisone (1 mg/kg per day) without improvement [4]. In the same period, he developed nosocomial pneumonia and septic shock and was managed with vasoactive amines and intravenous antibiotic therapy (meropenem combined with polymyxin B).

After three unsuccessful weaning trials, the patient was tracheotomised on the 14th day of intubation and transferred to the prolonged ventilation unit. Following hemodynamic stabilization and infection control, azathioprine 150 mg per day [4] was started in association with a inspiratory muscle training (IMT) program using an isokinetic electronic load device (POWERbreathe K-5, London, UK), 2 daily sessions of 30 respiratory cycles as previously described [9], with a load of 30% of the expected maximal inspiratory pressure as described elsewhere [10–12]. Load and intensity were reassessed weekly using commercial software (BreatheLink, POWERbreathe Co., London, UK). During the period of treatment, the patient comfortably remained under pressure support ventilation (frequency < 30). The IMT program was accompanied by an early mobilization protocol (active member exercising in bed followed by resistance exercising against gravity at the bedside, evolving to standing position and cycle ergometer activity) [13].

At the start of the new therapeutic program, the measured respiratory parameters of the patient were static compliance of 55 mL/cm H_2O, SpO_2 of 95% (FIO_2 35%), breathing frequency of 21 bpm, tidal volume of 0.390 L, an f/Vt index of 54 bpm/L, P0.1 of 4.66 cm H_2O, MIP of 20 cm H_2O (17% of the expected value of 118 cm H_2O), and timed inspiratory effort (TIE) index of 0.54 cm H_2O/sec (~50% of the expected value). The muscle function evaluation of the patient at the beginning of the training program showed an Medical Research Council (MRC) score of 22 (see Table 1), while the correspondent values for the degree of independence of the patient as assessed by the motor domain of the Functional Independence Measure (FIM) score was 14; see Table 2.

TABLE 1: Compromise of muscular force in the lower limbs by Medical Research Council (MRC).

Muscles	Before treatment Left/right	After treatment Left/right
Biceps brachii	3/3	5/5
Triceps brachii	1/1	4/4
Extensor carpi radialis	3/3	5/5
Iliopsoas	1/1	4/4
Quadriceps femoris	1/1	4/4
Tibialis anterior	2/2	4/4
Total	22	52

MRC scoring system. 0: no movement; 1: palpable contraction, no visible movement; 2: movement but only with gravity eliminated; 3: movement against gravity; 4: movement against resistance but weaker than normal; 5: normal power. [6].

After two weeks of IMT, the MIP increased to 28 cm H_2O, the TIE index to 1.09 cm H_2O/sec, and a partial respiratory independence was achieved (nocturnal pressure support ventilation was provided) [4]. After four weeks, MIP was 50 cm H_2O; see Figure 1. By that time, the load employed with the power breath device was 15 cm H_2O. He progressed to decannulation and was maintained on nocturnal noninvasive ventilation to avoid hypoventilation and carbonarcosis. By the time of hospital discharge, he was under IMT twice a day

Table 2: Evaluation of self-care, sphincters, and mobility by functional independence measure (FIM).

Parameters	Before treatment	After treatment
(1) Eating	1	7
(2) Grooming	1	7
(3) Bathing/showering	1	6
(4) Dressing upper body	1	6
(5) Dressing lower body	1	6
(6) Toileting	1	7
(7) Bladder management	2	7
(8) Bowel management mobility	2	7
(9) Transfers: bed/chair/wheelchair	1	7
(10) Transfers: toilet	1	7
(11) Locomotion: walking/wheelchair	1	7
(12) Locomotion: stairs	1	7
Total	14	81

FIM scoring. 7: complete independence, fully independent; 6: modified independence requiring the use of a device but no physical help; 5: supervision requiring only standby assistance or verbal prompting or help with setup; 4: minimal assistance requiring incidental hands-on help only (subject performs >75% of the task); 3: moderate assistance; subject still performs 50–75% of the task; 2: maximal assistance; subject provides less than half of the effort (25–49%); and 1: total assistance; subject contributes <25% of the effort or is unable to do the task [7, 8].

with a load of 17 cm H_2O and walking 380 m independently, but under supervision, and climbing a flight of stairs. His MRC score was 52 (see Table 1) and the motor FIM score was 81 (see Table 2). After 6 months of hospital discharge, the patient remains on a regular use of the inspiratory load device and continues to improve his muscle strength. He is now gradually coming back to his daily activities.

3. Discussion

We are reporting a case of body inclusion myositis in which the definite diagnosis was obtained early in the course of the disease. Following previous recommendations [1, 3–5], therapy was promptly started with intravenous immunoglobulin and steroids; the maintenance drug chosen was azathioprine. The experience with the treatment of this entity has been disappointing [1, 4, 5]. Unsuccessful weaning represents a major obstacle to patient recovery and is associated with a high rate of respiratory infection and a fatal outcome [2–4, 14]. Although effective in the management of the subjacent process that precipitated the disorder, immunosuppressive agents conceivably do not have any direct action upon the recovery of muscle function. It is plausible that the long period required for recovery of muscle strength may play a role in the weaning failure, emergency of infections, and the dismal prognosis of the disorder. Therefore, the use of a respiratory muscle training program could have a favourable impact on the outcome of the disease [9, 15, 16]. Indeed, the use of inspiratory muscle training has been found to be helpful in a variety of scenarios in which the mechanical ventilation weaning is troublesome [15, 17, 18].

We resorted to an isokinetic electronic load device using a protocol of endurance gain (higher number of repetitions using submaximal loads) given that the respiratory muscles display a large number of type I fibres, which are resistant to fatigue [9, 15, 16]. During the IMT program the patient showed no respiratory or hemodynamic changes that would prevent its continuation. The combination of the two strategies, one addressing the treatment of the acute immunological pathway and the other the recovery of muscle function, was associated with a successful weaning from mechanical ventilation, hospital discharge, and return to daily activities.

It is our view that the appropriate cleaning of the artificial airway, the correct positioning of the patient, and his collaboration were all essential to the success of the muscle training intervention.

In conclusion, the use of an inspiratory load device in association with the conventional therapy with immunosuppressive agents in the reported case was associated with an increase in the strength of the inspiratory muscles resulting in a favourable outcome. This is in line with previous reports above mentioned [15], but further studies are necessary to establish the exact role of IMT in the process of weaning from the ventilator these patients.

Authors' Contribution

Leonardo Cordeiro de Souza and Jocemir Ronaldo Lugon equally contributed to the design and paper preparation. Josué Felipe Campos, Leandro Possidente Daher, Priscila Furtado, Alex Ventura, Pollyana Zamborlini do Prado, Daniele Brasil, and Debora Mendonça helped regarding the patient care and the case report.

Acknowledgments

The authors are thankful to the respiratory physiotherapists (especially to Clarine Mendes, Erika Cristine Cordeiro, Monica Lourenço, Leandro Daher, Wanderlei Augusto Junior, Priscila Furtado, and Josué Felipe Campos) and physicians of the intensive care unit of the Hospital and Clínica São Gonçalo for their collaboration to our study.

References

[1] R. C. Griggs, V. Askanas, S. DiMauro et al., "Inclusion body myositis and myopathies," *Annals of Neurology*, vol. 38, no. 5, pp. 705–713, 1995.

[2] J. W. Teener and E. C. Raps, "Evaluation and treatment of respiratory failure in neuromuscular disease," *Rheumatic Disease Clinics of North America*, vol. 23, no. 2, pp. 277–292, 1997.

[3] I. Marie, P. Hatron, E. Hachulla, B. Wallaert, U. Michon-Pasturel, and B. Devulder, "Pulmonary involvement in polymyositis and in dermatomyositis," *Journal of Rheumatology*, vol. 25, no. 7, pp. 1336–1343, 1998.

[4] A. Selva-O'Callaghan, L. Sanchez-Sitjes, X. Muñoz-Gall et al., "Respiratory failure due to muscle weakness in inflammatory myopathies: maintenance therapy with home mechanical ventilation," *Rheumatology*, vol. 39, no. 8, pp. 914–916, 2000.

[5] R. Cohen, S. Lipper, and D. R. Dantzker, "Inclusion body myositis as a cause of respiratory failure," *Chest*, vol. 104, no. 3, pp. 975–977, 1993.

[6] Medical Research Council, *Aids to the Investigation of Peripheral Nerve Injuries. War Memorandum*, HMSO, London, UK, 2nd edition, 1943.

[7] C. V. Granger, B. B. Hamilton, J. M. Linacre, A. W. Heinemann, and B. D. Wright, "Performance profiles of the functional independence measure," *The American Journal of Physical Medicine and Rehabilitation*, vol. 72, no. 2, pp. 84–89, 1993.

[8] J. M. Linacre, A. W. Heinemann, B. D. Wright, C. V. Granger, and B. B. Hamilton, "The structure and stability of the functional independence measure," *Archives of Physical Medicine and Rehabilitation*, vol. 75, no. 2, pp. 127–132, 1994.

[9] S. R. Kulkarni, E. Fletcher, A. K. McConnell, K. R. Poskitt, and M. R. Whyman, "Pre-operative inspiratory muscle training preserves postoperative inspiratory muscle strength following major abdominal surgery—a randomised pilot study," *Annals of the Royal College of Surgeons of England*, vol. 92, no. 8, pp. 700–705, 2010.

[10] L. C. de Souza, C. T. da Silva Jr., and J. R. Lugon, "Evaluation of the inspiratory pressure using a digital vacuometer in mechanically ventilated patients: analysis of the time to achieve the inspiratory peak," *Respiratory Care*, vol. 57, no. 2, pp. 257–262, 2012.

[11] L. C. de Souza, C. T. da Silva Jr., J. R. Almeida, and J. R. Lugon, "Comparison of Maximal inspiratory pressure, tracheal airway occlusion pressure, and its ratio in the prediction of weaning outcome: impact of the use of a digital vacuometer and the unidirectional valve," *Respiratory Care*, vol. 57, no. 8, pp. 1285–1290, 2012.

[12] L. C. de Souza, F. S. Guimarães, and J. R. Lugon, "Evaluation of a new index of mechanical ventilation weaning: the timed inspiratory effort," *Journal of Intensive Care Medicine*, 2013.

[13] H. J. Engel, D. M. Needham, P. E. Morris, and M. A. Gropper, "ICU early mobilization: from recommendation to implementation at three medical centers," *Critical Care Medicine*, vol. 41, no. 9, supplement 1, pp. S69–S80, 2013.

[14] J.-M. Boles, J. Bion, A. Connors et al., "Weaning from mechanical ventilation," *European Respiratory Journal*, vol. 29, no. 5, pp. 1033–1056, 2007.

[15] A. D. Martin, B. K. Smith, P. D. Davenport et al., "Inspiratory muscle strength training improves weaning outcome in failure to wean patients: a randomized trial," *Critical Care*, vol. 15, no. 2, article R84, 2011.

[16] B. M. Bissett, I. A. Leditschke, J. D. Paratz, and R. J. Boots, "Protocol: Inspiratory muscle training for promoting recovery and outcomes in ventilated patients (IMPROVe): a randomised controlled trial," *BMJ Open*, vol. 2, no. 2, Article ID e000813, 2012.

[17] L. Moodie, J. Reeve, and M. Elkins, "Inspiratory muscle training increases inspiratory muscle strength in patients weaning from mechanical ventilation: a systematic review," *Journal of Physiotherapy*, vol. 57, no. 4, pp. 213–220, 2011.

[18] L. P. Cahalin, R. Arena, M. Guazzi et al., "Inspiratory muscle training in heart disease and heart failure: a review of the literature with a focus on method of training and outcomes," *Expert Review of Cardiovascular Therapy*, vol. 11, no. 2, pp. 161–177, 2013.

28

Rituximab Induced Pulmonary Edema Managed with Extracorporeal Life Support

Jacob R. Miller[1] **Warren Isakow,**[2] **Muhammad F. Masood,**[1] **Patrick Aguilar,**[2] **Kristen M. Sanfilippo,**[3] **Keki R. Balsara,**[1] **and Akinobu Itoh**[1]

[1] *Division of Cardiothoracic Surgery, Washington University, St. Louis, MO, USA*
[2] *Division of Pulmonary Critical Care, Washington University, St. Louis, MO, USA*
[3] *Division of Hematology, Washington University, St. Louis, MO, USA*

Correspondence should be addressed to Akinobu Itoh; akinobuitoh@wustl.edu

Academic Editor: Kurt Lenz

Though rare, rituximab has been reported to induce severe pulmonary edema. We describe the first report of ECLS utilization for this indication. A 31-year-old female with severe thrombotic thrombocytopenic purpura developed florid pulmonary edema after rituximab infusion. Despite advanced ventilatory settings, she developed severe respiratory acidosis and remained hypoxemic with a significant vasopressor requirement. Since her pulmonary insult was likely transient, ECLS was considered. Due to combined cardiorespiratory failure, she received support with peripheral venoarterial ECLS. During her ECLS course, she received daily plasmapheresis and high dose steroids. Her pulmonary function recovered and she was decannulated after 8 days. She was discharged after 23 days without residual sequelae.

1. Introduction

Rituximab, a monoclonal anti-CD20 antibody used in the treatment of hematologic and autoimmune diseases, though rare, has been reported to induce life-threatening pulmonary edema attributed to a large cytokine release [1, 2]. The management of severe noncardiogenic pulmonary edema with extracorporeal life support (ECLS) has been described [3]. Further, ECLS has been utilized for pulmonary edema secondary to cytokine release in the setting of transfusion-related acute lung injury [4] and tumor lysis syndrome [5]. We present here a case of acute florid pulmonary edema due to a rituximab infusion, the first reported successfully managed with ECLS. This case report was approved by the Washington University in St. Louis School of Medicine Internal Review Board with the patient's consent.

2. Case Presentation

This 31-year-old female suffered from thrombotic thrombocytopenic purpura (TTP) with multiple relapses requiring plasmapheresis, steroids, and rituximab. Two weeks prior to presentation, she was hospitalized for a TTP relapse with a platelet count of 17,000, hemoglobin of 7.9 g/dl, lactate dehydrogenase of 1,246 units/L, undetectable ADAMTS13 activity level, and ADAMTS13 inhibitor level greater than 8 inhibitor units. While admitted, she underwent seven rounds of plasmapheresis and was started on weekly low-dose rituximab (100 mg fixed dose) per clinical trial. She received two doses during admission, which she tolerated with only mild itching. At that time, she was receiving prednisone, 100 mg daily and premedication with diphenhydramine and acetaminophen. She presented 6 days after discharge for week three of low-dose rituximab, receiving the same premedications, during which she developed respiratory distress. The infusion was immediately stopped; however, she quickly deteriorated requiring intubation, producing copious white frothy sputum that required continuous suctioning. A chest radiograph confirmed severe bilateral pulmonary edema. Despite advanced ventilatory settings and inhaled nitric oxide (NO), she developed respiratory shock (pH: 7.19, pCO_2: 63 mm Hg, pO_2: 42 mm Hg). Her lactate peaked at

18.0 mmol/L and she became oliguric. A transthoracic echo (TTE) demonstrated grossly normal left ventricular (LV) and right ventricular (RV) function and ejection fraction (EF) of 70%, with pulmonary artery systolic pressures (PASP) of 36 mmHg. She became difficult to oxygenate requiring escalating ventilatory settings, pressure-control ventilation with a peak inspiratory pressure of 40 cm H_2O, and a plateau pressure of 20 cm H_2O giving a mean airway pressure of 26–30 cm H_2O, with a fraction of inspired oxygen of 100%. Her acidosis, elevated intrathoracic pressure, and increased pulmonary vascular resistance led to a significant vasopressor requirement. This was confirmed with a central venous catheter which measured her central venous pressure at 28 mmHg. Serial bedside ultrasounds were performed which showed a deterioration in left ventricular function with poor ventricular filling. An esophageal Doppler was placed which showed a cardiac output of 2.1 L/m for a cardiac index of 1.0 L/min/m^2 (body surface area: 2.2 m^2).

As this insult was anticipated to be transient and reversible, venoarterial (VA) ECLS was initiated. After 3,000 units of intravenous heparin, percutaneous cannulation was performed with a 25-French multistage cannula in the femoral vein and a 17-French arterial cannula in the common femoral artery. In addition, a 5-French vascular sheath was inserted into the superficial femoral artery for distal limb perfusion. All cannulas were placed with ultrasound guidance. The ECLS circuit initially provided a flow of 2.3–2.7 L/min/m^2 with a sweep gas flow rate of 8 L/min at 100% oxygen. Once the patient stabilized a repeat TTE was performed which showed severe LV dysfunction with an EF of 25% and PASP similar to the previous.

Vasopressors and NO were immediately weaned. With oliguria and pulmonary edema, continuous venovenous hemodialysis (CVVHD) was initiated. Despite a negative fluid balance, chest radiographs worsened until ECLS Day 3. By Day 5, the radiographs began to improve and she was able to be weaned to conventional pressure-control settings with 40% FiO_2. At this time, an echocardiogram demonstrated normal cardiac function. She received daily plasmapheresis and high dose steroids, methylprednisolone 1 mg/kg. As her acidosis corrected, the sweep speed was decreased. On Day 6, ECLS weaning was initiated gradually. She was decannulated on Day 8. After decannulation her pulmonary status continued to improve and she was extubated the next day.

Her course was well tolerated, without major complications. After decannulation she did well and was discharged after a total hospital stay of 23 days. She did develop acute kidney injury (AKI) prior to ECLS cannulation, further exacerbating her pulmonary edema. She received CVVHD with aggressive volume removal, net 300 ml/hour with plasmapheresis. Her renal function gradually improved and returned to baseline prior to discharge. Additionally, diffuse oral mucosal bleeding began immediately after cannulation. Though no intervention was necessary, due to this and her low platelet count, she was not anticoagulated. While maintained on ECLS, the initial goal platelet count was greater than 20,000/mm^3. However, once she developed oral mucosal bleeding, the goal was modified to greater than 40,000/mm^3. She received 9 platelet transfusions during her ECLS course.

When cannulated for ECLS her ADAMTS13 activity level was undetectable and her ADAMTS13 inhibitor level was 4.4 inhibitor units. Her platelet count reached a nadir of 12,000/mm^3. By ECLS Day 7 she improved to an ADAMTS13 activity level of 61% and an inhibitor level of 0.4 inhibitor units. In total, she received 13 rounds of plasmapheresis and was transitioned to 100 mg prednisone daily. Since she is no longer a candidate for rituximab and has a high probability of relapse, she has been referred for splenectomy.

3. Discussion

Rituximab decreases the production of antibodies to ADAMTS13, leading to increased ADAMTS13 activity and cleavage of the large von Willebrand Factor multimers, thus, preventing the multimer-induced platelet aggregation and microthrombi formation occurring with TTP [6]. Expansion of rituximab use has resulted in the reporting of rare adverse events in postmarketing surveillance [7]. Cytokine release syndrome (CRS) has been reported, though this typically occurs after the first infusion [2].

Initially, our patient had a broad differential diagnosis. Her rapid deterioration, frothy sputum, chest radiograph, and timing made pulmonary edema due to the rituximab infusion the most likely diagnosis. Rituximab induced pulmonary edema due to the fact that CRS has been previously reported and shown to be reversible [1]. Therefore, despite her grave condition, we anticipated that she had a potentially recoverable insult.

By the time ECLS was considered she required high levels of support, both respiratory and hemodynamic. At this time, the patient was on advanced ventilator settings with high peak inspiratory and mean airway pressures, which causes a decrease in left ventricular stroke volume and cardiac output [8]. Additionally, acidosis, metabolic or respiratory (our patient suffered from both), is known to lead to a decreased stroke volume due to the negative inotropic effects of the acidosis [9]. This likely resulted in her hemodynamic collapse, and, therefore, VA, rather than venovenous (VV) ECLS, was initiated. In this instance, the VA ECMO strategy allowed for decreased vasopressor requirements and helped to improve renal blood flow. However, if considered earlier, VV ECLS may have prevented her hemodynamic compromise by eliminating the respiratory acidosis, the elevated intrathoracic pressure and the increased pulmonary vascular resistance, and, therefore, the need for VA support.

As our patient's cardiac function improved such that she essentially had only respiratory failure, there was concern for differential hypoxia. As cardiac function recovered, due to her cannulation strategy, her cardiac output would consist of poorly oxygenated blood preferentially perfusing the coronaries and cerebral vessels. Further, a "dual circuit" can develop, such that deoxygenated blood recirculates from upper body (heart, brain, and upper extremities) through the superior vena cava (SVC), heart, lungs, and great vessels. A second circuit is established consisting of the descending aorta, lower body, inferior vena cava (IVC), and the

ECLS circuit [10]. To monitor for this, our patient had bilateral radial arterial access with arterial blood gas analysis from each. Had they demonstrated a developing differential hypoxia, alternative cannulation strategies would have been necessary, possibly including advancing the IVC catheter into the SVC or placing additional venous or arterial cannulas [11]. Placement of a subclavian arterial cannula in addition to, or rather than, a femoral cannula also would have abolished this phenomenon.

While the literature remains inconclusive, some suggest significant differences in survival based on cannulation strategy. Interestingly, veno-venoarterial (VVA) ECLS is touted by some as having superior survival, to both VV and VA, in patients with a primary pulmonary pathology [12]. This cannulation strategy utilizes a second outflow cannula, returning oxygenated blood to both the arterial and the venous system. If venous return is insufficient to support the increase in outflow, a second venous return cannula can be used. Indeed, despite the lack of differential hypoxia, our patient may have benefited from VVA ECLS by improving the oxygenation which would allow for lung protective ventilator settings earlier. Additionally, the preoxygenated blood flowing through the pulmonary system would lead to decreased pulmonary vascular resistance and further increase preload.

Since her hemodynamics continuously improved after VA ECLS initiation, though considered, the decision was made to not pursue a cannula reconfiguration. In addition to cannula reconfiguration, alternative therapies directed at the treatment of CRS could have been considered, rather than plasmapheresis. Recent literature has shown some promise with the anti-IL-6R mAb tocilizumab [13]. Though reports of its utilization are sparse, with only one report describing its utilization in 9 pediatric patients, the results are encouraging [14].

As new therapies are developed for hematologic, oncologic, and autoimmune diseases, the possibility of severe pulmonary edema related to CRS may become more frequent. Here, we demonstrate the utility of ECLS as a temporizing mechanism, though note that further research is necessary to determine optimal cannulation strategies.

Abbreviations

ECLS:	Extracorporeal life support
TTP:	Thrombotic thrombocytopenic purpura
TTE:	Transthoracic echocardiogram
LV:	Left ventricle
RV:	Right ventricle
EF:	Ejection fraction
PASP:	Pulmonary artery systolic pressure
NO:	Nitric oxide
VA:	Venoarterial
CVVHD:	Continuous venovenous hemodialysis
AKI:	Acute kidney injury
CRS:	Cytokine release syndrome
VV:	Venovenous
VVA:	Veno-venoarterial
SVC:	Superior vena cava
IVC:	Inferior vena cava.

Authors' Contributions

Jacob R. Miller was involved in the original procedure, data acquisition, interpretation, drafting the manuscript, and manuscript submission. Warren Isakow was involved in the care of the patient including original consideration of therapy in question. Muhammad F. Masood was involved in the care of the patient, data analysis, and manuscript revision. Patrick Aguilar was involved in manuscript revision and the submission process. Kristen M. Sanfilippo was involved in the care of the patient as well as manuscript revision. Keki R. Balsara was involved in the care of the patient, data interpretation, and manuscript revision. Akinobu Itoh was involved in all procedures, care of the patient, drafting of the manuscript, and manuscript revision.

References

[1] K. H. Chan and M. K. C. Ng, "Hyperacute pulmonary edema complicating rituximab infusion," *European Journal of Internal Medicine*, vol. 20, no. 1, 2009.

[2] U. Winkler, M. Jensen, O. Manzke, H. Schulz, V. Diehl, and A. Engert, "Cytokine-release syndrome in patients with B-cell chronic lymphocytic leukemia and high lymphocyte counts after treatment with an anti-CD20 monoclonal antibody (rituximab, IDEC-C2B8)," *Blood*, vol. 94, no. 7, pp. 2217–2224, 1999.

[3] Y.-W. Tung, F. Lin, M.-S. Yang, C.-W. Wu, and K.-S. Cheung, "Bilateral developing reexpansion pulmonary edema treated with extracorporeal membrane oxygenation," *The Annals of Thoracic Surgery*, vol. 89, no. 4, pp. 1268–1271, 2010.

[4] H. Kuroda, Y. Masuda, H. Imaizumi, Y. Kozuka, Y. Asai, and A. Namiki, "Successful extracorporeal membranous oxygenation for a patient with life-threatening transfusion-related acute lung injury," *Journal of Anesthesia & Clinical Research*, vol. 23, no. 3, pp. 424–426, 2009.

[5] E. Sanford, T. Wolbrink, J. Mack, and R. Grant Rowe, "Severe tumor lysis syndrome and acute pulmonary edema requiring extracorporeal membrane oxygenation following initiation of chemotherapy for metastatic alveolar rhabdomyosarcoma," *Pediatric Blood & Cancer*, vol. 63, no. 5, pp. 928–930, 2015.

[6] J.-P. Westwood, H. Webster, S. Mcguckin, V. Mcdonald, S. J. Machin, and M. Scully, "Rituximab for thrombotic thrombocytopenic purpura: benefit of early administration during acute episodes and use of prophylaxis to prevent relapse," *Journal of Thrombosis and Haemostasis*, vol. 11, no. 3, pp. 481–490, 2013.

[7] H. S. Kulkarni and P. M. Kasi, "Rituximab and cytokine release syndrome," *Case Reports in Oncology*, vol. 5, no. 1, pp. 134–141, 2012.

[8] T. Luecke, H. Roth, P. Herrmann, A. Joachim, G. Weisser, P. Pelosi et al., "Assessment of cardiac preload and left ventricular function under increasing levels of positive end-expiratory pressure," *Intensive Care Medicine*, vol. 30, no. 1, pp. 119–126, 2004.

[9] M. Stengl, L. Ledvinova, J. Chvojka et al., "Effects of clinically relevant acute hypercapnic and metabolic acidosis on the cardiovascular system: an experimental porcine study," *Critical Care*, vol. 17, no. 6, 2013.

[10] M. E. Cove, "Disrupting differential hypoxia in peripheral venoarterial extracorporeal membrane oxygenation," *Critical Care*, vol. 19, no. 1, 2015.

[11] X. Hou, X. Yang, Z. Du, J. Xing, H. Li, C. Jiang et al., "Superior vena cava drainage improves upper body oxygenation during veno-arterial extracorporeal membrane oxygenation in sheep," *Critical Care*, vol. 19, 2015.

[12] F. Stöhr, M. Y. Emmert, M. L. Lachat, R. Stocker, M. Maggiorini, V. Falk et al., "Extracorporeal membrane oxygenation for acute respiratory distress syndrome: Is the configuration mode an important predictor for the outcome?" *Interactive CardioVascular and Thoracic Surgery*, vol. 12, no. 5, pp. 676–680, 2011.

[13] S. A. Grupp et al., "Chimeric antigen receptor-modified T cells for acute lymphoid leukemia," *The New England Journal of Midicine*, vol. 368, no. 16, pp. 1509–1518, 2013.

[14] S. L. Maude et al., "Chimeric antigen receptor T cells for sustained remissions in leukemia," *The New England Journal of Midicine*, vol. 371, no. 16, pp. 1507–1517, 2014.

Severe Metformin Poisoning Successfully Treated with Simultaneous Venovenous Hemofiltration and Prolonged Intermittent Hemodialysis

Dovile Leonaviciute,[1] Bo Madsen,[2] Anne Schmedes,[3] Niels H. Buus,[2] and Bodil S. Rasmussen[1,4]

[1]*Department of Anaesthesiology and Intensive Care Medicine, Aalborg University Hospital, Aalborg, Denmark*
[2]*Department of Nephrology, Aalborg University Hospital, Aalborg, Denmark*
[3]*Department of Biochemistry and Immunology, Lillebaelt Hospital, Vejle, Denmark*
[4]*Department of Clinical Medicine, Aalborg University, Aalborg, Denmark*

Correspondence should be addressed to Dovile Leonaviciute; dole@rn.dk

Academic Editor: Anita J. Reddy

Metformin poisoning is a life-threatening condition with a high mortality rate. We present a patient case of metformin poisoning following intake of 80 g metformin resulting in severe lactate acidosis with a nadir pH of 6.73 and circulatory collapse, successfully treated with addition of prolonged intermittent hemodialysis (HD) to continuous venovenous hemofiltration (CVVH). The patient's pH became normal 48 hours after metformin ingestion during simultaneous CVVH and addition of 22 hours of intermittent HD in the ICU. The highest metformin level was found to be 991 μmol/L (therapeutic range 3.9–23.2 μmol/L). We conclude that in cases of severe metformin poisoning with circulatory shock and extreme lactic acidosis, the usual CVVH modality might not efficiently clear metformin. Therefore, additional prolonged HD should be considered even in the state of cardiovascular collapse with vasopressor requirement.

1. Introduction

Metformin is widely used and is the most frequently prescribed oral antidiabetic drug of the biguanide family [1]. Metformin inhibits hepatic gluconeogenesis and glycogenolysis and enhances peripheral glucose utilisation in patients with non-insulin-dependent diabetes [2, 3]. Metformin use is generally safe and well tolerated. However, lactic acidosis is a well-known complication to metformin treatment, especially in intentional overdose or in cases of renal insufficiency. Metformin poisoning is a life-threatening condition with a very high mortality rate. With the modern intensive care treatment, mortality ranges from 50% to 30% [4]. However, those intentional overdose patients with severe acidosis (pH less than 6.9) have a mortality rate as high as 83% [5]. We present a patient case of metformin poisoning following intake of 80 g metformin resulting in severe lactate acidosis with a nadir pH of 6.73 and circulatory collapse, successfully treated with addition of prolonged intermittent hemodialysis (HD) to continuous venovenous hemofiltration (CVVH).

2. Case Presentation

A 54-year-old patient with a body weight of 66 kg and a medical history of anxiety, type 2 diabetes, and previous stroke was admitted to the local hospital one hour after ingestion of 80 grams of metformin in a suicide attempt. At the Emergency Department, an aspiration of the gastric content was performed followed by administration of activated charcoal. The patient developed vomiting and diarrhoea. Arterial blood gas showed pH 7.33, $PaCO_2$ 4.8 kPa, PaO_2 12.8 kPa, bicarbonate 19.3 mmol/L, base deficit 7 mmol/L, lactate 5.9 mmol/L, and blood glucose 17.9 mmol/L. The patient was transferred to a university hospital. Three hours after ingestion of metformin, the metabolic acidosis had deteriorated with serum lactate 8.5 mmol/L and pH 7.23. Urgent hemodialysis (HD) was

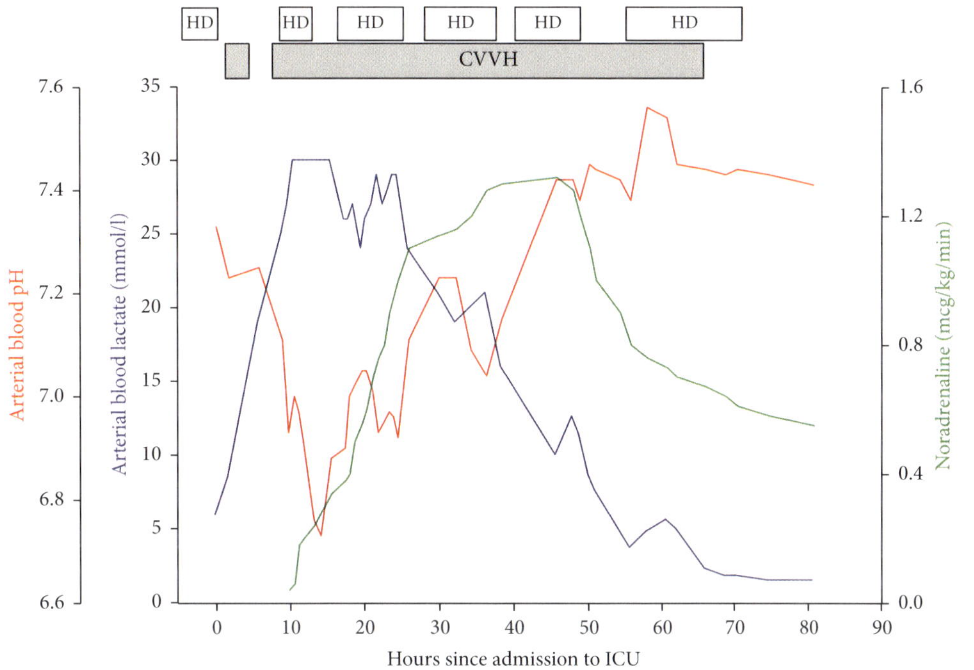

Figure 1: Measurements of arterial blood pH (red) and lactate (blue) together with the infusion rate of noradrenaline (green) in the hours following admission to the intensive care unit (ICU). HD denotes hemodialysis and CVVH continuous venovenous hemofiltration.

performed for 4 hours (h) by the nephrology department with a blood flow of 150 mL/min and a Fresenius FX60 dialyzer (Fresenius, Bad Homburg, Germany) with a surface area of 1.4 m^2. During HD, the patient became increasingly acidotic and circulatory unstable and was admitted to the intensive care unit (ICU) for circulatory support and continuous CVVH. CVVH (Aquarius, Edwards Lifesciences, Irvine, USA) was initiated with a blood flow of 300 mL/min and a replacement fluid rate of 2000 mL/h (30 mL/kg/h) with 35 mmol/L bicarbonate in Accusol 35 (Baxter Healthcare Ltd., Norfolk, United Kingdom) with 50% of the replacement fluid infused prefilter and 50% postfilter via a dialysis catheter placed in the right internal jugular vein. Dialyzer used was Aquamax HF 12 (Nikkiso, Bellco, Italy) with a surface area of 1,2 m^2. Because of filter clotting, CVVH stopped after one hour. The metabolic acidosis escalated further with a pH decreasing to 6.73 and a serum lactate above the upper measuring limit of 30 mmol/L (ABL800 Flex, Radiometer, Copenhagen, Denmark). The patient was less conscious but managed to hyperventilate to a $PaCO_2$ of 2.6 kPa and base deficit of 29 mmol/L. He developed severe hypotension, oliguria, hypothermia with core temperature 32.2°C, and hypoglycaemia with a nadir blood glucose of 2.3 mmol/L. Noradrenaline infusion was initiated with increasing dosage to keep mean arterial pressure above 60 mmHg. Bicarbonate 8.4% infusion was continued together with volume substitution with crystalloids. CVVH was restarted after 3 hours. Active external rewarming with forced-air warming blanket (Model 30000, 3M Health Care, St. Paul, USA) and maximal possible temperature of 39°C on CVVH was used to treat the hypothermia, but the temperature did not increase. As the patient's condition deteriorated, the hemodynamic instability progressed, cardiac arrhythmias occurred, and serum lactate remained immeasurably high. Focus Assessed Transthoracic Echocardiography (FATE) revealed a normal systolic function of both ventricles.

Because CVVH alone failed to stabilise the patient's condition and despite of hemodynamic instability and vasopressor requirement (noradrenaline infusion 0.4 mcg/kg/min), a decision was made to start HD simultaneously with CVVH. An extra dialysis catheter was placed in the left internal jugular vein and intermittent HD with a blood flow of 300 mL/min, Fresenius FX80 dialyzer (Fresenius, Bad Homburg, Germany) with a surface area of 1.8 m^2, with the highest possible concentration of bicarbonate buffer of 40 mmol/L on HD machine, was simultaneously performed for 4 h and repeated for 8 h on the first day. On the second day, HD was performed twice for 8 h and on the third day for 16.5 h, while CVVH was continued simultaneously for almost 58 h. Progression of the acidosis occurred with a drop in pH whenever HD was paused (Figure 1).

On the second day in the ICU, the patient was intubated and mechanical ventilation was initiated, because of respiratory insufficiency due to increasing $PaCO_2$. Only 48 h after metformin ingestion and 36 h in the ICU with cardiopulmonary support using very high doses of noradrenaline infusion (up to 1.4 mcg/kg/min) and CVVH combined with 22 h in total of intermittent HD with bicarbonate buffer, the patient's pH finally normalized. Serum lactate was still elevated but decreased very slowly to 2 mmol/L on the third day during the continued treatment with CVVH and intermittent HD. After 58 h on both CVVH and intermittent HD, the CVVH was discontinued and the patient remained on intermittent HD because of acute oliguric renal failure until day 15. The patient had an increase of international normalized ratio (INR) from 1.2 at the day of admission to a maximal value of 2.0 at day 2. The patient's condition improved gradually and he was discharged from the hospital after 7 weeks. At that time, the patient was still nourished via a percutaneous endoscopic gastrostomy tube due to dysphagia and used a walker due to polyneuropathy. The patient's renal function on discharge was normal.

A metformin plasma concentration, determined by high pressure liquid chromatography tandem mass spectrometry (Waters Acquity UPLC, Xevo TQ-S), was later measured from the plasma obtained 14 h after poisoning (after 4 h of HD and one hour of CVVH) and was found to be as high as 991 μmol/L (therapeutic range 3.9–23.2 μmol/L). 48 h after poisoning, remaining on CVVH and additional 20 hours of intermittent HD, metformin concentration was reduced to 327 μmol/L. After additional 8 hours of HD and CVVH, metformin concentration was further reduced to 84.4 μmol/L at 62 h after poisoning.

3. Discussion

Severe metformin poisoning often presents with a profound lactic acidosis followed by collapse of the cardiovascular system. Symptoms of metformin poisoning are diffuse with abdominal pain, nausea, vomiting, hypothermia, decreased level of consciousness, and circulatory instability leading to multiorgan failure. The circulatory instability is due to peripheral vasoplegia as described in many case reports where low systemic vascular resistance was measured [6]. We observed a clinical picture of a hyperdynamic circulatory state where FATE revealed normal contractility of the heart together with severe systemic hypotension. Vasoplegia and vasodilatation can explain hypothermia, which is a common symptom of metformin poisoning [6].

Treatment of metformin poisoning is symptomatic and supportive and there is no antidote available. Typical treatment strategies consist of correcting acidosis with intravenous sodium bicarbonate and decreasing the blood levels of metformin. Further prevention of gastrointestinal absorption can be achieved with activated charcoal. In case of renal insufficiency, renal replacement therapy is the only option for metformin removal and acidosis correction.

Metformin is readily dialyzable. It is a small molecule with a molecular weight of 165 Da, not protein bound, and after gastrointestinal absorption it rapidly moves into the tissue compartment and has a large volume of distribution of 63–276 L (1–5 L/kg) [1]. Lalau et al. previously demonstrated a biphasic pattern of metformin elimination according to a two-compartment model. This two-compartment model suggests that a brief hemodialysis session is not sufficient in eliminating metformin due to a rebound phenomenon [7]. These pharmacokinetic properties indicate a need of prolonged dialysis for metformin elimination. Several case reports describe favourable outcome after severe metformin poisoning treated with prolonged intermittent HD. These reports suggest that prolonged HD (>15 h) is needed and indicated in patients, who suffer from a severe overdose and who are able to tolerate HD [2, 8]. In our case, 62 h after ingestion and with ongoing treatment with CVVH and additional 32 h of intermittent HD, the metformin level was still elevated to 84.4 μmol/L, emphasizing the need for prolonged HD in severe metformin overdose.

Usually intermittent HD is poorly tolerated in critically ill patients with hemodynamic instability [9]. In the ICU setting CVVH or continuous venovenous hemodiafiltration (CVVHDF) is used because fluid shifts are less profound and therefore applicable in hemodynamic unstable patients. However, these modalities need high ultrafiltration rates for successful treatment in case of metformin intoxication [10], but clearance of metformin by continuous venovenous treatment modalities is still 3-4 times less than clearance by conventional HD [1, 11]. Panzer reported successful use of two CVVH machines simultaneously for hemodynamically unstable patient to facilitate high volume CVVH [12]. Friesecke has successfully applied the same approach with two dialysis catheters and used discontinuous hemofiltration (highflux) in addition to CVVH for severe circulatory unstable patient. To our knowledge, the use of intermittent HD in a patient with metformin poisoning with severe hemodynamic instability and such dependence on vasopressors is described only once [13]. However, the placement of two dialysis catheters in the jugular vein position may theoretically lead to a recirculation between them, if the tips of the catheters are placed close to each other. The jugular and femoral placement of the catheters will eliminate this possibility.

Substitution with bicarbonate in case of lactic acidosis is controversial as there are concerns that treatment with bicarbonate can increase intracellular acidosis [14]. However, bicarbonate treatment is widely used to stabilise metabolic acidosis in cases of metformin poisoning as described in the literature. We used high doses of bicarbonate as intravenous infusion and highest possible concentration of bicarbonate buffer in the HD machine simultaneously with CVVH with 35 mmol/L bicarbonate in the Accusol 35 (Baxter) replacement fluid. We observed worsening of the acidosis and cardiovascular status when HD was paused and we presume this deterioration to be due to lack of bicarbonate buffer. Renal replacement therapy, including conventional HD and CVVH, offers both theoretical and practical advantages over bicarbonate infusion. These allow for isovolemic correction of the metabolic acidosis while removing metformin and lactate [6].

Recent recommendations for metformin poisoning from the Extracorporeal Treatments in Poisoning Workgroup advocate for intermittent HD, but continuous renal replacement therapies may be considered if HD is unavailable [1]. Initiation of dialysis is suggested in very severe cases, when lactate concentration is >15 mmol/L and pH < 7.0 together with shock or organ failure [1]. In our opinion, these recommendations are more applicable in situations of metformin-associated lactic acidosis, as in acute high dose metformin poisoning the acidosis accelerates very fast and the patient's condition deteriorates dramatically with development of circulatory collapse.

We therefore suggest that in cases of acute high dose metformin poisoning HD should be initiated earlier than that stated in the recommendations.

4. Conclusion

In cases of severe metformin poisoning with shock and extreme lactic acidosis usual CVVH modality might not effectively clear metformin and additional prolonged intermittent HD should be considered instead or together with CVVH, even in the state of cardiovascular collapse with vasopressor requirement.

References

[1] D. P. Calello, K. D. Liu, T. J. Wiegand et al., "Extracorporeal treatment for metformin poisoning: Systematic review and recommendations from the extracorporeal treatments in poisoning workgroup," *Critical Care Medicine*, vol. 43, no. 8, pp. 1716–1730, 2015.

[2] P. Y. F. Guo, L. J. Storsley, and S. N. Finkle, "Severe lactic acidosis treated with prolonged hemodialysis: Recovery after massive overdoses of metformin," *Seminars in Dialysis*, vol. 19, no. 1, pp. 80–83, 2006.

[3] C. J. Bailey and R. C. Turner, "Metformin," *The New England Journal of Medicine*, vol. 334, no. 9, pp. 574–579, 1996.

[4] N. Peters, N. Jay, and D. Barraud, "Metformin-associated lactic acidosis in an intensive care unit," *Critical Care*, vol. 12, no. 6, article R149, 2008.

[5] D. M. Dell'Aglio, L. J. Perino, Z. Kazzi, J. Abramson, M. D. Schwartz, and B. W. Morgan, "Acute metformin overdose: examining serum pH, lactate level, and metformin concentrations in survivors versus nonsurvivors: a systematic review of the literature," *Annals of Emergency Medicine*, vol. 54, no. 6, pp. 818–823, 2009.

[6] K. F. H. Teale, A. Devine, H. Stewart, and N. J. H. Harper, "The management of metformin overdose," *Anaesthesia*, vol. 53, no. 7, pp. 698–701, 1998.

[7] J. D. Lalau, M. Andrejak, P. Moriniere, and et al., "Hemodialysis in the treatment of lactic acidosis in diabetics treated by metformin: a study of metformin elimination," *International Journal of Clinical Pharmacology, Therapy, and Toxicology*, vol. 27, pp. 285–288, 1989.

[8] A. Seidowsky, S. Nseir, N. Houdret, and F. Fourrier, "Metformin-associated lactic acidosis: A prognostic and therapeutic study," *Critical Care Medicine*, vol. 37, no. 7, pp. 2191–2196, 2009.

[9] L. Brochard, F. Abroug, M. Brenner et al., "An official ATS/ERS/ESICM/SCCM/SRLF statement: prevention and management of acute renal failure in the ICU patient: an international consensus conference in intensive care medicine," *American Journal of Respiratory and Critical Care Medicine*, vol. 181, no. 10, pp. 1128–1155, 2010.

[10] B. Harvey, C. Hickman, G. Hinson, T. Ralph, and A. Mayer, "Severe lactic acidosis complicating metformin overdose successfully treated with high-volume venovenous hemofiltration and aggressive alkalinization," *Pediatric Critical Care Medicine*, vol. 6, no. 5, pp. 598–601, 2005.

[11] F. Barrueto, W. J. Meggs, and M. J. Barchman, "Clearance of metformin by hemofiltration in overdose," *Journal of Toxicology - Clinical Toxicology*, vol. 40, no. 2, pp. 177–180, 2002.

[12] U. Panzer, S. Kluge, G. Kreymann, and G. Wolf, "Combination of intermittent haemodialysis and high-volume continuous haemofiltration for the treatment of severe metformin-induced lactic acidosis [5]," *Nephrology Dialysis Transplantation* , vol. 19, no. 8, pp. 2157-2158, 2004.

[13] S. Friesecke, P. Abel, M. Kraft, A. Gerner, and S. Runge, "Combined renal replacement therapy for severe metformin-induced lactic acidosis [18]," *Nephrology Dialysis Transplantation* , vol. 21, no. 7, pp. 2038-2039, 2006.

[14] S. Sabatini and N. A. Kurtzman, "Bicarbonate therapy in severe metabolic acidosis," *Journal of the American Society of Nephrology*, vol. 20, no. 4, pp. 692–695, 2009.

30

Flucytosine Pharmacokinetics in a Critically Ill Patient Receiving Continuous Renal Replacement Therapy

Megan E. Kunka,[1] Elizabeth A. Cady,[1]
Heejung C. Woo,[2] and Melissa L. Thompson Bastin[1]

[1] *University of Kentucky HealthCare, 800 Rose Street, H110, Lexington, KY 40536, USA*
[2] *University of Kentucky, Lexington, KY 40506, USA*

Correspondence should be addressed to Megan E. Kunka; m-kunka@onu.edu

Academic Editor: Caterina Mammina

Purpose. A case report evaluating flucytosine dosing in a critically ill patient receiving continuous renal replacement therapy. *Summary*. This case report outlines an 81-year-old male who was receiving continuous venovenous hemofiltration (CVVH) for acute renal failure and was being treated with flucytosine for the treatment of disseminated *Cryptococcus neoformans* infection. Due to patient specific factors, flucytosine was empirically dose adjusted approximately 50% lower than intermittent hemodialysis (iHD) recommendations and approximately 33% lower than CRRT recommendations. Peak and trough levels were obtained, which were supratherapeutic, and pharmacokinetic parameters were calculated. The patient experienced thrombocytopenia, likely due to elevated flucytosine levels, and flucytosine was ultimately discontinued. *Conclusion*. Despite conservative flucytosine dosing for a patient receiving CVVH, peak and trough serum flucytosine levels were supratherapeutic (120 μg/mL at 2 hours and 81 μg/mL at 11.5 hours), which increased drug-related adverse effects. The results indicate that this conservative dosing regimen utilizing the patient's actual body weight was too aggressive. This case report provides insight into flucytosine dosing in CVVH, a topic that has not been investigated previously. Further pharmacokinetic studies of flucytosine dosing in critically ill patients receiving CVVH are needed in order to optimize pharmacokinetic and pharmacodynamic parameters while avoiding toxic flucytosine exposure.

1. Background

Amphotericin and flucytosine are the first-line agents for the treatment of cryptococcal meningoencephalitis [1]. Dosing of flucytosine is weight based and is typically 25 mg/kg/dose every 6 hours for at least 4 weeks for cryptococcal meningoencephalitis in non-HIV infected, nontransplant patients. A shorter, two-week course of induction therapy may be considered for patients who have low risk of therapeutic failure, who were previously healthy with no underlying, uncontrolled disease states, and who have had an excellent clinical response to the initial two-week combination. Six weeks of induction therapy may be required in patients with neurological complications. Consolidation and then maintenance therapy are recommended following the induction stage, for a total of 6–12 months of treatment. The Infectious Diseases Society of America (IDSA) Guidelines elaborate on numerous caveats in the event that patients are unable to tolerate the first-line antifungal combination for cryptococcal infections.

Regarding flucytosine dosing in patients with severe renal impairment requiring renal replacement therapy, limited evidence exists regarding the appropriate dosing. In fact, a boxed warning, a caution issued by the U.S. Food and Drug Administration (FDA) regarding serious adverse drug reactions, suggests extreme caution be utilized if flucytosine is warranted in patients with renal dysfunction [2].

Flucytosine (5-fluorocytosine; 5-FC) is one of the oldest antifungal agents on the market. Initially synthesized in 1957 as a potential antitumor agent, flucytosine was later approved to treat human candidiasis and cryptococcosis [3]. Flucytosine penetrates susceptible fungal cells where it is converted to fluorouracil (5-FU) via the enzyme cytosine deaminase [2–4]. Fluorouracil is converted into several active metabolites

TABLE 1: Flucytosine dosing recommendations in renal impairment[a] [3, 5, 8–10].

Flucytosine dosing of 100 mg/kg/day (normal renal function)		Flucytosine dosing of 150 mg/kg/day (normal renal function)	
CrCL (mL/min)	Dose	CrCL (mL/min)	Dose
>50	25 mg/kg every 6 hours	>40, >50	37.5 mg/kg every 6 hours
10–50	25 mg/kg every 12–24 hours	20–40, 10–50	37.5 mg/kg every 12–24 hours
<10	25 mg/kg every 24–48 hours	<20, <10	37.5 mg/kg every 24–48 hours
Hemodialysis	Single, supplemental doses of 20–50 mg/kg after dialysis sessions	Hemodialysis	Single, supplemental doses after dialysis sessions
CRRT	No specific recommendations	CRRT	CVVHD/CVVH: 37.5 mg/kg every 12–24 hours

[a]CrCL: creatinine clearance, CRRT: continuous renal replacement therapy, and CVVHD/CVVH: continuous venovenous hemodialysis/continuous venovenous hemofiltration.

that falsely incorporate into the fungal RNA or interfere with fungal DNA, ultimately inhibiting fungal protein synthesis [2]. Flucytosine is readily absorbed with a bioavailability of 75–90% following oral administration [5, 6]. In the United States, flucytosine is only available in oral capsule dosage form (250 mg, 500 mg capsules) [2]. Due to the high water solubility, flucytosine is not well distributed into adipose tissues, with a volume of distribution range of 0.6–0.9 L/kg at steady state [6–9]. Due to the limited distribution, dosing in obese patients should be based upon ideal body weight [4]. Distribution sites of flucytosine include the cerebrospinal fluid (CSF), aqueous humor, joints, and peritoneal fluid. In fact, CSF concentrations can reach up to 60–90% of serum flucytosine concentrations [5]. Flucytosine is minimally protein bound, approximately 2–4%, and it undergoes minimal hepatic metabolism with more than 90% of the drug excreted unchanged in the urine, resulting in the need for renal dosage adjustments [4, 5]. The elimination half-life of flucytosine is typically 2–5 hours in patients with normal renal function; however, the half-life can increase up to 250 hours in patients with end stage renal disease or patients who are anuric [9]. No specific renal dose adjustment is recommended per the package insert directly, but the manufacturer recommends dose reduction in patients with impaired renal function. In patients receiving intermittent hemodialysis (iHD), it is recommended to administer flucytosine after dialysis, as flucytosine is dialyzable [8, 9]. Data for dosing flucytosine in continuous renal replacement therapy are scarce. See Table 1 for flucytosine dosing recommendations, which are dependent upon flucytosine total daily dose of either 100 mg/kg or 150 mg/kg [8, 9]. Utilizing recommended dose adjustments is pertinent, as flucytosine is associated with potentially severe adverse effects. Hepatotoxicity and bone marrow suppression (agranulocytosis, aplastic anemia, leukopenia, pancytopenia, and thrombocytopenia) are life-threatening conditions that can occur as a result of flucytosine therapy, which limits use in certain patients. Additional adverse effects of flucytosine include cardiac toxicity, central nervous system toxicity, and renal abnormalities.

In vivo studies indicate time above minimum inhibitory concentration (MIC) is the pharmacodynamic parameter most correlated to outcome with flucytosine monotherapy [3, 4]. Peak flucytosine efficacy has been reported at serum concentrations four times the MIC [6, 7]. The standard flucytosine dose of 100–150 mg/kg/day in non-HIV infected patients targets serum concentrations of ten times the MIC breakpoint of 4 μg/mL. This suggests that much higher serum flucytosine concentrations are being obtained than required for optimal efficacy.

Current data suggest obtaining a peak flucytosine level once at steady state (after 3-5 doses), 2 hours after the oral dose [6]. Based on available literature, the peak flucytosine level should be 30–100 μg/mL for the treatment of cryptococcal infections, and target flucytosine trough levels should be 25–50 μg/mL [3, 4]. Flucytosine concentrations above 100 μg/mL should be avoided, as levels that elevated have been associated with a greater incidence of thrombocytopenia and elevated liver enzymes [3, 4]. A general recommendation is to maintain flucytosine levels above 25 μg/mL, but under 100 μg/mL, in order to optimize pharmacodynamic parameters and avoid toxicity, although other sources suggest steady-state serum flucytosine goal ranges of 50–100 μg/mL [4, 5].

The mode of renal replacement therapy plays a major role in the amount and type of medications that are removed during the dialysis session.

Key factors that determine the amount of drug removed by CVVH are surface area of the filter, type of filter, blood flow rate, replacement fluid rate, and location of replacement fluid entry, prefilter or postfilter [10]. Drugs that are readily cleared by CVVH are of low molecular weight, <500 Daltons, and low protein binding, <80% protein bound, with a small volume of distribution (Vd) ≤0.7 L/kg [11]. Flucytosine's pharmacokinetic properties mostly match that of drugs readily cleared by dialysis, as it is 129.1 Daltons in molecular weight and only 3-4% protein bound; however, the Vd has been reported as up to 0.9 L/kg in some studies (0.6–0.9 L/kg), which may limit the amount of drug available to be removed by convection.

2. Case Report

An 81-year-old Caucasian male presented to the emergency department with shortness of breath and hemoptysis. Over the previous one to two months, the patient experienced fatigue and increasing shortness of breath. Episodes of hemoptysis were two to four times per day. His past medical history included ureteral and bladder cancer, recurrence of papillary tumor and prostatic urethra status after right nephroureterectomy and chemotherapy, deep vein thrombosis, hypertension, type 2 diabetes mellitus, and hypothyroidism. Regarding social history, the patient farmed full-time in his retirement, and he had recently cleaned out his chicken coop, which contained several months of built-up feces and straw bedding.

Upon admission, initial laboratory values included sodium 143 mEq/L, potassium 4.2 mEq/L, chloride 106 mEq/L, blood urea nitrogen 58 mg/L, creatinine 4.29 mg/dL, glucose 118 mg/dL, white blood cell count $9.7 \times 10^3/mm^3$, hemoglobin 6.4 g/dL, and platelet count $169 \times 10^3/mm^3$. Liver function test values were alanine aminotransferase 6 U/L, aspartate aminotransferase 13 U/L, and alkaline phosphatase 55 U/L. The patient was on warfarin for deep vein thrombosis, and anticoagulation results indicated prothrombin time (PT) 108.2 seconds, international normalized ratio (INR) 9.6, and activated partial thromboplastin time (aPTT) 49 seconds.

Numerous other laboratory tests were completed, including cytoplasmic anti-neutrophil cytoplasmic antibodies (c-ANCA), perinuclear anti-neutrophil cytoplasmic antibodies (p-ANCA), glomerular basement membrane antibody IgG, urine *Histoplasma*/*Legionella*/*Streptococcus pneumoniae* antigens, QuantiFERON tuberculosis gold, and beta-glucan. All of these tests were negative. Of note, beta-glucan test does not reliably detect *Cryptococcus*, Zygomycetes, or *Blastomyces dermatitidis*. Abnormal laboratory values included c-reactive protein 8.9 mg/dL, automated sedimentation rate >120 mm/hr, N-terminal pro-brain natriuretic peptide (NT-proBNP) 9,789 pg/mL, and troponin T 0.106 ng/mL.

The initial differential diagnosis and assessment included inflammatory pneumonitis, infection, and immunologic pathology. The patient was initiated on ceftriaxone and azithromycin, and a respiratory culture was obtained. Throughout the initial hospital course, his oxygen saturation dropped on a nonrebreather mask, and the patient was agreeable to elective intubation with bronchoscopy. Antibiotics were broadened to levofloxacin, piperacillin/tazobactam, and vancomycin, and corticosteroids were added. Cystogram was completed per urology which showed reflux with nonobstructive hydronephrosis, and nephrology was consulted to rule out other causes of the patient's acute kidney injury, none of which were definitive diagnoses. On hospital day 19, the patient's blood cultures were positive for yeast, which was presumed to be *Cryptococcus neoformans*, and liposomal amphotericin B 300 mg (3.1 mg/kg actual body weight) daily was initiated. On hospital day 23, *Cryptococcus neoformans* was identified in the blood via matrix assisted laser desorption/ionization-time-of-flight (MALDI-TOF) mass spectrometry and confirmed via a biochemical method (API 20C strip). A lumbar puncture was completed which also grew *Cryptococcus neoformans*. Flucytosine was initiated on day five of liposomal amphotericin B treatment (hospital day 23).

As the patient was receiving intermittent hemodialysis at the time of flucytosine initiation, a dose of 2,500 mg (25.8 mg/kg actual body weight) every Tuesday, Thursday, and Saturday after dialysis sessions was chosen. See Table 2 for a schedule of the hemodialysis sessions the patient received. On hospital day 27, the patient was initiated on continuous renal replacement therapy due to hemodynamic instability with the addition of multiple vasopressors (norepinephrine, phenylephrine, and vasopressin). The patient remained intubated, sedated, and paralyzed for facilitation of mechanical ventilation. Continuous venovenous hemofiltration (CVVH) was initiated (with citrate for anticoagulation) as the primary mode of dialysis and was maintained on the following settings: total replacement fluid rate, 2,500 mL/hr; blood flow rate, 300 mL/min; preblood pump rate (PBP) (citrate flow rate), 450 mL/hr; and ultrafiltration rate, 100–400 mL/hr. Our institution utilizes the Gambro PrismaSATE system with the PrismaSATE HF 1400 polyarylethersulfone filter. Due to inability to ultrafiltrate with CRRT at all times, the average fluid removal rate was 265 mL/day (11 mL/hr) over 3 days (hospital days 27–29).

Table 2: Hemodialysis sessions and corresponding flucytosine administrations.

Hospital day	Event
14	Intermittent hemodialysis session
18	Intermittent hemodialysis session
20	Partial intermittent hemodialysis session
22	Intermittent hemodialysis session
23	Flucytosine 2,500 mg given
25	Intermittent hemodialysis session Flucytosine 2,500 mg given

As a result of the dialysis change to CVVH, the flucytosine dose was increased to 2,500 mg (25.8 mg/kg actual body weight) by mouth every 12 hours. Of note, this flucytosine dose was significantly conservative, as it utilized a total daily dose of 50 mg/kg/day, as compared to some literature that recommends up to 150 mg/kg/day divided. The choice for conservative flucytosine dosing was made based on the patient's baseline thrombocytopenia; the patient's platelet count was $39 \times 10^3/mm^3$ the day CVVH was initiated. Over the 3 days of CVVH, the patient had a mean urine output of approximately 0.21 mL/kg/day, classified as nonoliguric renal failure.

Flucytosine was discontinued on hospital day 29 due to thrombocytopenia, and high dose fluconazole was added. Liposomal amphotericin was replaced with conventional amphotericin on hospital day 37. The patient had negative blood cultures on hospital days 32 and 34.

The patient passed away on hospital day 47 from refractory hypoxemic respiratory failure, as life prolonging efforts were withdrawn per family request.

3. Methods

As the patient was overweight and not quite obese (body mass index, 29.7 kg/m^2), flucytosine dosing was based upon the patient's actual body weight of 97 kg. The patient was initiated on flucytosine 2,500 mg by mouth every 12 hours on hospital day 27. An initial flucytosine level was ordered without regard to scheduled flucytosine doses (2 hours prior to the dose while the patient was receiving CVVH), and it resulted at 90 μg/mL (hospital day 28). Peak and trough flucytosine levels were obtained after the fifth dose of the CVVH flucytosine regimen. Of note, prior to that, the patient had received three doses of flucytosine 2,500 mg after intermittent hemodialysis sessions. The peak level was obtained two hours after the fifth dose of flucytosine, and the trough level was obtained 30 minutes prior to the next scheduled dose of flucytosine (11.5 hours after the previously administered dose). These peak and trough levels were obtained on hospital day 29, but the results were not reported until hospital day 38. Due to the thrombocytopenic toxicity of flucytosine experienced by the patient, flucytosine was discontinued on hospital day 29, prior to the results of the peak and trough levels.

4. Results

The patient's flucytosine peak level resulted at 120 μg/mL, and the flucytosine trough level was 81 μg/mL. Pharmacokinetic calculations indicate an elimination rate constant (ke) of 0.04 hr^{-1}, with a half-life ($t1/2$) of 16.75 hours [12]. The volume of distribution was 48.1–57.7 L (0.50–0.59 L/kg, range based on bioavailability of 75–90%), the area under the curve (AUC) was 2,980 μg·hr/mL, and the total clearance was 1,924–2,308 mL/hr (range based on bioavailability of 75–90%). The minimum inhibitory concentration (MIC) for flucytosine was reported as 2 μg/mL; however, it was noted that no Clinical Laboratory Standards Institute (CLSI) range exists for flucytosine and *Cryptococcus neoformans* for susceptibility interpretation. Results of the MIC are for research use only. The patient's serum flucytosine concentrations were well above the concentration associated with peak flucytosine efficacy, four times the MIC or 8 μg/mL.

Figure 1 depicts the patient's flucytosine concentrations.

As a result of the patient's declining platelet count, flucytosine was discontinued on hospital day 29 (platelet count of 26 × 10^3/mm^3), 48 hours after CVVH was initiated. Figure 2 depicts the platelet count trend for the patient. The nadir platelet count was 15 × 10^3/mm^3, which occurred on hospital day 31, 9 days after initiation of flucytosine. The patient was receiving concomitant medications that could contribute to thrombocytopenia during this time, including amphotericin, cefepime, famotidine, metronidazole, and vancomycin.

Despite the elevated flucytosine levels, the patient did not experience any hepatotoxicity. In fact, the patient's liver function tests throughout the course of his stay were lower than or within normal range.

5. Discussion

The patient described above had a supratherapeutic flucytosine peak concentration of >100 μg/mL and higher than expected levels overall. Potential reasons for the higher flucytosine levels include potential accumulation of flucytosine during the hemodialysis period, limited fluid removal from CVVH, and limited time receiving CVVH before flucytosine discontinuation (<72 hours). The initial flucytosine level of

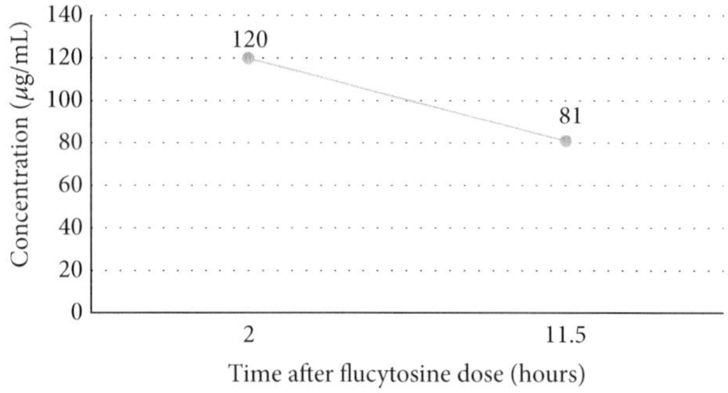

FIGURE 1: Flucytosine concentration versus time.

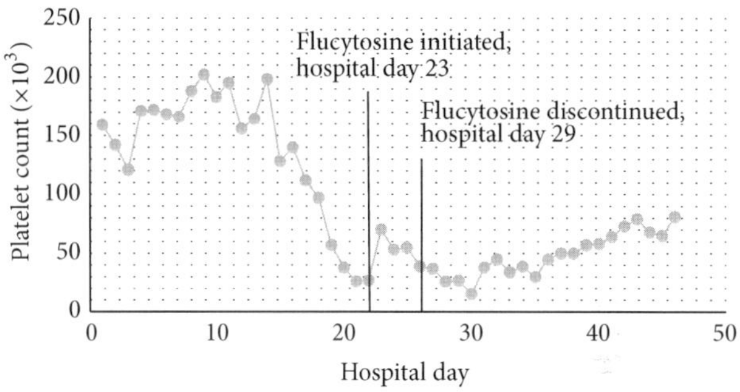

FIGURE 2: Platelet count trend.

90 μg/mL, albeit drawn 2 hours prior to the flucytosine dose, indicates that the patient was likely accumulating flucytosine while receiving intermittent hemodialysis, as this level was obtained after only 4 flucytosine doses (2 iHD doses and 2 CRRT doses). As the method of CVVH utilizes a convection-only method of solute removal, this may have limited the flucytosine removal and resulted in higher than expected flucytosine levels. Flucytosine has a small molecular weight (129.1 Daltons), which could explain the lower flucytosine clearance seen with convection, as low molecular weight solute is more efficiently removed by diffusion modalities such as continuous venovenous hemodialysis (CVVHD) or iHD.

Another potential reason for the flucytosine toxicity is the use of the patient's actual body weight for flucytosine dosing. Although the patient was not technically obese, the patient was overweight, and potentially utilizing adjusted (80 kg) or ideal body weight (75 kg) would have resulted in therapeutic flucytosine levels. Dodds and colleagues suggest utilizing ideal body weight in obese patients; however, limited literature exists regarding the weight utilized for flucytosine dosing in patients who are overweight, and consensus does not exist.

The patient was receiving multiple vasopressors as well as trophic tube feeds during the time of flucytosine administration and CVVH. Food decreases the rate of flucytosine absorption, but it does not impact the extent of absorption [5]. Therefore, we believe the trophic tube feeds had minimal impact on the patient's flucytosine concentrations.

In comparing the patient-specific flucytosine pharmacokinetics to what is documented in the literature, the patient had a lower volume of distribution (0.50–0.59 L/kg) than the general population (0.6–0.9 L/kg). Our observed reduced volume of distribution offers no explanation as to the reduced flucytosine clearance.

As this is the first published case of its kind regarding flucytosine dosing in CVVH, we believe our findings make a significant contribution to the critical care literature.

6. Conclusion

Flucytosine is recommended as a component of the first-line antifungal combination for the treatment of cryptococcal infections. Despite its use for many years, optimizing flucytosine dosing in critically ill patients on renal replacement therapy remains difficult, as clinical data are lacking in this patient population. In our patient summarized above, the total clearance of flucytosine by CVVH was less than expected and resulted in significant hematologic toxicities, warranting drug discontinuation. Our patient experienced significant toxicities related to the supratherapeutic flucytosine levels, even though the empiric dosing regimen was conservative, approximately 1/2 the recommended iHD dose and 1/3 the recommended CRRT dose [3, 5, 8–10]. As the patient was overweight, yet not obese, potentially utilizing a lower dosing regimen with the patient's adjusted or ideal body weight would have resulted in therapeutic serum levels and reduced the risk of toxicity. As flucytosine is a mainstay of treatment for patients with severe cryptococcal disease, it is paramount that dosing recommendations more accurately reflect the real world experience with CRRT dosing. This case report provides insight into flucytosine dosing in CVVH, a topic that has not been investigated previously in the literature. Additional pharmacokinetic studies are needed to further explore the pharmacokinetics of flucytosine removal with CVVH, as the dosing regimens currently recommended may be supratherapeutic and result in unwanted toxicities.

References

[1] J. R. Perfect, W. E. Dismukes, F. Dromer et al., "Clinical practice guidelines for the management of cryptococcal disease: 2010 update by the infectious diseases society of America," *Clinical Infectious Diseases*, vol. 50, no. 3, pp. 291–322, 2010.

[2] *Ancobon (Flucytosine) Package Insert*, Valeant Pharmaceuticals, Bridgewater, NJ, USA, 2013.

[3] A. Vermes, H.-J. Guchelaar, and J. Dankert, "Flucytosine: a review of its pharmacology, clinical indications, pharmacokinetics, toxicity and drug interactions," *Journal of Antimicrobial Chemotherapy*, vol. 46, no. 2, pp. 171–179, 2000.

[4] M. I. Goodwin and R. H. Drew, "Antifungal serum concentration monitoring: an update," *Journal of Antimicrobial Chemotherapy*, vol. 61, no. 1, pp. 17–25, 2008.

[5] *Clinical Pharmacology [Online Database]*, Gold Standard, Tampa, Fla, USA, 2014.

[6] E. S. Dodds, R. H. Drew, and J. R. Perfect, "Antifungal pharmacodynamics: review of the literature and clinical applications," *Pharmacotherapy*, vol. 20, no. 11, pp. 1335–1355, 2000.

[7] J. W. Baddley and P. G. Pappas, "Antifungal combination therapy: clinical potential," *Drugs*, vol. 65, no. 11, pp. 1461–1480, 2005.

[8] Truven Health Analytics, "Flucytosine [monograph]," in *Micromedex Drudex [Online Database]*, Truven Health Analytics, Greenwood Village, Colo, USA, 2014.

[9] Lexi-Comp, "Flucytosine [monograph]," in *Lexicomp Online [Online Database]*, Lexi-Comp, Hudson, Ohio, USA, 2014.

[10] D. Kuang and C. Ronco, "Adjustment of antimicrobial regimen in critically ill patients undergoing continuous renal replacement therapy," in *Intensive Care Medicine*, vol. 2007 of *Yearbook of Intensive Care and Emergency Medicine*, pp. 592–606, Springer, Berlin, Germany, 2007.

[11] B. H. Heintz, G. R. Matzke, and W. E. Dager, "Antimicrobial dosing concepts and recommendations for critically Ill adult patients receiving continuous renal replacement therapy or intermittent hemodialysis," *Pharmacotherapy*, vol. 29, no. 5, pp. 562–577, 2009.

[12] M. E. Winter, *Basic Clinical Pharmacokinetics*, Lippincott Williams & Wilkins, Philadelphia, Pa, USA, 4th edition, 2004.

31

Anabolic Steroid use for Weight and Strength Gain in Critically Ill Patients

Matthew Anstey,[1,2] Shilpa Desai,[1] Luke Torre,[1] Bradley Wibrow,[1,2] Jason Seet,[1] and Emma Osnain[1]

[1] *Sir Charles Gairdner Hospital, Nedlands, WA, Australia*
[2] *School of Medicine, University of Western Australia, Crawley, WA, Australia*

Correspondence should be addressed to Matthew Anstey; matthew.anstey@health.wa.gov.au

Academic Editor: Petros Kopterides

Background. An important long-term complication of critical illness is significant weakness and its resulting functional impairment. Recent advances have aimed to prevent critical illness weakness via early mobilisation of patients, minimising sedation, and optimising nutrition. One other potential treatment may be to provide anabolic support in the recovery phase, especially as patients have decreased levels of anabolic hormones. *Case Presentation.* We describe a case series of 4 patients who had either (1) profound critical illness myopathy and (2) profound weight loss. All patients were already receiving appropriate nutritional support and physiotherapy. All patients had functional improvements in their muscle strength. *Conclusions.* For patients in the recovery phase of critical illness, we provide examples of when anabolic steroid supplementation may assist the treating clinicians in rehabilitating their patients who are still in the Intensive Care Unit. We discuss patient selection and the current supporting literature for anabolic supplementation in critically ill patients.

1. Background

An important long-term complication of critical illness is significant weakness and its resulting functional impairment [1]. The mechanisms leading to profound weakness are diverse but include catabolism due to caloric deficits, increased stress hormone production, prolonged immobility, and inflammation causing myoneuropathy [2]. These result in structural changes that include axonal nerve degeneration, muscle myosin loss, and muscle necrosis [3]. Recent advances have aimed to prevent critical illness weakness via early mobilisation of patients, minimising sedation, and optimising nutrition [2, 4–6]. One other potential treatment may be to provide anabolic support in the recovery phase [4]. Low testosterone levels are frequent in critically ill patients [5, 7, 8]. This may reflect hormonal dysregulation in acute illness, as is seen with other hormones (insulin, cortisol). However, hypotestosteronaemia after acute illness may contribute to impaired recovery and rehabilitation. Testosterone supplementation in older healthy men has been shown to have benefits on physical functioning, including improved fat-free mass and muscle strength [9, 10].

We describe a case series of patients for whom we prescribed a course of anabolic steroids for one of the following indications: (1) profound weakness or (2) significant weight loss. All patients were already receiving sufficient nutritional support (at least 3 days of caloric intake at estimated goal) and were engaging in physiotherapy (graded rehabilitation according to optimal mobility scale) [11].

Anabolic steroids have two main properties: androgenic and anabolic effects. The different mechanisms include modulation of androgen receptor expression and interference of glucocorticoid receptor expression, which results in an anti-catabolic effect. The most common androgen is testosterone, which exerts its effects by directly binding with the androgen receptors. Testosterone also undergoes metabolism via the aromatase or 5-α reductase enzymes to convert to oestradiol and 5-α-dihydrotestosterone, respectively. Many synthetic or designer anabolic steroids have had modifications to the testosterone structure to maximise the anabolic properties,

Table 1: Overview of indications and results of anabolic steroid supplementation.

	Indication for anabolic steroids	Date of first dose administered	Testosterone level before administration	Weight change after administration	Grip strength change	Strength change
Patient 1	Profound critical illness weakness	Day 32 of ICU stay	0.6 nmol/L (<2.0 nmol/L)	*+7.3 kg* 45 kg (22/4) → 52.3 (15/5)	(L) +4.4 kg (R) +6 kg	*From* 1/5 power globally *to* ambulation with minimal assist on discharge
Patient 2	Profound critical illness weakness	Day 82 of ICU stay	5.7 nmol/L (1035 nmol/L)	*−3.8 kg* 115.8 kg (3/9) → 112 (17/9)	(L) −0.6 kg (R) +5.7 kg	*From* profound generalised weakness (0-1/5) *to* multiple repetitions of assisted sitting to stand exercises and tracheostomy decannulation
Patient 3	Profound critical illness weakness	Day 30 of ICU stay	Not available	*+1.5 kg* 72.5 kg (23/5) → 74 kg (26/5)	Grip strengths not assessed	*From* profound weakness (flicker contraction 1/5) *to* increased strength in all muscle groups (3-4/5)
Patient 4	Long-term malnutrition and inability to gain weight or strength	Day 70 of admission and ICU review for ongoing TPN/nutritional advice	6.5 nmol/L (10–35 nmol/L)	*+4.4 kg*	(L) −3.6 kg (R) −3.4 kg	Power globally 3/5. *From* fatigue on transfers *to* ambulating independently for very short distances with frame

Handgrip threshold of 11 kg force in males and 7 kg force in females for the diagnosis of ICU acquired weakness (sensitivity 80.6%, specificity 83.2%, NPV 92.3%, and PPV 63.0%) [13].

while attempting to eliminate the androgenic effects. Such changes enhance protein anabolic effects and thus present themselves as potential therapeutic options for the restoration of fat-free muscle mass, and strength in chronic illnesses or conditions including critical illness related myopathy. In our first patient, we used testosterone due to an inability to obtain nandrolone. Testosterone possesses a relatively balanced ratio of myotrophic to androgenic activity (0.7–1.3), which means more virilizing effects for women, potential aggression, and negative impact on cholesterol levels. Danazol is an isoxazole of testosterone with weak androgenic activity and no oestrogenic activity. Alternative anabolic agents such as nandrolone or oxandrolone exhibit significantly greater selectivity for myotropic properties, with minimal androgenic effects (myotrophic : androgenic activity ratio of 12 and 13, resp.) [12]. Consequently, the potential for adverse outcomes including aromatization and virilizing effects in women is minimised.

Patients were considered for participation if they had profound weight loss or muscle loss as a result of their illness or Intensive Care Unit (ICU) admission and were in the recovery phase and failing to make progress. Consent to receive the medication was obtained from the patient, and an individual patient approval was obtained for our hospital pharmacy. All patients consented to publication of these results. Table 1 outlines the indications and results of anabolic steroid supplementation for these patients.

2. Case Presentations

2.1. Patient 1. A 23-year-old lady was admitted to the ICU with respiratory distress requiring emergent intubation on 25 March 2014. She was being managed on the ward for bilateral infected leg ulcers, on a background of systemic lupus erythematous (SLE), hypertension, rheumatic fever, chronic renal failure, microscopic haemolytic anaemia, and extensive oesophageal ulceration. Her admission weight was 60.5 kg.

The cause of her respiratory failure was invasive aspergillosis and CMV pneumonitis. This was further complicated by microangiopathic haemolytic anaemia and thrombocytopenia thrombotic purpura requiring plasmapheresis, liver dysfunction, and renal failure requiring continuous renal replacement therapy. A percutaneous tracheostomy was performed on day 10 of her ICU admission. By day 22, she had lost > 25% weight from admission despite provision of enteral nutritional support aimed at 120% of predicted caloric requirements. She was clinically severely deconditioned (serum albumin 22) with evidence of fat and muscle wasting, undergoing a protracted wean from the ventilator (on day 30 she was still receiving pressure support ventilation 12/5 and transitioned to T-piece ventilation trials on day 31), and globally weak with 1-2/5 power throughout.

She was commenced on testosterone (Sustanon®) 250 mg IM on day 32. Subjectively her appetite improved as did her ventilator weaning and she was decannulated 3 days after the first dose. After further consultation with the immunology team, the Sustanon was replaced by 200 mg danazol daily from day 43 due to improved safety in SLE. Upon discharge to the ward (day 46), her upper limb strength had improved to 3-4/5 bilaterally and 2/5 power in the lower limbs. She was able to move from supine to standing with minimal assistance and continued with tilt table for strengthening and stretching. After 3 weeks of rehabilitation on the ward, she could walk approximately 20 m unassisted with a frame. She was subsequently transferred to a rehabilitation unit on day 62 and discharged home on day 73, after 30 doses of danazol.

2.2. Patient 2. A 62-year-old male presented to the Emergency Department on 14 June 2015 with fevers and rigors, 5 days after a complex transoesophageal AF ablation (admission weight 139 kg). Following a brief cardiac arrest on the coronary care unit, a CT chest revealed an oesophageal perforation and atrio-oesophageal fistula. He underwent urgent repair of the left atrio-oesophageal fistula. Postoperatively he developed mediastinitis and vasopressor dependent shock. On day 8, he developed severe abdominal pain and had a right hemicolectomy and ileostomy for caecal perforation. Following these complications, he was severely deconditioned (critical illness myopathy was evident from day 9) and received a tracheostomy on day 16. Despite optimal nutritional supplementation, he was losing weight (at one point he lost 6 kg weight in one week, and from admission weight to time of administration he had lost 16.6% of admission weight) with evidence of fat and muscle wasting. Due to the profound weakness in all limbs, an electromyogram (EMG) was performed on day 39, which was consistent with severe critical illness myopathy and mild axonal degeneration neuropathy.

He was prescribed nandrolone 50 mg IMI on day 82. At this point, despite daily physiotherapy throughout his stay, he required full hoist transfers. At the time of his second injection (day 90) his strength was dramatically improving with 3-4/5 power throughout. Serial testosterone measurements decreased from 10 before first dose to 5.7 before the second dose and 7.3 before the third dose. Although he still required full hoist for transfers, he could perform up to 6 reps of sitting to standing with ArjoHoist®. He was also able to sit unassisted for 30 minutes. On day 95 he was transferred to a rehabilitation unit and received his third dose of nandrolone the following day. He eventually flew back to Queensland (his home) and received ongoing rehabilitation and strengthening at a local hospital.

2.3. Patient 3. A 49-year-old male was admitted on 7 April 2015 with worsening abdominal pain on a background of known diverticulitis and colovesical fistula. After an initial anterior resection and cystectomy, he returned to theatre a further 5 times due to anastomotic breakdown and faecal peritonitis. He also developed multiorgan failure as a result of septic shock.

During his ICU stay, he lost approximately 16 kg (17% of admission weight) over 2 months, despite adequate parenteral and enteral feeding. In addition, he had overwhelming critical illness weakness with severe limb weakness. On day 29 after admission, he required pressure support ventilation via his tracheostomy and had only a flicker of movement in his limbs distally. He was given 50 mg IMI of nandrolone. One week later prior to receiving his second dose, he no longer required ventilatory assistance, and his power was measured at 2/5 on the left side of his body and 2+ on the right. He received subsequent doses on days 36 and 48.

At day 46, he was sitting on the edge of the bed with assistance and on day 48 he could walk a few assisted steps with a frame. His tracheostomy was removed on day 51. He was discharged from ICU on the 2 June (54 days after admission) with muscle power measured at 4/5 bilaterally (3/5 ankle/toes). On discharge from hospital on day 85 he was able to independently move, including up and down a flight of stairs.

2.4. Patient 4. A 70-year-old male, with a background of colonic cancer resection (1997) and recurrent small bowel obstructions (SBO), was admitted on 10 July 2015 with another SBO. During this admission, his weight dropped to 42 kg (BMI 13.5 kg/m2) with evidence of severe fat and muscle wasting. The weight loss was attributed to severe malnutrition related to chronic poor oral intake. He was commenced on total parenteral nutrition (TPN) after failed enteral feeding. Dexamethasone and mirtazapine were trialled as appetite stimulants, but he developed further obstruction which was managed conservatively.

He was severely deconditioned and had not been able to move out of bed for the first 20 days of admission due to profound weakness. He was not receiving mechanical ventilation. He was severely fatigued on transfer to the commode or shower and had 3/5 power throughout his limbs. He was able to ambulate less than 10 m with a frame. Nandrolone 50 mg IMI was prescribed to assist predominantly with weight gain, but also with deconditioning. He received his first dose on day 60 and a subsequent dose on day 69. He gained 4.5 kg following his first dose and was able to ambulate independently for gradually increasing short distances with a frame. He was discharged on day 89 with home TPN and rehabilitation in the home.

3. Discussion and Conclusions

In each of the cases presented, despite attempts to optimise their nutrition and physical rehabilitation, there was limited improvement. As a result, the treating team chose to trial anabolic steroids as an adjunct to standard care. The loss of lean body mass in critical illness is associated with misalignment between catabolic and anabolic hormones. Correcting this imbalance with hormonal therapy such as anabolic steroids could increase weight and improve nitrogen balance, respiratory muscle strength, and potential survival. It is important to note that the types of patients described, although not frequent in the Intensive Care Unit, do have extremely long stays in the ICU and use a large number of resources. Reducing that burden has significant implications for the ICU, its staff, and the patient.

For all of the patients involved, we were careful to ensure that the patient was in the recovery phase of illness. We defined this as no ongoing organ support (such as needing vasopressors or inotropes), with no increasing inflammatory markers. Low testosterone levels, while frequently seen, may actually serve as an energy conservation mechanism for the body under stress. In addition, we are aware that most patients in the recovery phase after critical illness will regain their muscle strength, especially with the addition of early mobility programs, but this can be an extremely slow process [11, 14, 15]. For this reason, we would also consider using anabolic steroids to assist with patients suffering a protracted ventilator wean.

As a caution, the literature suggests that there may be several contraindications to hormonal supplementation in the critically ill, apart from the listed contraindications (prostate cancer, liver disease, pregnancy, prepubescent). A previous randomised controlled trial using growth hormone found an increased mortality [16]. It may be that, during the state of critical illness, hormonal supplementation may be proinflammatory or misdirects protein synthesis to protein building rather than immune function. Furthermore, an observational study suggests an association between testosterone supplementation and increased cardiac events [17]. Just as athletes have used performance enhancing supplements in conjunction with strength training and nutritional supplementation, it is essential that our patients have sufficient nutritional stores to build muscle and that they are able to interact with a rehabilitation program. Thus, we selected our patients for anabolic steroid therapy if they were stable, which was defined as having no evidence of ongoing sepsis (no fevers, increasing inflammatory markers, or broad spectrum antibiotics) or heart disease (no recent myocardial infarction and ejection fraction > 35%); myopathic; adequately awake to participate in rehabilitation/physiotherapy; and receiving sufficient nutrition to make muscle.

The choice of dose was based on a literature review. Nandrolone has been used in a variety of doses and settings. Outpatient HIV patients with HIV wasting syndrome were given 150 mg fortnightly in one study and 200/400/600 mg weekly in another study for 12 weeks. In both studies the intervention was associated with weight gain [18, 19]. A randomised comparison of nandrolone, testosterone, or placebo for adult HIV patients with HIV wasting syndrome showed superior weight gain and improvement in BMI and quality of life from nandrolone [20]. Patients with COPD were given 50 mg fortnightly for 4 doses with improvement of muscle function and exercise capacity. Patients with chronic renal failure on haemodialysis were given nandrolone (100 mg females, 200 mg males) and undertook resistance training weekly for 6 months with improvement in functional activities (walking and stair-climbing), but no difference in grip strength between groups [21]. The study closest to our case series was a pilot study giving 50 mg of nandrolone weekly for 3 weeks to critically ill patients which resulted in positive nitrogen balance in 8/10 patients [22]. Interestingly, in patient 2 we were able to measure sequential testosterone levels, which actually showed a decrease in levels, which has been previously shown, as nandrolone may reduce endogenous testosterone production [20].

Our results need to be interpreted with caution. There are multiple factors at play in the recovery of a critically ill patient, such as nutritional supplementation, ongoing low grade illness, dose of physical rehabilitation, and the patient's baseline health. While most of our outcome indicators suggest an improvement, it may be that these achievements would have happened regardless of the anabolic supplementation. For instance, patient 1 was undergoing a protracted ventilatory wean but was making some progress and while the anabolic supplementation may have accelerated this, it is also possible it made no difference. Changes in weight in these patients may reflect fluid shifts (especially in those on dialysis), and lean body mass or estimation of muscle thickness may have been better outcome variables [23]. Handgrip strength is independently associated with poor hospital outcome and serves as a simple test to identify ICU acquired weakness, but with asymmetric weakness it may not be the best measure [13, 24]. Grip strength did not improve in all our patients. Furthermore, timing of administration of anabolic supplementation is important, as administering it too early before neuronal injury has improved may prevent optimal results. The duration of therapy may also be of importance and most of the outpatient studies gave the therapy for a longer duration, which we elected not to do, as the patients were no longer in our unit. However, we did not detect any significant adverse effects of the anabolic supplementation. Finally, there was one other patient who we considered for a course of anabolic steroids, but after the first dose and recurrence of sepsis we elected not to give ongoing doses.

Critical illness weakness is an important patient outcome that is associated with medical, economical, and psychosocial adverse outcomes for the patient, the patient's family, and the community [2]. There are limited medical interventions that have shown promise in this important condition. This case series suggests a possible role for stimulation of muscle growth using anabolic steroids. Amongst long stay ICU survivors, it is estimated that one-quarter to one-half or more will suffer from significant weakness and impaired mobility and function. While the absolute numbers of patients this affects is low, the consequences of a prolonged ICU stay, deconditioning, and muscle loss have significant implications on their ability to return to a functional quality of life [25, 26]. We have commenced a pilot randomised controlled trial to explore these results further (the GAINS trial ACTRN12616000835448), including ultrasound measurements of quadriceps thickness as a surrogate for muscle strength as an outcome and functional activity levels using the Chelsea critical care physical assessment tool [23, 27].

Abbreviations

ICU: Intensive Care Unit

SBO: Small bowel obstruction

SLE: Systemic lupus erythematous.

Authors' Contributions

Matthew Anstey, Luke Torre, and Bradley Wibrow were responsible for the design of the case series. All authors contributed to the data collection and to the development and final approval of the manuscript.

References

[1] M. S. Herridge, C. M. Tansey, A. Matté et al., "Functional disability 5 years after acute respiratory distress syndrome," *The New England Journal of Medicine*, vol. 364, no. 14, pp. 1293–1304, 2011.

[2] J. P. Kress and J. P. Hall, "ICU-acquired weakness and recovery from critical illness," *The New England Journal of Medicine*, vol. 370, no. 17, pp. 1626–1635, 2014.

[3] N. Latronico and C. F. Bolton, "Critical illness polyneuropathy and myopathy: A major cause of muscle weakness and paralysis," *The Lancet Neurology*, vol. 10, no. 10, pp. 931–941, 2011.

[4] L.-R. B. Weitzel, P. A. Sandoval, W. J. Mayles, and P. E. Wischmeyer, "Performance-enhancing sports supplements: Role in critical care," *Critical Care Medicine*, vol. 37, no. 10, pp. S400–S409, 2009.

[5] K. F. Almoosa, A. Gupta, C. Pedroza, and N. B. Watts, "Low testosterone levels are frequent in patients with acute respiratory failure and are associated with poor outcomes," *Endocrine Practice*, vol. 20, no. 10, pp. 1057–1063, 2014.

[6] T. Strøm, T. Martinussen, and P. Toft, "A protocol of no sedation for critically ill patients receiving mechanical ventilation: a randomised trial," *The Lancet*, vol. 375, no. 9713, pp. 475–480, 2010.

[7] D. M. Nierman and J. I. Mechanick, "Hypotestosteronemia in chronically critically ill men," *Critical Care Medicine*, vol. 27, no. 11, pp. 2418–2421, 1999.

[8] A. Bech, H. Van Leeuwen, and H. De Boer, "Etiology of low testosterone levels in male patients with severe sepsis requiring mechanical ventilation," *Critical Care*, vol. 17, 448 pages, 2013.

[9] T. W. Storer, S. Basaria, T. Traustadottir et al., "Effects of testosterone supplementation for 3 years on muscle performance and physical function in older men," *The Journal of Clinical Endocrinology & Metabolism*, vol. 102, no. 2, pp. 583–593, 2017.

[10] J. W. Skinner, D. M. Otzel, A. Bowser et al., "Muscular responses to testosterone replacement vary by administration route: a systematic review and meta-analysis," *Journal of Cachexia, Sarcopenia and Muscle*.

[11] S. J. Schaller, M. Anstey, M. Blobner et al., "Early, goal-directed mobilisation in the surgical intensive care unit: a randomised controlled trial," *The Lancet*, vol. 388, no. 10052, pp. 1377–1388, 2016.

[12] A. T. Kicman, "Pharmacology of anabolic steroids," *British Journal of Pharmacology*, vol. 154, no. 3, pp. 502–521, 2008.

[13] N. A. Ali, J. M. O'Brien Jr., S. P. Hoffmann et al., "Acquired weakness, handgrip strength, and mortality in critically Ill patients," *American Journal of Respiratory and Critical Care Medicine*, vol. 178, no. 3, pp. 261–268, 2008.

[14] D. M. Needham, R. Korupolu, J. M. Zanni et al., " Early physical medicine and rehabilitation for patients with acute respiratory failure: a quality improvement project," *Archives of Physical Medicine and Rehabilitation*, vol. 91, no. 4, pp. 536–542, 2010.

[15] W. D. Schweickert, M. C. Pohlman, A. S. Pohlman et al., "Early physical and occupational therapy in mechanically ventilated, critically ill patients: a randomised controlled trial," *The Lancet*, vol. 373, no. 9678, pp. 1874–1882, 2009.

[16] J. Takala, E. Ruokonen, N. R. Webster et al., "Increased mortality associated with growth hormone treatment in critically ill adults," *The New England Journal of Medicine*, vol. 341, no. 11, pp. 785–792, 1999.

[17] W. D. Finkle, S. Greenland, and G. K. Ridgeway, "Increased risk of non-fatal myocardial infarction following testosterone therapy prescription in men," *PLoS ONE*, vol. 9, no. 1, Article ID e85805, 2014.

[18] J. Gold, M. Batterham, H. Rekers et al., "Effects of nandrolone decanoate compared with placebo or testosterone on HIV-associated wasting," *HIV Medicine*, vol. 7, no. 3, pp. 146–155, 2006.

[19] F. R. Sattler, S. V. Jaque, E. T. Schroeder et al., "Effects of pharmacological doses of nandrolone decanoate and progressive resistance training in immunodeficient patients infected with human immunodeficiency virus," *The Journal of Clinical Endocrinology & Metabolism*, vol. 84, no. 4, pp. 1268–1276, 1999.

[20] P. Sardar, A. Jha, D. Roy et al., "Therapeutic effects of nandrolone and testosterone in adult male HIV patients with AIDS wasting syndrome (AWS): A randomized, double-blind, placebo-controlled trial," *HIV Clinical Trials*, vol. 11, no. 4, pp. 220–229, 2010.

[21] K. L. Johansen, K. Mulligan, and M. Schambelan, "Anabolic effects of nandrolone decanoate in patients receiving dialysis: A randomized controlled trial," *Journal of the American Medical Association*, vol. 281, no. 14, pp. 1275–1281, 1999.

[22] J. Pikul and MD. Sharpe, "Use of anabolic steroid therapy in critically ill ICU patients," *Critical Care*, p. P014, 2003.

[23] M. Tillquist, D. J. Kutsogiannis, P. E. Wischmeyer et al., "Bedside ultrasound is a practical and reliable measurement tool for assessing quadriceps muscle layer thickness," *Journal of Parenteral and Enteral Nutrition*, vol. 38, no. 7, pp. 886–890, 2014.

[24] R. W. Bohannon, "Hand-grip dynamometry predicts future outcomes in aging adults," *Journal of Geriatric Physical Therapy*, vol. 31, no. 1, pp. 3–10, 2008.

[25] T. J. Iwashyna, E. W. Ely, D. M. Smith, and K. M. Langa, "Long-term cognitive impairment and functional disability among survivors of severe sepsis," *Journal of the American Medical Association*, vol. 304, no. 16, pp. 1787–1794, 2010.

[26] A. M. Cheung, C. M. Tansey, G. Tomlinson et al., "Two-year outcomes, health care use, and costs of survivors of acute respiratory distress syndrome," *American Journal of Respiratory and Critical Care Medicine*, vol. 174, no. 5, pp. 538–544, 2006.

[27] E. J. Corner, H. Wood, C. Englebretsen et al., "The Chelsea Critical Care Physical Assessment Tool (CPAx): Validation of an innovative new tool to measure physical morbidity in the general adult critical care population; An observational proof-of-concept pilot study," *Physiotherapy (United Kingdom)*, vol. 99, no. 1, pp. 33–41, 2013.

32

Rhabdomyolysis and Acute Kidney Injury due to Severe Heat Stroke

Máximo H. Trujillo[1,2] and Carlos Fragachán G.[1,2]

[1] *Critical Care Department, ICU, Instituto Médico La Floresta (IMLF), Caracas 1060, Venezuela*
[2] *Critical Care Department, University Hospital of Caracas, Caracas 1050, Venezuela*

Correspondence should be addressed to Máximo H. Trujillo, maximotrujillo@gmail.com

Academic Editor: F. Mariano

We present a case of heat stroke (HS) and acute kidney injury (AKI) due to severe rhabdomyolysis in a 14-year-old previously healthy female patient. When she was practicing strenuous exercise she suffered acute seizures and high fever. These symptoms were followed by coma and multiple organ failure (MOF), which included AKI, encephalopathy, fulminant hepatic failure (FHF), and disseminated intravascular coagulation (DIC). The patient was managed in the ICU with renal replacement therapy, ventilatory support, and other vital supporting measures. After three weeks of ICU treatment she made a full recovery.

1. Introduction

Rhabdomyolysis is a syndrome characterized by the leakage of muscle-cell contents into the circulation. Strenuous exercise and HS are the most common causes of rhabdomyolysis. The severity of illness ranges from asymptomatic elevations of the serum levels of muscle enzymes to life-threatening cases associated with extreme elevations of creatine kinase (CK) and liver enzymes (ALT, AST), electrolyte imbalances, and AKI. There are two forms of rhabdomyolysis: traumatic, often resulting from crush injuries and extensive trauma sustained in natural disasters and wars and nontraumatic, which include, among other causes, excessive physical exertion, HS, exogenous toxins, usage of illicit drugs, malignant hyperthermia, alcohol, and prescription medications. The risk of AKI in rhabdomyolisis is usually low when CK levels on admission are less than 20000 U/L. Nevertheless, AKI is still at risk with values of CK as low as 5000 U/L when other coexisting conditions occurs such as sepsis, severe dehydration, and acidosis [1–4]. In addition to rhabdomyolisis, all three risk factors may coexist in severe HS. Usually the cause of rhabdomyolysis is evident from the patient's history or from circumstances immediately preceding the disorder, and only occasionally the precipitant cause will not be obvious.

The classic presentation of rhabdomyolysis includes myalgias, limb weakness, and pigmenturia due to myoglobinuria without hematuria. AKI is a potential complication of severe rhabdomyolysis independently of its etiology, which accounts for 8–15% of all cases of AKI in the US. The mortality rate of HS can be as high as 70%, especially when treatment is delayed, and the presence of MOF [5–9]. Elevated serum creatinine and oliguria associated with rhabdomyolysis and coagulopathy in HS further increase the rate of AKI and mortality [8].

2. Report of the Case

On admission to the ICU her physical examination revealed a temperature of 38°C, blood pressure of 160/90 mmHg, pulse rate of 150/min, and respiratory rate of 35/min. Oxygen saturation was 90%. Except for dry mucous membranes, the rest of her physical examination was unremarkable. Soon after admission to the ICU she became unconscious, requiring tracheal intubation and ventilatory support. A chest X-ray and EKG were normal. A cerebral CT scan revealed mild cerebral edema in both hemispheres.

Laboratory testing revealed serum creatinine 2.4 mg/dL, blood urea nitrogen (BUN) 104 mg/dL, potassium 3 mEq/L, sodium 150 mEq/L, CPK level 24,385 U/L, serum myoglobin >3000 ng/mL, total bilirubin 3.12 mg/dL (d/i: 1.49/1.71), ALAT 382 U/L and AST of 282 U/L, and LDH of 1,376 U/L; serum ammonium 16 mmol/L (reference values 10–80 mmol/L); INR 2.73, and serum fibrinogen of 203 mg/dL. The urinalysis revealed reddish brown urine highly positive for myoglobin. The diagnosis of severe exertional HS and rhabdomyolysis with ensuing AKI was established. The patient received IV hydration, ventilatory support, sodium bicarbonate, corticosteroids, and enteral nutrition. During the next 3 days, her CPK level increased to 36,423 U/L, the serum myoglobin >3000 ng/mL, ALAT 9,942 U/L, AST 5,910 U/L, and LDH to 4,623 U/L. Serum ammonium 117 mmol/L, INR 4.7, and the total bilirubin 11.9 mg/dL (d/i: 9.6/2.3). These last laboratory findings and the onset of encephalopathy and coagulopathy in a patient with not known previous liver disease were consistent with the diagnosis of FHF.

The platelet count decreased to 18,000/mm^3, the plasma fibrinogen to 104 mg/dL, and the fibrinogen split products were 20 μg/mL (<10 μg/mL), supporting the diagnosis of DIC without evidence of active bleeding. On the fourth day, the patient became oliguric (<20 mL/h) and the serum creatinine increased to 5.6 mg/dL with BUN of 118 mg/dL. The diagnosis of AKI was definitively established, and daily hemodialysis was started and maintained for 17 days. By the 5th hospitalization day she had a maximum APACHE II and SAPS scores of 37 and 78 points, respectively. By the 12th day in the ICU, the urine flow started a progressive increase, reaching a maximum of 5 L/24 h. This was accompanied by a decrease of serum creatinine to 2.3 mg/dL and BUN to 38 mg/dL. Hemodialysis was then discontinued. Simultaneously, serum levels of bilirubin, ammonium, ALAT, AST, CK, and myoglobin showed a progressive decrease to normal values. The patient was weaned from the ventilator and extubated on her 14th day of admission to the ICU. Her CNS involvement improved steadily, and complete recovery was attained by the 25th day of hospitalization. Further recovery was uneventful, and she was discharged home. After 3 weeks, she returned to school and normal activities.

3. Discussion

Two forms of HS have been described: the classic or nonexertional HS, which occurs frequently during environmental heat waves, and exertional HS, which usually occurs in healthy, young, and physically active people who engage in strenuous exercise. Renal dysfunction is a well-documented feature in HS that occurs in 30% of cases approximately. The etiology is multifactorial, and this includes direct thermal injury, rhabdomyolysis, DIC, and renal hypoperfusion due to volume depletion and arterial hypotension [10–13]. AKI associated with myoglobinuria is the most serious complication of both traumatic and nontraumatic rhabdomyolysis and may be life threatening. AKI as a complication of rhabdomyolysis is quite common, representing about 7–10% of all cases of AKI in the United States [14], but the incidence of AKI in rhabdomyolysis may be as high as 50% [3, 4, 14].

In spite of early volume replacement and correction of transient arterial hypotension, AKI was an early feature in the present case, suggesting that rhabdomyolysis played a central role in the pathophysiology of this complication. Massive rhabdomyolysis may follow strenuous physical exertion, particularly when associated with other risk factors such as extremely hot and humid conditions, poor physical fitness, and hypokalemia [5, 15]. Apart from severe dehydration and fluid sequestration in injured muscles, AKI in the context of rhabdomyolysis results from a combination of factors. These include direct tubular toxicity, ischemia caused by circulating vasoconstrictors, activation of the sympathetic nervous system, antidiuretic hormone, and the renin-angiotensin system [16]. Myoglobin itself seems to have no marked nephrotoxic effect on the tubules unless the urine is acid. In which case it is reasonable to consider alkalinization of urine as a therapeutic measure, especially in patients with metabolic acidosis [14, 16]. When serum myoglobin levels reach 100 mg/dL, the urine becomes reddish-brown in color. In establishing a differential diagnosis of myoglobinuria, other causes of pigmenturia should be considered (Table 1).

One of the first steps in managing patients with HS in addition to rapid body cooling is prompt IV repletion of fluids. However, once renal damage supervenes, as occurred with our patient, renal replacement therapy is required to control hyperkalemia, fluid overload, and uremia. The outcome of rhabdomyolysis is usually good provided there is no renal failure. Mortality data vary widely according to severity and coexisting conditions. In cases of rhabdomyolysis secondary to limb ischemia (crush injury) mortality can be as high as 32% [17], and among patients hospitalized in intensive care units mortality has been reported to be as high as 59% when AKI is present and 22% when it is not [18]. In contrast, long-term survival among patients with AKI due to rhabdomyolysis is close to 80%, and the majority of them usually recover full renal function [19].

Liver dysfunction and increased serum levels of liver enzymes are commonly observed in HS, whereas FHF is a rare event FHF, defined as "the onset of encephalopathy and coagulopathy in patients with no known previous liver disease," is very uncommon in HS, and only three reports of such cases have been previously published. Two of them recovered completely with conservative ICU treatment [20, 21]. Our patient also made a full recovery from FHF, suggesting that both liver injury and AKI in exertional HS may be reversible.

The severity and complications of exertional HS correlate with the temperature duration curve, suggesting that a rapid reduction in the core temperature by any cooling method (immersion in iced water, iced peritoneal, or gastric lavage) as early as possible should have a positive effect on prognosis. In fact, this single measure seems to be the most effective way of preventing MOF in HS patients. Unfortunately, the "golden hour" for our patient had probably passed by the time she arrived at the ICU [22]. We believe that had she received rapid cooling measures immediately on admission to the suburban hospital, the extent of organ damage may have been limited.

Table 1: Differential diagnosis of pigmenturia.

	Hematuria	Hemoglobinuria	Myoglobinuria	Bile pigments	Porphyria	Alkaptonuria
Pigment	RBC*	Hemoglobin	Myoglobin	Bilirubin/Urobilin	Porphobilinogen	Homogentisinic acid
Urine color	Red	Pink	Red to brown	Brown	Turns brown, red, purple or black on standing at sunlight. Fluoresces with UV light	Turns dark in alkaline solutions. Darkens on standing at sunlight.
Urine Sedi-ment***	RBC and RBC casts	Normal**	Normal	Normal	Normal	Normal
Supernatant urine color	Yellow	Red to brown	Red to brown	Brown	Red. (Watson-Schwartz test positive)	Normal (Ferric chloride test positive)
Urine dipstick test****	1 to 4 +	1 to 4 +	1 to 4 +	Normal	Normal	Normal
Serum	Normal	Pink (low haptoglobin)	Normal (increase ofmyo-globin,creatinine kinase, and liverenzymes inrhabdomyolysis)	Icteric	Normal	Normal
Muscle symptoms	No	No	Myalgias	No	Abdominal cramps.	No (ochronosis and arthritis)

*RBC red blood cells.
**Normal refers to white or yellow in color.
***The sediment and supernatant urine examined after centrifugation.
****Semiquantitative test (orthotolidine or peroxidase) detects heme peroxidase activity in RBC, hemoglobin or myoglobin with reported sensitivity of 91–100%. (1 + = 5–10 RBC/μL, 4+ = approx. 250 RBC/μL).

Although rapid reduction of body temperature and repletion of body fluids remain the vital first priority in the treatment of HS, this together with vigorous intensive care management and vital supporting measures may result in patient survival and complete recovery. Nevertheless, to date little is known about the prognosis of patients with HS, and more data are needed to determine the most appropriate and effective management strategies for these cases.

Acknowledgment

The authors are indebted to Mr. Michael Bench for his assistance in the preparation of the paper.

References

[1] P. A. Gabow, W. D. Kaehny, and S. P. Kelleher, "The spectrum of rhabdomyolysis," *Medicine*, vol. 61, no. 3, pp. 141–152, 1982.

[2] R. L. Mehta, J. A. Kellum, S. V. Shah et al., "Acute Kidney Injury Network: report of an initiative to improve outcomes in acute kidney injury.," *Critical Care*, vol. 11, no. 2, article R31, 2007.

[3] G. Melli, V. Chaudhry, and D. R. Cornblath, "Rhabdomyolysis: an evaluation of 475 hospitalized patients," *Medicine*, vol. 84, no. 6, pp. 377–385, 2005.

[4] M. M. Ward, "Factors predictive of acute renal failure in rhabdomyolysis," *Archives of Internal Medicine*, vol. 148, no. 7, pp. 1553–1557, 1988.

[5] A. Bouchama and J. P. Knochel, "Medical progress: heat stroke," *The New England Journal of Medicine*, vol. 346, no. 25, pp. 1978–1988, 2002.

[6] J. P. Knochel and G. Reed, "Disorders of heat regulation," in *Maxwell and Kleeman's Clinical Disorders of Fluid and Electrolytes Metabolism*, R. G. Narins, Ed., pp. 1549–1590, McGraw-Hill, New York, NY, USA, 5th edition, 1994.

[7] G. H. Clowes Jr. and T. F. O'Donnell, "Heat stroke," *The New England Journal of Medicine*, vol. 291, no. 11, pp. 564–567, 1974.

[8] B. Misset, B. De Jonghe, S. Bastuji-Garin et al., "Mortality of patients with heatstroke admitted to intensive care units during the 2003 heat wave in France: a national multiple-center risk-factor study," *Critical Care Medicine*, vol. 34, no. 4, pp. 1087–1092, 2006.

[9] F. LoVecchio, A. F. Pizon, C. Berrett, and A. Balls, "Outcomes after environmental hyperthermia," *American Journal of Emergency Medicine*, vol. 25, no. 4, pp. 442–444, 2007.

[10] P. Dennen, I. S. Douglas, and R. Anderson, "Acute kidney injury in the intensive care unit: an update and primer for the intensivist," *Critical Care Medicine*, vol. 38, no. 1, pp. 261–275, 2010.

[11] D. J. Buggy and A. W.A. Crossley, "Thermoregulation, mild perioperative hypothermia and post-anaesthetic shivering," *British Journal of Anaesthesia*, vol. 84, no. 5, pp. 615–628, 2000.

[12] J. E. Dematte, K. O'Mara, J. Buescher et al., "Near-fatal heat stroke during the 1995 heat wave in Chicago," *Annals of Internal Medicine*, vol. 129, no. 3, pp. 173–181, 1998.

[13] S. F. Raju, G. H. Robinson, and J. D. Bower, "The pathogenesis of acute renal failure in heat stroke," *Southern Medical Journal*, vol. 66, no. 3, pp. 330–333, 1973.

[14] W. H. Bagley, H. Yang, and K. H. Shah, "Rhabdomyolysis," *Internal and Emergency Medicine*, vol. 2, no. 3, pp. 210–218, 2007.
[15] S. G. Holt and K. P. Moore, "Pathogenesis and treatment of renal dysfunction in rhabdomyolysis," *Intensive Care Medicine*, vol. 27, no. 5, pp. 803–811, 2001.
[16] X. Bosch, E. Poch, and J. M. Grau, "Rhabdomyolysis and acute kidney injury," *The New England Journal of Medicine*, vol. 361, no. 1, pp. 62–72, 2009.
[17] J. Veenstra, W. M. Smit, R. T. Krediet, and L. Arisz, "Relationship between elevated creatine phosphokinase and the clinical spectrum of rhabdomyolysis," *Nephrology Dialysis Transplantation*, vol. 9, no. 6, pp. 637–641, 1994.
[18] A. R. de Meijer, B. G. Fikkers, M. H. De Keijzer, B. G. M. van Engelen, and J. P. H. Drenth, "Serum creatine kinase as predictor of clinical course in rhabdomyolysis: a 5-year intensive care survey," *Intensive Care Medicine*, vol. 29, no. 7, pp. 1121–1125, 2003.
[19] G. Woodrow, A. M. Brownjohn, and J. H. Turney, "The clinical and biochemical features of acute renal failure due to rhabdomyolysis," *Renal Failure*, vol. 17, no. 4, pp. 467–474, 1995.
[20] F. V. Schiødt and W. M. Lee, "Fulminant liver disease," *Clinics in Liver Disease*, vol. 7, no. 2, pp. 331–349, 2003.
[21] M. A. Pastor, F. Perez-Aguilar, V. Ortiz, D. Nicolas, and J. Berenguer, "Acute hepatitis due to heatstroke," *Gastroenterología y Hepatología*, vol. 22, no. 8, pp. 398–399, 1999.
[22] Y. Heled, M. Rav-Acha, Y. Shani, Y. Epstein, and D. S. Moran, "The "golden hour" for heatstroke treatment," *Military Medicine*, vol. 169, no. 3, pp. 184–186, 2004.

33

Nuclear Imaging to Detect Diaphragmatic Perforation as a Rare Complication of Microwave Ablation

Stephanie Cull,[1] Gebran Khneizer,[1] Abhishek Krishna,[2] Razi Muzaffar,[3] Sameer Gadani,[3] and Zafar Jamkhana[1,2]

[1]*Department of Internal Medicine, Saint Louis University School of Medicine, St. Louis, MO, USA*
[2]*Division of Pulmonary, Critical Care and Sleep Medicine, Saint Louis University School of Medicine, St. Louis, MO, USA*
[3]*Radiology Department, Saint Louis University, St. Louis, MO, USA*

Correspondence should be addressed to Stephanie Cull; culls@slu.edu

Academic Editor: Kenneth S. Waxman

Acquired diaphragmatic perforation leading to massive hepatic hydrothorax and respiratory failure is a rare complication of microwave ablation (MWA) of hepatocellular carcinoma (HCC). Imaging modalities to detect pleuroperitoneal communication remain poorly described. We report a nuclear imaging technique used to efficiently diagnose and locate diaphragmatic defects. A 57-year-old male with cirrhosis and HCC presented with respiratory distress after undergoing MWA of a HCC lesion. He was admitted to the intensive care unit for noninvasive positive pressure ventilator support. Chest radiography revealed a new large right pleural effusion. Large-volume thoracentesis was consistent with hepatic hydrothorax. The fluid reaccumulated within 24 hours; therefore an acquired diaphragmatic perforation induced by the ablation procedure was suspected. To investigate, ^{99m}Technetium-labeled albumin was injected into the peritoneal cavity. The tracer accumulated in the right hemi thorax almost immediately. The patient then underwent transjugular intrahepatic portosystemic shunting in efforts to relieve portal hypertension and decrease ascites volume. Unfortunately, the patient deteriorated and expired after few days. Although diaphragmatic defects develop in cirrhotic patients, such small fenestrations do not normally lead to rapid development of life-threatening pleural effusion. MWA procedures can cause large diaphragmatic defects. Immediate detection of this complication is essential for initiating early intervention.

1. Introduction

Hepatic hydrothorax is defined as a pleural effusion volume greater than 500 mL in a patient with liver cirrhosis, not otherwise explained by a cardiopulmonary or primary pleural process [1–3]. Only 1-2% of pleural effusions are secondary to cirrhosis and only 5–10% of patients with cirrhosis are affected by hepatic hydrothorax [3]. The exact pathogenesis of such effusions remains poorly understood. Many agree upon the theory that ascitic fluid passes directly through diaphragmatic defects (either congenital or acquired), which constitute direct pleuroperitoneal communications in the form of holes or blebs [3–5]. The condition may even occur in patients with minimal ascites [6]. Negative intrathoracic pressure draws ascitic fluid directly into the pleural space, more commonly to the right thorax considering the right hemidiaphragm is thinner and less muscular than the left counterpart. These pleuroperitoneal communications are often small fenestrations through which fluid slowly accumulates in the thorax. However, literature describes cases of large diaphragmatic defects which lead to accumulation of massive fluid volume in the pleural space with subsequent respiratory failure, often requiring daily thoracentesis or chest tube placement [4, 6]. Chest tube placement is relatively contraindicated in hepatic hydrothorax as it leads to rapid fluid depletion and electrolyte imbalance [3]. Although this patient population may benefit from transjugular intrahepatic portosystemic shunting (TIPS), there are many cases where the patient cannot tolerate this procedure due to rapid clinical decompensation.

Acquired diaphragmatic defect is a rare complication of microwave ablation (MWA), a form of thermal ablation

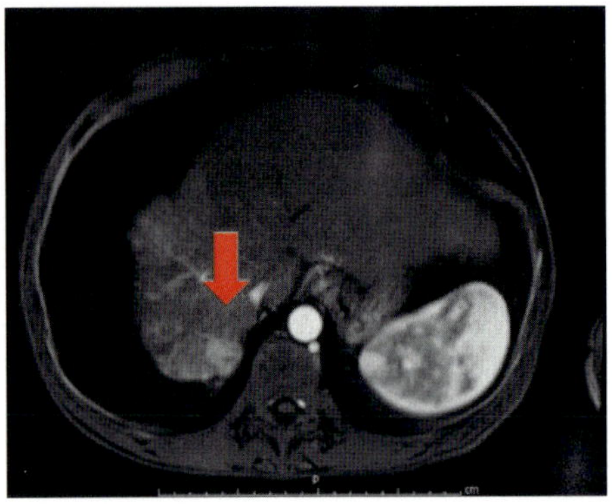

Figure 1: MRI image of an arterially enhanced lesion representing hepatocellular carcinoma seen with washout and delayed capsular enhancement. The tumor measures 2.2 cm in diameter and is located on segment 7 of the liver in close proximity to the tendinous portion of the right hemidiaphragm.

treatment for cancer, commonly hepatocellular carcinoma (HCC) [7, 8]. If the tumor is located on segment seven or eight in close proximity to the diaphragm, the heat deployed during ablation may lead to thinning of the diaphragm and widening of preexisting fenestrations or perforation of blebs [9]. Despite the ability to discover diaphragmatic defects through thoracoscopy and even autopsy [5], imaging techniques to visualize these defects remain uncommon and not well described. We report a simple and efficient nuclear imaging technique to diagnose significant diaphragmatic defects.

2. Case Presentation

A 57-year-old male with a past medical history of cirrhosis and HCC secondary to chronic alcohol abuse and hepatitis C infection was undergoing serial transarterial chemoembolization (TACE) procedures. He also had recurrent ascites refractory to both low sodium diet restriction and diuretic therapy. Prior to admission and in addition to TACE, the patient underwent MWA for an enlarging HCC lesion located on segment 7 of the liver (see Figure 1). A 20 cm probe (with a 3-4 cm ablation zone) was advanced under CT guidance and deployed across the lesion. After confirming the position of the probe, ablation was performed per protocol (65 watts for 10 minutes). An overlapping session was also performed. Immediately after the MWA procedure, the patient underwent therapeutic large-volume paracentesis (8 L), without complication, and was discharged home afterwards.

Three days after procedure, the patient presented to the emergency department with respiratory distress reporting progressive shortness of breath which began the day after MWA. Vital signs were significant for a respiratory rate of 33 breaths per minute and oxygen saturation of 87% while breathing ambient air. Physical exam revealed a cachectic-appearing man in respiratory distress using accessory muscles of respiration. There were diminished breath sounds on auscultation of the right lung fields. The patient was admitted directly to the intensive care unit for noninvasive positive pressure ventilation support. Chest radiography showed a large right-sided pleural effusion. Computed tomography of the chest confirmed the effusion and ruled out pulmonary embolism and lipiodol embolism. The patient had no prior history of pleural effusion or evidence of such on previous imaging studies. Thoracentesis was performed and pleural fluid analysis revealed a transudative fluid consistent with hepatic hydrothorax. Pleural fluid microbiology was negative for infection and cytology studies were negative for malignancy. The effusion reaccumulated within 24 hours with associated atelectasis of the right lung. A bedside ultrasound revealed minimal ascitic fluid, even though the patient was known to have significant refractory ascites. With careful consideration of the clinical timeline, an acquired diaphragmatic perforation induced by MWA therapy was suspected. Therefore, a nuclear medicine peritoneal shunt study was performed whereby 4.0 mCi Technetium-99m mixed with albumin was injected into the peritoneal cavity under sterile conditions. Planar nuclear images of the chest and abdomen were obtained immediately and at intervals of 15 minutes and 90 minutes after radiotracer administration (see Figure 2). Tracer accumulation in the right hemi thorax was evident on the image taken immediately after injection (see Figure 2(a)). The patient later required frequent thoracenteses and therefore a chest tube was necessary (weighing the benefits against the known risks associated with placing a chest tube). The decision was then taken to pursue TIPS in an effort to relieve portal hypertension and decrease the volume of ascitic fluid formation. Intubation was required for the procedure with subsequent inability to extubate afterwards. The patient's clinical status declined further as he developed atrial fibrillation and distributive shock. Upon discussion with the family and thoracic surgery service, together it was decided to not pursue a surgical evaluation of the diaphragmatic perforation. Furthermore, the decision was made to pursue comfort care measures as per the patient's previously stated wishes to the family. The patient passed away.

3. Discussion

MWA has become widely utilized as a form of cancer treatment in multiple medical disciplines with the advances in interventional technology. Recently, such modules became an alternative treatment for liver malignancy, particularly for those who are poor surgical candidates. Postprocedure complications are uncommon and include hemorrhage, bile leak, fluid collection/abscess formation, cholangitis, tumor seeding, and abdominal pain [10].

Acquired diaphragmatic perforation has been reported as a rare complication of MWA for the treatment of HCC [8, 9]. Although diaphragmatic defects are seen in patients with cirrhosis who develop hepatic hydrothorax, they are usually described as small fenestrations that do not lead to rapid development of pleural effusion [5]. It is hypothesized that the heat generated from the ablation procedure stretches the small fenestrations or leads to perforation of preexisting blebs of the diaphragm [9]. Another potential explanation for

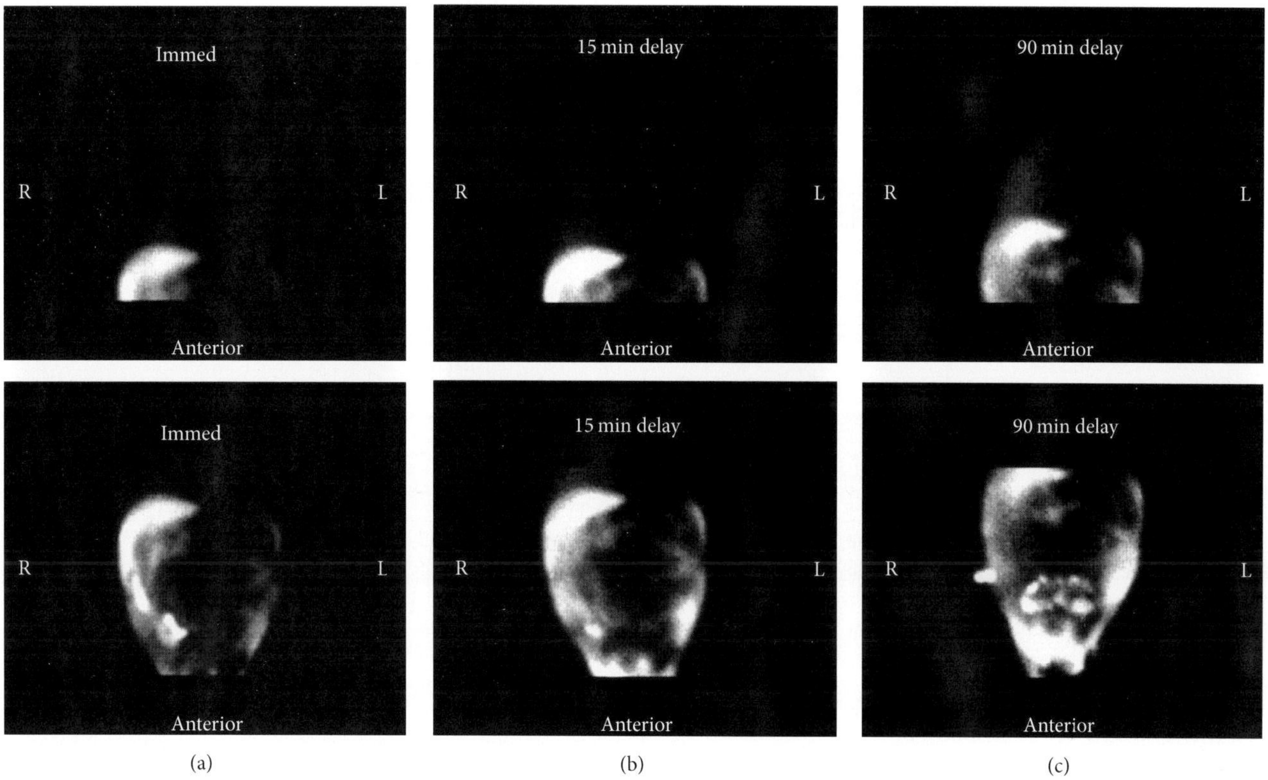

FIGURE 2: Anterior planar nuclear images of the thorax (upper images) and abdomen (lower images) obtained after radiotracer administration with ^{99m}Technetium-labeled albumin into the peritoneal cavity. Images were obtained immediately after tracer injection (a) and at intervals of 15 minutes (b) and 90 minutes (c). Very faint radiotracer accumulation is evident in the right hemi thorax immediately (a) and is more pronounced at 15 minutes (b) and at 90 minutes (c). Radiotracer is seen to equalize in the abdomen over time (bottom images of (a), (b), and (c)). There is no visible tracer in the left hemi thorax.

such large defects is the microwave needle penetrating the diaphragm. As a result, large amount of ascitic fluid is drawn into the pleural space secondary to the negative intrathoracic pressure.

Even though multiple imaging modalities have been reported for indirect measurement of pleuroperitoneal communication across the diaphragm, such imaging techniques remain uncommon and not well reported. First, an indirect visualization of colored dyes such as methylene blue and indocyanine green was injected into the peritoneal space and migrated into the pleural space [4, 11]. Then MRI has been used to visualize a hypointense jet across the diaphragm in both T1- and T2-weighted sagittal scans [11]. But this modality is both time consuming and heavily dependent on patient participation. Furthermore, contrast-enhanced ultrasound detects such diaphragmatic defects by injecting the peritoneum with perflubutane microbubbles, an imaging agent that is safely eliminated from the lung. The patient then undergoes postural changes which elicits a jet-like flow of tracer-enhanced ascitic fluid into the hemithorax [8, 12]. These postural changes may not be clinically practical in critically ill patients. Another example is injecting radioisotope (such as ^{99m}Tc-sulfur colloid) into the peritoneum and then visualizing the tracer in the hemithorax [13, 14].

The imaging modality that we employed offers several unique advantages in critically ill patients. First, it is time efficient and inexpensive. Second, it requires minimal patient participation and thus it can be performed on critically ill patients in contrast to previously described modalities such as MRI and contrast-enhanced ultrasound. Moreover, the low cost of such modalities is also promising. But availability of the nuclear agent, namely, ^{99m}Technetium mixed with albumin, is the imaging technique's main limitation.

Identifying the diaphragmatic perforations early in the clinical course is essential to evaluate life-saving intervention and potential repair. Repair would include procedures such as chemical pleurodesis [6, 11] or video-assisted thoracoscopic surgery (VATS) [8]. Matono et al. described the clinical outcome of a patient who remained free of pleural effusion for over a year after closure of the diaphragmatic defect with sutures via VATS [8]. Liang et al. used a Dacron heart patch trimmed to appropriate size to close the lesion with minimal pleural effusion afterwards [9]. Such potential repair techniques offer a promising future for patient population with large diaphragmatic defects.

In conclusion, following MWA if a patient develops respiratory distress and a significant pleural effusion, early detection of diaphragmatic perforation using a nuclear peritoneal shunt study can be life-saving. This imaging is possibly the essential step between diagnosis and immediate intervention to avoid fluid and electrolyte depletion and respiratory clinical deterioration.

References

[1] R. M. Strauss and T. D. Boyer, "Hepatic hydrothorax," *Seminars in Liver Disease*, vol. 17, no. 3, pp. 227–232, 1997.

[2] C. S. Morrow, M. Kantor, and R. N. Armen, "Hepatic hydrothorax," *Annals of Internal Medicine*, vol. 49, no. 1, pp. 193–203, 1958.

[3] A. Cardenas, T. Kelleher, and S. Chopra, "Review article: hepatic hydrothorax," *Alimentary Pharmacology and Therapeutics*, vol. 20, no. 3, pp. 271–279, 2004.

[4] A. Chen, Y.-S. Ho, Y.-C. Tu, H.-S. Tang, and T.-C. Cheng, "Diaphragmatic defect as a cause of massive hydrothorax in cirrhosis of liver," *Journal of Clinical Gastroenterology*, vol. 10, no. 6, pp. 663–666, 1988.

[5] P.-M. Huang, Y.-L. Chang, C.-Y. Yang, and Y.-C. Lee, "The morphology of diaphragmatic defects in hepatic hydrothorax: thoracoscopic finding," *Journal of Thoracic and Cardiovascular Surgery*, vol. 130, no. 1, pp. 141–145, 2005.

[6] D. Rubinstein, I. E. McInnes, and F. J. Dudley, "Hepatic hydrothorax in the absence of clinical ascites: diagnosis and management," *Gastroenterology*, vol. 88, no. 1, part 1, pp. 188–191, 1985.

[7] J. Ding, X. Jing, J. Liu et al., "Comparison of two different thermal techniques for the treatment of hepatocellular carcinoma," *European Journal of Radiology*, vol. 82, no. 9, pp. 1379–1384, 2013.

[8] T. Matono, M. Koda, and Y. Murawaki, "Right diaphragmatic defect in hepatic hydrothorax exposed by contrast-enhanced ultrasonography after radiofrequency ablation," *Hepatology*, vol. 56, no. 2, pp. 784–785, 2012.

[9] Q.-C. Liang, Y.-J. Tian, and X.-T. Jiang, "Laparoscopic repair of diaphragm perforation with heart patch after microwave ablation," *Saudi Medical Journal*, vol. 37, no. 3, pp. 320–323, 2016.

[10] T. Livraghi, F. Meloni, L. Solbiati, and G. Zanus, "Complications of microwave ablation for liver tumors: results of a multicenter study," *CardioVascular and Interventional Radiology*, vol. 35, no. 4, pp. 868–874, 2012.

[11] T. Zenda, S. Miyamoto, S. Murata, and H. Mabuchi, "Detection of diaphragmatic defect as the cause of severe hepatic hydrothorax with magnetic resonance imaging," *American Journal of Gastroenterology*, vol. 93, no. 11, pp. 2288–2289, 1998.

[12] M. Tamano, T. Hashimoto, K. Kojima, C. Maeda, and H. Hiraishi, "Diagnosis of hepatic hydrothorax using contrast-enhanced ultrasonography with intraperitoneal injection of Sonazoid," *Journal of Gastroenterology and Hepatology*, vol. 25, no. 2, pp. 383–386, 2010.

[13] A. Serena, L. Aliaga, J. A. Richter, R. Calderon, L. Sanchez, and M. A. Charvet, "Scintigraphic demonstration of a diaphragmatic defect as the cause of massive hydrothorax in cirrhosis," *European Journal of Nuclear Medicine*, vol. 11, no. 1, pp. 46–48, 1985.

[14] A. Bhattacharya, B. R. Mittal, T. Biswas et al., "Radioisotope scintigraphy in the diagnosis of hepatic hydrothorax," *Journal of Gastroenterology and Hepatology (Australia)*, vol. 16, no. 3, pp. 317–321, 2001.

34

DRESS Syndrome in the ICU: When a Patient is Treated with Multiple Drugs

Florent Moriceau,[1] Johanne Prothet,[1] Benjamin J. Blaise,[2] Benoit Ben Said,[3] Mathieu Page,[1] Charles-Eric Ber,[1] Jullien Crozon,[1] and Thomas Rimmelé[1,4]

[1] *Département d'Anesthésie-Réanimation, Hôpital Edouard Herriot, 5 place d'Arsonval, 69003 Lyon, France*
[2] *Département de Néonatologie et de Réanimation Néonatale, Hôpital Femme Mère Enfant, 32 Avenue Doyen Jean Lépine, 69500 Bron, France*
[3] *Département d'Allergologie et d'Immunologie Clinique, Centre Hospitalier de Lyon-Sud, 165 Chemin du Grand Revoyet, 69310 Pierre-Bénite, France*
[4] *Université Claude Bernard Lyon 1, 43 Boulevard du 11 Novembre 1918, 69100 Villeurbanne, France*

Correspondence should be addressed to Florent Moriceau; flo.moriceau@gmail.com

Academic Editor: Caterina Mammina

The Drug Reaction with Eosinophilia and Systemic Symptoms (DRESS) syndrome is life-threatening. It associates a skin condition with hematological and visceral disorders. The DRESS syndrome diagnosis in the intensive care unit (ICU) is difficult as clinical features are nonspecific. Furthermore, the need to treat patients with multiple drugs usually prevents the identification of the causative drug. We report the case of a patient who developed two bouts of DRESS caused by piperacillin-tazobactam, the first being complicated with a distributive shock. Cases of DRESS occurring inside ICU are seldom reported. However, any intensivist may encounter this situation during his career and should be aware of its diagnostic and management specific aspects.

1. Introduction

The DRESS (Drug Reaction with Eosinophilia and Systemic Symptoms) syndrome is a severe drug hypersensitivity reaction. Although it is less known than Lyell or Stevens-Johnson syndromes and less striking than anaphylactic shock, it can result in a dreadful prognosis, with a mortality rate of 2 to 45% [1–3]. DRESS occurring in an intensive care unit (ICU) is a complex situation. It can mimic more usual causes of shock and organ failure, such as sepsis. Furthermore, identifying the responsible treatment may not be straightforward due to the multiple drugs use in the intensive care unit. Finally, the necessity to remove any suspected treatment will make the patient's management more complicated. We report the case of DRESS induced by piperacillin-tazobactam initially identified as a septic shock and reoccurring after the inappropriate reintroduction of a suspected treatment. The patient's family gave a written consent to report this case.

2. Case Report

A 53-year-old woman was admitted to the ICU due to angiocholitis complicated by a septic shock. She had a medical history of high blood pressure and, despite two episodes of kidney transplantation, she had recently reached end-stage renal disease. She was under antihypertensive therapy and immunosuppressant drugs (prednisolone, mycophenolate, and cyclosporine).

The early evolution was positive with a probabilistic antibiotherapy associating piperacillin-tazobactam and amikacin. It was decreased to ceftriaxone alone on the fifth day, after the identification of a biliary *Klebsiella pneumoniæ pneumoniæ* (Figure 1). On the 21st day after the ICU admission, the patient developed another septic shock due to angiocholitis, forcing the reintroduction of the initial probabilistic antibiotherapy. On the 23rd day, the antibiotherapy was modified again to ceftriaxone and vancomycin, after

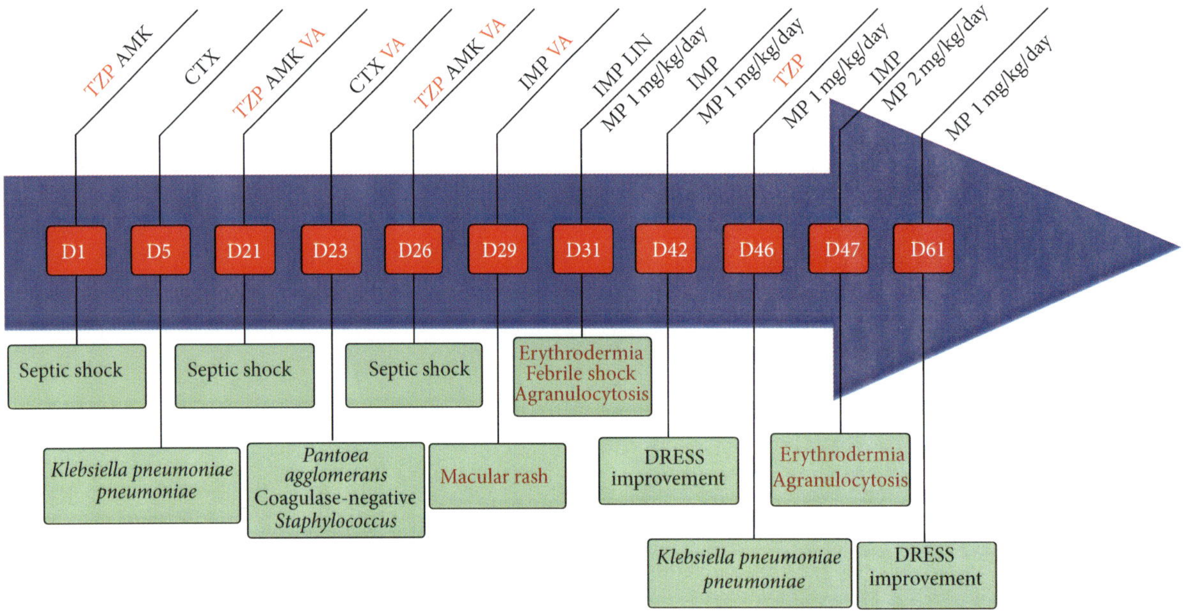

Figure 1: The chronology of events and drugs use related to DRESS occurrences. D: day; TZP: piperacillin-tazobactam; AMK: amikacin; CTX: ceftriaxone; VA: vancomycin; IMP: imipenem; LIN: linezolid; MP: methylprednisolone. Day 1: admission to the ICU.

the bloodstream identification of a *Pantoea agglomerans* and a coagulase-negative *Staphylococcus*. A third round of septic shock occurred on the 26th day leading us to widen the antibiotherapy, associating piperacillin-tazobactam and amikacin to the already administered vancomycin (Figure 1).

Following this last modification, a benign-looking rash appeared on the patient's chest on the 29th day. After 48 h of hemodynamic stability, a high fever and a distributive shock requiring consequent norepinephrine infusion (1 μg/kg/min) emerged. The procalcitonin measurement reached a high level (2.98 μg/L), which was compatible with sepsis. However, the rash evolved into erythrodermia (Figure 2), associated with enlarged cervical and inguinal lymph nodes, eosinophilia (absolute eosinophil count of 1.0×10^9/L), agranulocytosis (absolute neutrophil count of 0.4×10^9/L), and activated circulating T-lymphocytes. These elements led to the diagnosis of DRESS syndrome.

All drugs introduced at least ten days before the rash were interrupted, except for vasopressors. Vancomycin was replaced by linezolid. A systemic corticotherapy with methylprednisolone (1 mg/kg/d) was initiated, along with the use of granulocyte colony-stimulating factors (G-CSF).

Eosinophilia reached a maximum of 4.2×10^9/L on the 32nd day, associated with a thrombocytopenia and a nonregenerative anemia. A myelogram revealed a hypoplastic bone marrow, mostly composed of eosinophils (30%) without hemophagocytic lymphohistiocytosis. A skin biopsy showed basal membrane vacuoles, spongiosis, and an inflammatory infiltration of dermis, described as activated lymphocytes and eosinophils. The Epstein-Barr Virus (EBV) load was found elevated at 700 copies/mL. No differential diagnosis was identified.

The cutaneous condition improved within 10 days, from the chest to the limbs, with a reepithelialization following a desquamation and blisters. Eosinophilia and agranulocytosis normalized within five days. However, the nonregenerative anemia and the thrombocytopenia remained.

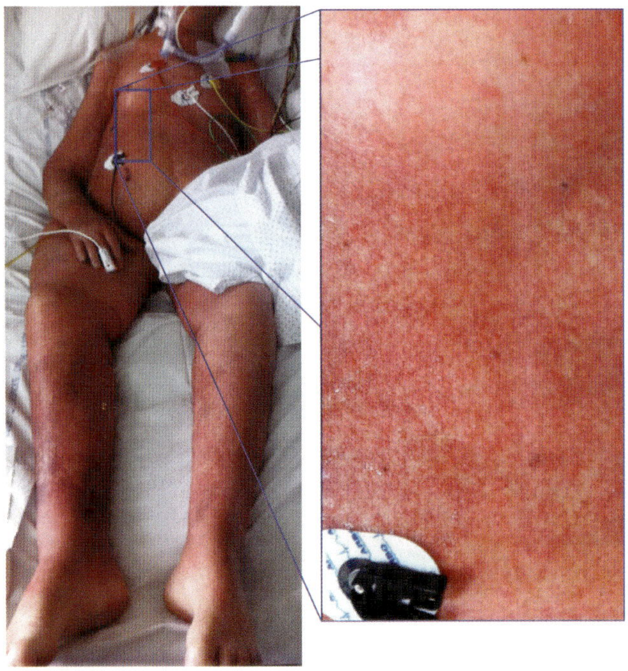

Figure 2: Erythrodermia in ICU ventilated patient. Focus on the chest showing a maculopapular rash.

Vancomycin was initially suspected. Therefore, piperacillin-tazobactam was used again during another bout of sepsis, after the identification of a sensitive *Klebsiella pneumoniæ pneumoniæ* (Figure 1). Erythrodermia reoccurred immediately following this reintroduction, with early eosinophilia (absolute eosinophil count of 1.0×10^9/L), deep agranulocytosis (undetectable neutrophils), and hyperlactatemia (3.2 mmol/L), but without hemodynamic instability. This new DRESS was associated with EBV reactivation (viral load of 5,200 copies/mL). A new myelogram reported a highly hypoplastic bone marrow, with more eosinophils (40%) than previously counted, and the noticeable absence of neutrophilic cells. We thus interrupted the piperacillin-tazobactam administration and increased methylprednisolone up to 2 mg/kg/d. Cutaneous and hematological conditions improved within two weeks. This recurrence clearly incriminated piperacillin-tazobactam.

Later evolution was unfortunately negative, with numerous ICU-associated adverse events (ventilator-associated pneumonia, neuromyopathy, and severe malnutrition). The patient died of septic shock complications triggered by pneumonia, on day 102 after ICU admission.

3. Discussion

An occurrence of DRESS inside the ICU is difficult to diagnose, and its management is not obvious. In addition, the intensive care specific aspects are seldom mentioned in the literature.

The DRESS syndrome is a delayed hypersensitivity reaction. Its clinical features include a cutaneous reaction (almost 100% of cases, usually maculopapular, often itchy and extensive to the whole body), a facial edema (76%), a polyadenopathy (54%), a fever (90%), and an organ involvement (91%, either liver, lung, brain, kidney, or heart) [2, 4, 5]. Mortality ranges from 2 to 45% depending on the severity of the organ involvement [1–3, 6]. Few cases of shock have recently been reported, highlighting the need to mention the DRESS syndrome in the diagnosis algorithm of a distributive shock [6]. Hematological abnormalities include a possible eosinophilia (95%) which can be delayed, with either lymphopenia (5%) or lymphocytosis, and often circulating activated T-lymphocytes (67%), as observed in infectious mononucleosis [2]. A hemophagocytic lymphohistiocytosis is not uncommon. It is associated with a worse prognosis and sometimes preceded by biological marker raises (hyperferritinemia, hypertriglyceridemia, and elevated lactate dehydrogenase levels). Procalcitonin can rise regardless of any sepsis [5].

The pathophysiology of the organ involvement is multifactorial and still not fully understood. Human herpesvirus family reactivations, their local proliferation, and the cytotoxic immune response they induce may be involved. Indeed, viral DNAs have been identified in affected organs, but no causal link has yet been established [3, 7, 8]. The viral load is a diagnosis criterion in some countries [9]. Descamps and Ranger-Rogez also reported a genetic predisposition that influences cytotoxic T-lymphocytes response [5].

The list of medications that may potentially induce DRESS keeps growing and includes more than 40 drugs. The most frequent triggers are (in descending order) anticonvulsants (carbamazepine, lamotrigine, phenobarbital, phenytoin, and sodium valproate), allopurinol, psychotropic drugs, sulfonamides (dapsone, sulfasalazine, and sulfamethoxazole), antiviral therapies, and antibiotics (mostly vancomycin and beta-lactam antibiotics) [2, 4, 10, 11]. The DRESS syndrome is a relatively rare drug reaction with an incidence of 1/5000 for anticonvulsants [12]. It occurs with a median delay of 22 days after the administration of the causal treatment [2]. Any drug initiated one to four weeks before the rash must be suspected. In the intensive care unit, the use of multiple medications may prevent the identification of the responsible drug. This is usually achieved after full recovery, through further allergological investigations such as skin or immunobiological tests (lymphocytes proliferation and cytokine production assays). In this case, the antibiotic changes increased the number of potential causal drugs. Vancomycin was the initial main suspect as it is the most common trigger for DRESS among antibiotics [2], and as the 10-day delay between introduction and symptoms was compatible with the pathophysiology of the DRESS. Furthermore, piperacillin-tazobactam had seldom been related to DRESS at that time, with only three cases reported [13–15]. Since then, Cabañas et al. have added 8 more [16]. Interestingly, piperacillin-tazobactam had been used only 24 hours before the last onset of symptoms. The delay of the symptoms onset can indeed be dramatically shortened in the case of a previous exposure, as the sensitized antigen-specific T-lymphocytes can remain activated for years [17, 18]. Thus, we observed a shortened delay and an intensified reaction when DRESS reoccurred.

Ruling out the differential diagnoses is an additional difficulty in the ICU. DRESS can indeed complicate an underlying condition, such as sepsis with which it shares many clinical features. Kardaun et al. [4] suggested a score that classifies cases as definite, probable, possible, or no case. Relevant clinical features were fever, enlarged lymph nodes, a skin condition, and a late resolution (more than 15 days). Additional criteria were hematological abnormalities (eosinophilia, activated circulating lymphocytes), a compatible skin biopsy, and organ involvement. They also considered the unfruitful research of differential diagnoses, after ruling out autoimmune diseases (lupus, Kawasaki disease), infectious diseases (mononucleosis or other viral exanthems, toxic shock syndrome), and hematological diseases (angioimmunoblastic lymphoma, hypereosinophilic syndrome), to be relevant. In the present case, Kardaun's score reached 8 points, making the diagnosis of DRESS syndrome certain.

The key element in the management of a patient with DRESS is the early and permanent withdrawal of every suspected medication. The use of strong topical steroids is sufficient for mild cases. Severe cases will require the use of a systemic corticotherapy (methylprednisolone 1-2 mg/kg/d). In our case, the early corticotherapy initiated with 1 mg/kg/d of methylprednisolone allowed a general improvement but did not prevent the recurrence. Full recovery will generally be obtained after weeks, even with an early and optimal management [5]. Intravenous immunoglobulins are no longer recommended due to their frequent secondary effects and lack of benefit compared to corticotherapy [19]. A granulopoietic stimulant (G-CSF) can be discussed. On one hand, it may shorten the duration of agranulocytosis. On the other hand, it may redirect the immune response of T4 lymphocytes from the hyperactivated T helper 1 (Th-1) response to the Th-2 response [20, 21]. Viral reactivations may benefit from a specific treatment.

4. Conclusion

Any intensivist may encounter or may have to manage a patient with DRESS syndrome. In the ICU, clinical features and organ involvement have a poor specificity. The suspicious drugs are often numerous due to the many treatments used. The prognosis relies on organ failure and delay to the treatment initiation. The early and permanent withdrawal of every suspected causal agent is of primary importance. Any reintroduction of a drug exposes the patient to the risk of a more severe recurrence.

Disclosure

All the authors have approved the final paper.

References

[1] H. Bocquet, M. Bagot, and J. C. Roujeau, "Drug-induced pseudolymphoma and drug hypersensitivity syndrome (Drug Rash with Eosinophilia and Systemic Symptoms: DRESS)," *Seminars in Cutaneous Medicine and Surgery*, vol. 15, no. 4, pp. 250–257, 1996.

[2] S. H. Kardaun, P. Sekula, L. Valeyrie-Allanore et al., "Drug reaction with eosinophilia and systemic symptoms (DRESS): an original multisystem adverse drug reaction. Results from the prospective RegiSCAR study," *British Journal of Dermatology*, vol. 169, no. 5, pp. 1071–1080, 2013.

[3] M. Eshki, L. Allanore, P. Musette et al., "Twelve-year analysis of severe cases of drug reaction with eosinophilia and systemic symptoms: a cause of unpredictable multiorgan failure," *Archives of Dermatology*, vol. 145, no. 1, pp. 67–72, 2009.

[4] S. H. Kardaun, A. Sidoroff, L. Valeyrie-Allanore et al., "Variability in the clinical pattern of cutaneous side-effects of drugs with systemic symptoms: does a DRESS syndrome really exist?" *British Journal of Dermatology*, vol. 156, no. 3, pp. 609–611, 2007.

[5] V. Descamps and S. Ranger-Rogez, "DRESS syndrome," *Joint Bone Spine*, vol. 81, no. 1, pp. 15–21, 2014.

[6] A. Kimmoun, E. Dubois, P. Perez, A. Barbaud, and B. Levy, "Shock state: an unrecognized and underestimated presentation of drug reaction with eosinophilia and systemic symptoms," *Shock*, vol. 40, no. 5, pp. 387–391, 2013.

[7] L. Mardivirin, V. Descamps, A. Lacroix, S. Delebassée, and S. Ranger-Rogez, "Early effects of drugs responsible for DRESS on HHV-6 replication *in vitro*," *Journal of Clinical Virology*, vol. 46, no. 3, pp. 300–302, 2009.

[8] L. Mardivirin, L. Valeyrie-Allanore, E. Branlant-Redon et al., "Amoxicillin-induced flare in patients with DRESS (Drug Reaction with Eosinophilia and Systemic Symptoms): report of seven cases and demonstration of a direct effect of amoxicillin on human herpesvirus 6 replication in vitro," *European Journal of Dermatology*, vol. 20, no. 1, pp. 68–73, 2010.

[9] T. Shiohara, M. Iijima, Z. Ikezawa, and K. Hashimoto, "The diagnosis of a DRESS syndrome has been sufficiently established on the basis of typical clinical features and viral reactivations," *British Journal of Dermatology*, vol. 156, no. 5, pp. 1083–1084, 2007.

[10] P. Cacoub, P. Musette, V. Descamps et al., "The DRESS syndrome: a literature review," *American Journal of Medicine*, vol. 124, no. 7, pp. 588–597, 2011.

[11] S. J. Um, S. K. Lee, Y. H. Kim et al., "Clinical features of drug-induced hypersensitivity syndrome in 38 patients," *Journal of Investigational Allergology and Clinical Immunology*, vol. 20, no. 7, pp. 556–562, 2010.

[12] P. Tennis and R. S. Stern, "Risk of serious cutaneous disorders after initiation of use of phenytoin, carbamazepine, or sodium valproate: a record linkage study," *Neurology*, vol. 49, no. 2, pp. 542–546, 1997.

[13] J. Jurado-Palomo, R. Cabañas, N. Prior et al., "Use of the lymphocyte transformation test in the diagnosis of DRESS syndrome induced by ceftriaxone and piperacillintazobactam: two case reports," *Journal of Investigational Allergology and Clinical Immunology*, vol. 20, no. 5, pp. 433–436, 2010.

[14] R. Cabañas, L. Muñoz, C. López-Serrano et al., "Hypersensitivity to piperacillin," *Allergy*, vol. 53, no. 8, pp. 819–820, 1998.

[15] S. Fahim, V. Jain, G. Victor, and T. Pierscianowski, "Piperacillin-tazobactam-induced drug hypersensitivity syndrome," *Cutis*, vol. 77, no. 6, pp. 353–357, 2006.

[16] R. Cabañas, O. Calderón, E. Ramírez et al., "Piperacillin-induced DRESS: distinguishing features observed in a clinical and allergy study of 8 patients," *Journal of Investigational Allergology and Clinical Immunology*, vol. 24, no. 6, pp. 425–430, 2014.

[17] Y. Wu, J. Farrell, M. Pirmohamed, B. K. Park, and D. J. Naisbitt, "Generation and characterization of antigen-specific $CD4^+$, $CD8^+$, and $CD4^+CD8^+$ T-cell clones from patients with carbamazepine hypersensitivity," *Journal of Allergy and Clinical Immunology*, vol. 119, no. 4, pp. 973–981, 2007.

[18] A. Rozieres, M. Vocanson, B. B. Saïd, A. Nosbaum, and J.-F. Nicolas, "Role of T cells in nonimmediate allergic drug reactions," *Current Opinion in Allergy and Clinical Immunology*, vol. 9, no. 4, pp. 305–310, 2009.

[19] P. Joly, B. Janela, F. Tetart et al., "Poor benefit/risk balance of intravenous immunoglobulins in DRESS," *Archives of Dermatology*, vol. 148, no. 4, pp. 543–544, 2012.

[20] D. Nishio, K. Izu, K. Kabashima, and Y. Tokura, "T cell populations propagating in the peripheral blood of patients with drug eruptions," *Journal of Dermatological Science*, vol. 48, no. 1, pp. 25–33, 2007.

[21] A. Franzke, W. Piao, J. Lauber et al., "G-CSF as immune regulator in T cells expressing the G-CSF receptor: implications for transplantation and autoimmune diseases," *Blood*, vol. 102, no. 2, pp. 734–739, 2003.

Acute-Onset Panhypopituitarism Nearly Missed by Initial Cosyntropin Testing

Claudine A. Blum,[1] Daniel Schneeberger,[1] Matthias Lang,[1] Janko Rakic,[1,2] Marc Philippe Michot,[1] and Beat Müller[1]

[1] *Medical University Clinic, Kantonsspital Aarau, Aarau, Switzerland*
[2] *Department of Pneumology, Medical Clinic, Kantonsspital Baden, Baden, Switzerland*

Correspondence should be addressed to Claudine A. Blum; claudine.blum@ksa.ch

Academic Editor: Kurt Lenz

Introduction. Diagnosis of adrenal crisis and panhypopituitarism in patients with septic shock is difficult but crucial for outcome. *Case.* A 66-year-old woman with metastasized breast cancer presented to the ED with respiratory insufficiency and septic shock after a 2-day history of the flu. After transfer to the ICU, corticosteroids were started in addition to antibiotics, as the patient was vasopressor-nonresponsive. Diabetes insipidus was diagnosed due to polyuria and treated with 4 mg desmopressin. Thereafter, norepinephrine could be tapered rapidly. On day 2, basal cortisol was 136 nmol/L with an increase to 579 nmol/L in low-dose cosyntropin testing. Polyuria had not developed again. Therefore, corticosteroids were stopped. On day 3, the patient developed again nausea, vomiting, and polyuria. Adrenal crisis and diabetes insipidus were postulated. Corticosteroids and desmopressin were restarted. Further testing confirmed panhypopituitarism. MRI showed a new sellar metastasis. After 2 weeks, stimulated cortisol in cosyntropin testing reached only 219 nmol/l, confirming adrenal insufficiency. *Discussion.* The time course showed that the adrenal glands took 2 weeks to atrophy after loss of pituitary ACTH secretion. Therefore, a misleading result of the cosyntropin test in the initial phase with low basal cortisol and allegedly normal response to exogenous ACTH may be seen. Cosyntropin testing in the critically ill should be interpreted with caution and in the corresponding clinical setting.

1. Introduction

We present the case of acute-onset panhypopituitarism due to a rapid growing sellar metastasis of breast cancer, where adrenal crisis and manifest diabetes insipidus were triggered by a lower respiratory tract infection.

2. Case Presentation

A 66-year-old woman presented to the emergency department with a two-day history of fever, cough, vomiting, and lethargy. Past medical history revealed a recently diagnosed recurrence of breast cancer with diffuse bone and mediastinal metastases. The patient was hypotensive (RR 85/55 mmHg, HR 105/min) and febrile (39.3°C). Arterial blood gas analysis showed global respiratory insufficiency. A chest computed tomography revealed an infiltrate in the left lower lobe. Fluid resuscitation and treatment with broad spectrum antibiotics were begun for presumed community-acquired pneumonia with septic shock. The patient was admitted to the ICU, where she required high doses of intravenous fluids and circulatory support with norepinephrine up to 0.4 ug/kgKG/min. Adjunct treatment with corticosteroids was started after obtaining a random cortisol of 258 nmol/L. The clinical condition of the patient stabilized rapidly, and norepinephrine was tapered within 8 hours after beginning of corticosteroid therapy. Confusingly, cosyntropin testing 14 hours later showed a basal cortisol of 136 nmol/L with an adequate absolute and relative (>250 nM) increase of cortisol after 30 minutes to 579 nmol/L.

The presence of polyuria (600–800 ml/hr) despite septic shock raised the suspicion of diabetes insipidus, which was

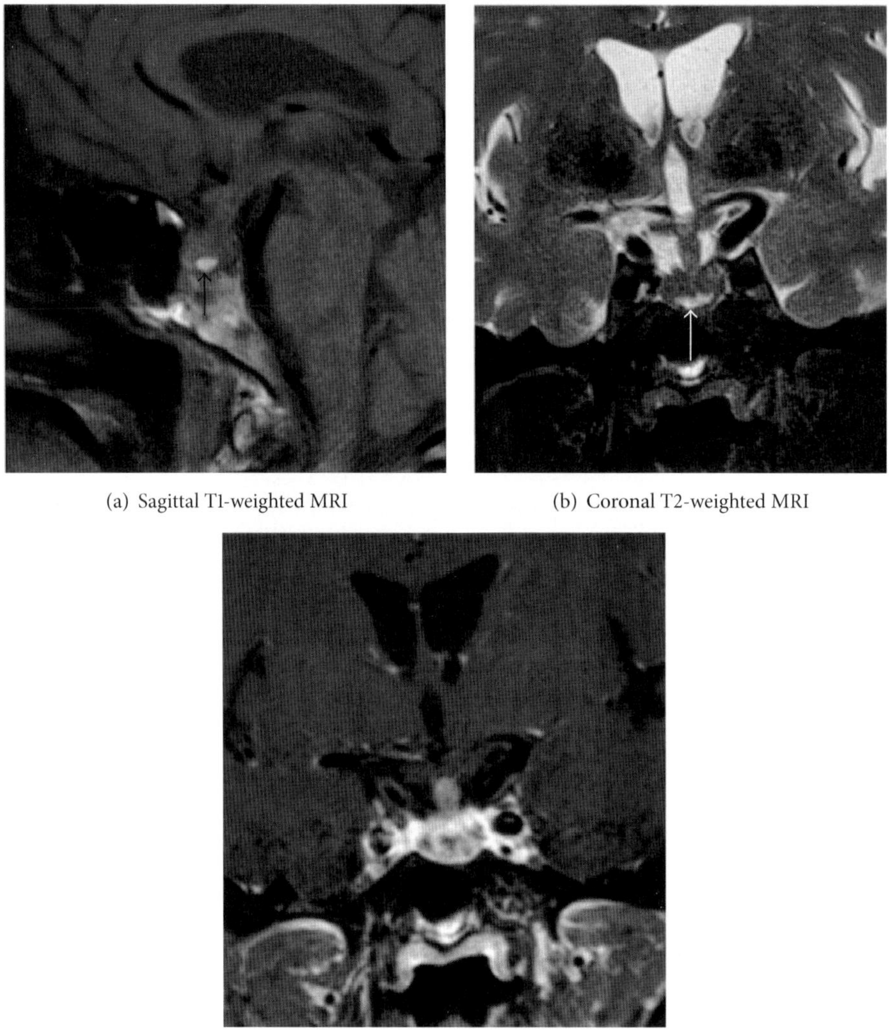

(a) Sagittal T1-weighted MRI

(b) Coronal T2-weighted MRI

(c) Coronal T1-weighted MRI

FIGURE 1: Inhomogeneity of the pituitary indicative of local metastases. Sagittal T1-weighted MRI (a) and coronal T2-weighted MRI (b) of the pituitary showed signal increase suggesting hemorrhage (arrows). Coronal T1-weighted MRI (c) with contrast shows inhomogeneous enhancement of pituitary with metastasis.

confirmed with a serum osmolality of 320 mosm/kg and a urine osmolality of 148 mosm/kg. Consequently, four ug of desmopressin was administered intravenously.

After 36 hours, corticosteroid infusion was stopped, as the formal requirements for adrenal insufficiency and critical-illness-related corticosteroid insufficiency [1, 2] were only marginally met. Furthermore, as only one dose of desmopressin had been given and polyuria had not developed again, desmopressin was paused as well. The patient was then discharged from the ICU.

The following day, the patient complained of nausea, vomiting, and polyuria again. Vital signs were stable, but due to the clinical presentation, adrenal crisis was postulated and methylprednisolone 40 mg intravenously every 8 hours was administered. Furthermore, the patient failed to concentrate urine with a urine osmolality of 146 mmol/l and hypernatremia of 151 mmol/l. Manifest central diabetes insipidus was diagnosed and desmopressin treatment was restarted.

The diagnosis of acute septic shock due to influenza A/H1N1-pneumonia was made retrospectively due to positive nasopharyngeal swabs.

Further exploration of pituitary axis testing confirmed panhypopituitarism with a low FSH level in a post-menopausal patient and low serum levels of TSH, free T4, growth hormone, and IGF-1. Also, posterior lobe pituitary insufficiency was confirmed with levels of vasopressin and copeptin [3] in the low-normal range at the presence of high urine output with a low urine osmolality and high serum sodium (for detailed laboratory values, see Table 1).

Pituitary MRI showed signal increase suggesting hemorrhage in sagittal T1-weighted and coronal T2-weighted MRI, but coronal T1-weighted MRI with contrast showed inhomogeneous enhancement of pituitary with metastasis. The concluding diagnosis was a sellar metastasis (Figure 1) of the known metastasizing breast cancer. This lesion was new, as it had not been present in a PET scan 2 months earlier.

Table 1: Laboratory values.

Variable	Reference range, adults	One week before admission	Day 1, 10 a.m.	Day 1, 10 p.m.	Day 2	Day 3	Day 4	Day 8	Day 15	Day 32
Hematocrit (%)	36.0–45.0	0.423	0.433	0.353	0.372	0.297				0.384
Hemoglobin (g/l)	120–155 g/l	140	137	107	118	97				118
White cell count (per mm^3)	4000–10000	5700	9500	9400	6400	7000				7390
Thrombocytes (G/l)	140–400	234	287	277	292	243				306
Sodium (mmol/l)	136–146	148	139	153	147	147	151		143	144
Potassium (mmol/l)	3.6–5.0	3.6	3.9		3.8	4.3	4.2		4.3	4.3
Osmolality (mosmol/kg)	280–300		298	320			310		298	
Urine osmolality (mosmol/kg)	100–1200			148	274		146	271		
Urea (mmol/l)	2–7		8.1		4.6	4.9			5.7	7
Creatinine (umol/l)	53–94	61	170		120	91	83		90	55
Procalcitonin (ug/l)	<0.5	0.18	0.47		3.88					
C-reactive protein mg/l	<3.0	15.8	79.2		71.3	100	47.3			
Copeptin (pmol/l)	<31		4.8		2.3					
Vasopressin (ADH) (pmol/l)	1.0–4.2			<0.90						
TSH (mU/l)	0.4–4.0		0.14		0.05		0.07	0.1		
T3 (nmol/l)	0.90–2.60				2.05		0.91			
fT4 (nmol/l)	9.9–19.3						10.1	8.71		
HGH (ug/l)	<7				0.23					
IGF1 (ug/l)	59–195				64.7					105
FSH (U/l)	19–140				1.08					1.77
Prolactin (ug/l)	2.2–28						73.6			94.3
Morning cortisol (nmol/l)	140–700		258							
Cosyntropin test (low dose)										
Cortisol 0′ (nmol/l)				136				292	122	67
Cortisol 30′ (nmol/l)	>500			579				497	356	219

After 2 weeks, stimulated cortisol levels in the repeated low-dose cosyntropin test reached only 219 nmol/l.

3. Discussion

Acute panhypopituitarism is rare and mostly due to acute ischemia or hemorrhage of the pituitary. In our patient, the reason for panhypopituitarism was a fast expanding sellar metastasis, with a pulmonary infection as a trigger for an adrenal crisis and manifest diabetes insipidus. The time course of the low-dose cosyntropin testing showed that it took two weeks for the adrenal glands to atrophy after loss of pituitary ACTH stimulation. Importantly, as exemplified in our patient, a misleading result of the cosyntropin testing in the initial phase with allegedly normal response to exogenous ACTH may be seen. The clinical presentation and suspicion in these patients are crucial together with the correct interpretation of an inadequately low random cortisol. Random serum cortisol and the response to cosyntropin test depend on the individual stress level [4, 5] and have to be interpreted with caution in critically ill patients with acute onset of a disease. Importantly, the critical care setting already represents a major stress stimulus for serum cortisol. Therefore, cosyntropin testing should not be routinely performed in the critical care setting [6, 7]. If adrenal failure in addition to septic shock or critical illness is suspected despite a borderline random cortisol, failure to stimulate after cosyntropin testing may help to diagnose primary adrenal insufficiency [8]. However, the present case shows that a high stimulated cortisol level does not rule out secondary adrenal insufficiency.

Disclosure

This case was presented as a poster abstract at the annual meeting of the Swiss Society for Endocrinology and Diabetology (SGED/SSED) in Bern in November 2013 [9].

Authors' Contributions

Daniel Schneeberger, Matthias Lang, Claudine A. Blum, Janko Rakic, Marc Philippe Michot, and Beat Müller looked after the patient. Daniel Schneeberger, Janko Rakic, and Claudine A. Blum wrote the report.

Acknowledgments

The authors gratefully thank Professor Dr. Luca Remonda from the Department of Neuroradiology, Kantonsspital Aarau, Switzerland, for the kind permission to use the radiologic image.

References

[1] R. B. Moraes, M. A. Czepielewski, G. Friedman, and E. L. Borba, "Diagnosis of adrenal failure in critically ill patients," *Arq Bras Endocrinol Metabol*, vol. 55, pp. 295–302, 2011.

[2] P. E. Marik, "Glucocorticoids in sepsis: Dissecting facts from fiction," *Critical Care*, vol. 15, article 158, no. 3, 2011.

[3] N. Nigro, B. Muller, NG. Morgenthaler, F. Fluri, and P. Schutz, "The use of copeptin, the stable peptide of the vasopressin precursor, in the differential diagnosis of sodium imbalance in patients with acute diseases," *Swiss Med Wkly*, vol. 141, article w13270, 2011.

[4] I. E. Widmer, J. J. Puder, C. König et al., "Cortisol response in relation to the severity of stress and illness," *Journal of Clinical Endocrinology and Metabolism*, vol. 90, no. 8, pp. 4579–4586, 2005.

[5] G. Dickstein, "On the term "relative adrenal insufficiency"—Or what do we really measure with adrenal stimulation tests?" *Journal of Clinical Endocrinology and Metabolism*, vol. 90, no. 8, pp. 4973-4974, 2005.

[6] B. Venkatesh and J. Cohen, "The utility of the corticotropin test to diagnose adrenal insufficiency in critical illness: An update," *Clinical Endocrinology*, vol. 83, no. 3, pp. 289–297, 2015.

[7] A. Rhodes, L. E. Evans, W. Alhazzani, M. M. Levy, and M. Antonelli, "Surviving Sepsis Campaign," in *Proceedings of the International Guidelines for Management of Sepsis and Septic Shock*, vol. 45, pp. 486–552, 2017.

[8] M. S. Cooper and P. M. Stewart, "Adrenal insufficiency in critical illness," *Journal of Intensive Care Medicine*, vol. 22, no. 6, pp. 348–362, 2007.

[9] C. A. Blum, D. Schneeberger, M. Lang, J. Rakic, M. P. Michot et al., *Acute-onset panhypopituitarismus nearly missed by initial ACTH testing*, Bern, Switzerland, 2013.

36

Anoxic Brain Injury Presenting as Pseudosubarachnoid Hemorrhage in the Medical Intensive Care Unit

O'Dene Lewis, Samina Afreen, Supo Folaranmi, Marie Fidelia-Lambert, Vishal Poddar, and Alicia Thomas

Howard University Hospital, 2041 Georgia Ave. NW, Washington, DC 20060, USA

Correspondence should be addressed to O'Dene Lewis; odene_lewis@yahoo.com

Academic Editor: Gerhard Pichler

Anoxic encephalopathy is frequently encountered in the medical intensive care unit (ICU). Cerebral edema as a result of anoxic brain injury can result in increased attenuation in the basal cisterns and subarachnoid spaces on computerized tomography (CT) scans of the head. These findings can mimic those seen in acute subarachnoid hemorrhage (SAH) and are referred to as pseudosubarachnoid hemorrhage (pseudo-SAH). Pseudo-SAH is a diagnosis critical care physicians should be aware of as they treat and evaluate their patients with presumed SAH, which is a medical emergency. This lack of awareness could have important clinical implications on outcomes and impact management decisions if patients with anoxic brain injury are inappropriately treated for SAH. We describe three patients who presented to the hospital with anoxic brain injury. Subsequent CT head suggested SAH, which was subsequently proven to be pseudo-SAH.

1. Introduction

Subarachnoid hemorrhage (SAH) is often a devastating clinical event with high mortality. An accurate diagnosis in patients with neurological impairment is essential [1]. In patients suspected of having SAH, nonenhanced computed tomography of the brain is the diagnostic imaging of choice. It has a high sensitivity for the detection of SAH, up to 98% [2] in patients scanned within 24 hours of symptom onset. CT head finding of high attenuation areas (HDAs) along the basal cisterns or cortical sulci is thought to be specific for SAH [3]. A similar appearance in the CT of the head may occur in the absence of blood in the subarachnoid spaces. This distinct finding is referred to as pseudosubarachnoid hemorrhage (pseudo-SAH).

Mimics of SAH include diffuse cerebral edema and purulent meningitis [3]. Spiegel et al. first described these findings in 1986 [4]. They reported that 10 patients with marked brain edema associated with a brain tumor or cerebral infarction showed SAH-like HDAs along the interhemispheric fissure and tentorium cerebelli on CT head. Autopsy done on all 10 patients showed no intracranial hemorrhage. In 1998, on reviewing head CT examinations of 100 comatose patients with brain edema, Avrahami et al. [5] found SAH-like findings along the cisterns and sulci in all of them and concluded that a CT diagnosis of SAH was unlikely. They proposed the term "pseudosubarachnoid hemorrhage" (pseudo-SAH) for this phenomenon.

In this report, we describe three patients with pseudo-SAH associated with diffuse cerebral edema and reviewed the literature regarding this imaging finding.

2. Patient 1

A 25-year-old African American female with an unknown past medical history was found unresponsive in her apartment. The patient was found to be severely hypoglycemic and was intubated for airway protection. She was admitted to the intensive care unit with a primary diagnosis of acute encephalopathy due to metabolic and/or septic etiology. On examination, she had a Glasgow Coma Scale (GCS) of 6T/15 with preserved brainstem reflexes and no lateralizing signs. An initial CT scan of her head appeared to be normal. A repeat CT scan of her head was performed in response to minimal improvement in the patient's

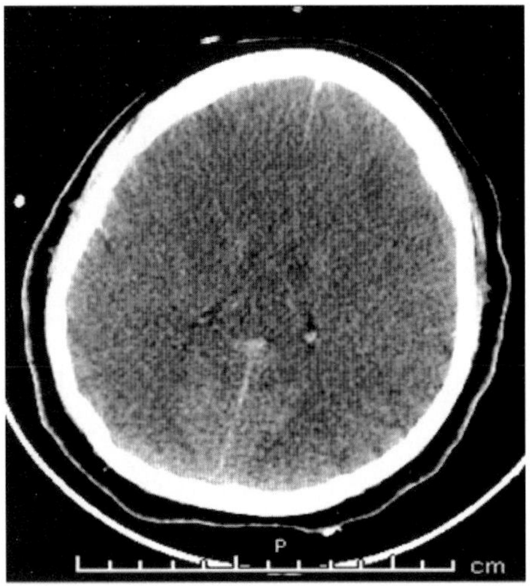

Figure 1: Noncontrast head computed tomography (CT) showing diffuse sulcal effacement and obliterated basal cisterns.

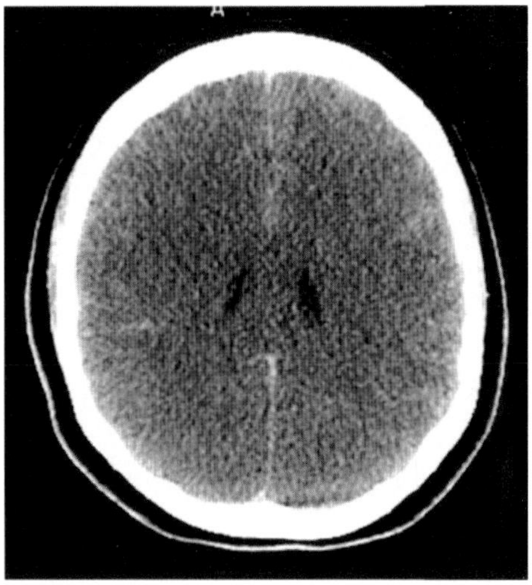

Figure 2: Noncontrast head computed tomography (CT) showing diffuse sulcal effacement, obliterated basal cisterns, and hyperdensity in the interhemispheric fissure.

neurological status. This revealed diffuse sulcal effacement and obliterated basal cisterns suggestive of SAH (Figure 1). Lumbar puncture showed an opening pressure of 29 cm and closing pressure of 25 cm. Cerebrospinal fluid (CSF) revealed the following: leucocytes $13/mm^3$ with a lymphocytic predominance, erythrocytes $10/mm^3$ without xanthochromia, normal protein and glucose, and negative Gram stain. Cerebral angiography was not performed. Lumbar puncture results were inconsistent with a diagnosis of SAH; thus, a diagnosis of SAH was rejected. Over the course of the hospital stay, there was a slight improvement in the patient's mental status to GCS of 8T/15. She subsequently had tracheostomy and percutaneous endoscopic gastrostomy (PEG) tube placement and was transferred to a long-term acute care hospital.

3. Patient 2

A 62-year-old African American female with a past medical history of tobacco abuse (no home medication) was brought in by an ambulance after a cardiac arrest. Her husband, a witness, reported generalized tonic-clonic seizure lasting approximately 5 minutes and she subsequently became unresponsive. The Emergency Medical Services (EMS) were called and cardiopulmonary resuscitation (CPR) was initiated. The patient had a return of spontaneous circulation after approximately 10 minutes and was intubated in the emergency vehicle and brought to the emergency room. On examination, the patient had a GCS of 3T/15. CT scan of the head showed diffuse sulcal effacement, obliterated basal cisterns, and hyperdensity in the interhemispheric fissure suggestive of SAH (Figure 2). The patient subsequently demised. Autopsy done revealed that the cause of death was a large inferior wall myocardial infarction with no evidence of SAH.

4. Patient 3

A 20-year-old African American female with a complaint of progressive shortness of breath 1 week earlier was brought in by an ambulance to the hospital after a cardiac arrest after she collapsed and lost consciousness in her room. Her roommate, who immediately called the EMS, witnessed the syncope. CPR was initiated, which continued en route to the hospital. After approximately 15 minutes of advance cardiac life support (ACLS), there was a return of spontaneous circulation. The patient was admitted to the ICU for post-cardiac arrest care. Based on the brief history, there was a high clinical index of suspicion for massive pulmonary embolism. An echocardiogram showed a dilated right ventricle suggestive of increased pulmonary artery pressure. CT angiography of the chest was not done due to hemodynamic instability and renal impairment. Based on the evidence highly suggestive of a massive pulmonary embolism, tissue plasminogen activator (TPA) infusion was started. She remained in a comatose state with no neurological response. CT scan of her head was performed which showed diffuse cerebral edema, with hyperattenuated cisterns and cerebral sulci, compatible with diffuse SAH (Figure 3). The patient at that time was too unstable to perform lumbar puncture or cerebral angiography. The TPA was stopped due to findings suggestive of SAH. A neurosurgery consult was requested, and the consultant reviewed the CT scan of the head with the radiologist. The attenuation coefficient at the basal cistern was 25–40 HU (Hounsfield unit) with a mean of 30–35 HU consistent with pseudo-SAH. The patient subsequently demised, thought to be due to a massive pulmonary embolism.

5. Discussion

A pseudo-SAH is a brain CT finding that is seen as high attenuation areas (HDAs) along the basal cisterns, the sylvian

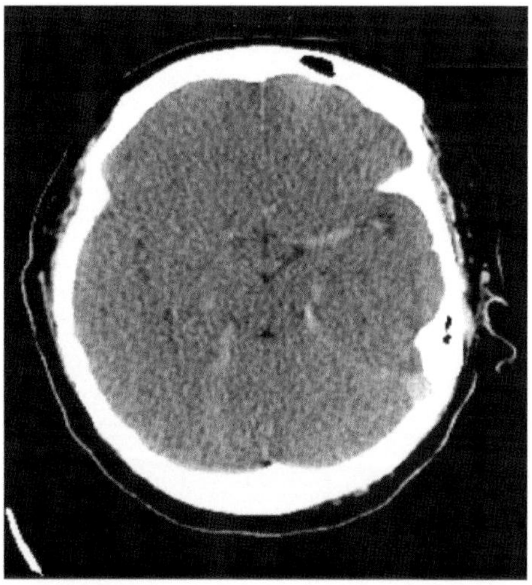

Figure 3: Noncontrast head computed tomography (CT) showing diffuse cerebral edema, with hyperattenuated cisterns and cerebral sulci.

fissure, the tentorium cerebelli, or the cortical sulci in patients with severe brain edema, where no SAH is seen at autopsy or lumbar puncture [6].

To explain the origin of pseudo-SAH in association with cerebral edema, we considered the proposed causes of pseudo-SAH in other diseases. In purulent meningitis, bacterial toxins lead to the breakdown of the brain-blood barrier (BBB). The resultant BBB disruption allows proteinaceous material to leak into the subarachnoid space. However, CSF protein concentrations are sufficiently elevated to cause appreciable changes in CSF attenuation only in the most severe cases of meningitis [7–9]. The proteinaceous material in the subarachnoid space leads to vasogenic and cerebral edema, which contribute to the appearance of pseudo-SAH. Clinical history, CSF analysis, and enhancement of the basal cistern in postcontrast CT head can help differentiate between SAH and pseudo-SAH in this case [3].

Cerebral edema can lead to the cerebral cortex being displaced into the cerebrospinal fluid space and veins become congested due to the brain edema compressing the dural sinuses. The resultant subarachnoid spaces become relatively devoid of the hypoattenuated CSF and fill with a larger fraction of meninges and blood vessels than in the normal state, potentially increasing their CT attenuation [10]. With the development of cerebral edema, the attenuation of the brain parenchyma decreases concurrently [11, 12]. The decreased attenuation in brain parenchyma contributes to the pseudo-SAH appearance by increasing the conspicuity of the distended vasculature within the basal cisterns. Hypoxic ischemic encephalopathy after resuscitation from cardiopulmonary arrest, toxic encephalopathy due to valproate poisoning or bee sting, cerebral infarction, and/or severe head trauma can lead to cerebral edema and hence to the imaging finding of pseudo-SAH. In cases of cerebral edema, pseudo-SAH can be differentiated from SAH based on the attenuation coefficient in the basal cisterns. Attenuation coefficient is 21 to 44 Hounsfield units (HU) in case of pseudo-SAH, while it is 60–70 HU in cases with SAH. This difference was used to identify pseudo-SAH in our third patient in the absence of a lumbar puncture or autopsy findings. Following cardiopulmonary resuscitation, pseudo-SAH may develop within 3 days in approximately 20% of patients [6]. This indicates severe brain damage and suggests a poor prognosis, providing important information for deciding treatment strategies [6].

Agha and Al-Hakami described a young man with chronic renal failure who suddenly collapsed after starting hemodialysis. CT scan of the head showed severe brain edema and loss of sulci with hyperattenuated cisterns, suggestive of SAH. However, a four-vessel angiography did not show SAH. Further testing confirmed that the patient was brain-dead [13]. Given et al. described seven patients with diffuse cerebral edema and the appearance of SAH in the basal cisterns [10]. True SAH was excluded by lumbar puncture in four of the cases and by autopsy in three of the cases. Of the seven cases, only one patient survived. Al-Yamany et al. reported a case of a young man who suddenly collapsed after a drug overdose. CT scan showed an appearance of diffuse SAH, but autopsy performed 40 hours after his seizure revealed anoxic encephalopathy with no evidence of SAH [5]. Like these previously reported patients, our three cases exhibited clinical and radiological evidence of cerebral edema and increased intracranial pressure. In all three cases, the cisterns were effaced and the gray-white matter differentiation was obscured, compatible with diffuse cerebral edema. In the first case, CSF was not purulent and showed no evidence of hemorrhage. In the second case, autopsy did not show SAH similar to Al-Yamany et al. There was no definitive diagnostic test done on the third case. However, the imaging met criteria for pseudo-SAH based on the HDAs. Similar to the previously reported series, all of our patients had poor outcomes including 2 deaths and 1 with permanent neurologic sequelae.

Pseudosubarachnoid hemorrhage is considered a rare finding. It is important to recognize pseudo-SAH as it can lead to other diagnostic tests being performed, including angiographic studies to rule out vascular lesions and influence therapeutic decision-making in critically ill patients. Pseudo-SAH should be considered in patients with suspected SAH on CT scan of the head whose lumbar puncture does not demonstrate xanthochromia or in whom the clinical history is atypical for SAH but suggestive of another diagnosis, such as infection. However, due to the high morbidity and mortality from undiagnosed aneurysmal SAH, angiography should always be performed, unless a clear alternative diagnosis can be made.

Disclosure

The abstract was presented at the American Thoracic Society 2017 international conference.

References

[1] M. Al-Yamany, J. Deck, and M. Bernstein, "Pseudo-subarachnoid hemorrhage: A rare neuroimaging pitfall," *Canadian Journal of Neurological Sciences*, vol. 26, no. 1, pp. 57–59, 1999.

[2] J. J. Perry, I. G. Stiell, M. L. A. Sivilotti et al., "Sensitivity of computed tomography performed within six hours of onset of headache for diagnosis of subarachnoid haemorrhage: Prospective cohort study," *BMJ (Online)*, vol. 343, no. 7817, Article ID d4277, 2011.

[3] C.-Y. Lin, P.-H. Lai, J.-H. Fu, P.-C. Wang, and H.-B. Pan, "Pseudo-subarachnoid hemorrhage: A potential imaging pitfall," *Canadian Association of Radiologists Journal*, vol. 65, no. 3, pp. 225–231, 2014.

[4] S. M. Spiegel, A. J. Fox, F. Vinuela, and D. M. Pelz, "Increased density of tentorium and falx: A false positive CT sign of subarachnoid hemorrhage," *Canadian Association of Radiologists Journal*, vol. 37, no. 4, pp. 243–247, 1986.

[5] E. Avrahami, R. Katz, A. Rabin, and V. Friedman, "CT diagnosis of non-traumatic subarachnoid haemorrhage in patients with brain edema," *European Journal of Radiology*, vol. 28, no. 3, pp. 222–225, 1998.

[6] H. Yuzawa, S. Higano, S. Mugikura et al., "Pseudo-subarachnoid hemorrhage found in patients with postresuscitation encephalopathy: Characteristics of CT findings and clinical importance," *American Journal of Neuroradiology*, vol. 29, no. 8, pp. 1544–1549, 2008.

[7] D. B. Mendelsohn, M. L. Moss, D. P. Chason, S. Muphree, and S. Casey, "Acute purulent leptomeningitis mimicking subarachnoid hemorrhage on ct," *Journal of Computer Assisted Tomography*, vol. 18, no. 1, pp. 126–128, 1994.

[8] T. Chatterjee, J. R. Gowardman, and T. D. Goh, "Pneumococcal meningitis masquerading as subarachnoid haemorrhage," *Medical Journal of Australia*, vol. 178, no. 10, pp. 505–507, 2003.

[9] D. Norman, D. Price, D. Boyd, R. Fishman, and T. H. Newton, "Quantitative aspects of computed tomography of the blood and cerebrospinal fluid," *Radiology*, vol. 123, no. 2, pp. 335–338, 1977.

[10] C. A. Given, J. H. Burdette, A. D. Elster, and D. W. Williams, "Pseudo-subarachnoid hemorrhage: A potential imaging pitfall associated with diffuse cerebral edema," *American Journal of Neuroradiology*, vol. 24, no. 2, pp. 254–256, 2003.

[11] K. G. Rieth, K. Fujiwara, G. Di Chiro et al., "Serial measurements of CT attenuation and specific gravity in experimental cerebral edema," *Radiology*, vol. 135, no. 2, pp. 343–348, 1980.

[12] R. A. Clasen, M. S. Huckman, K. A. Von Roenn, S. Pandolfi, I. Laing, and J. J. Lobick, "A Correlative Study Of Computed Tomography And Histology In Human And Experimental Vasogenic Cerebral Edema," *Journal of Computer Assisted Tomography*, vol. 5, no. 3, pp. 313–327, 1981.

[13] A. Agha and M. Al-Hakami, "A case report of pseudo-subarachnoid hemorrhage," *Maedica*, vol. 6, no. 3, pp. 210–212, 2011.

37

Ethylene Glycol Poisoning: An Unusual Cause of Altered Mental Status and the Lessons Learned from Management of the Disease in the Acute Setting

R. Singh, E. Arain, A. Buth, J. Kado, A. Soubani, and N. Imran

Detroit Medical Center/Wayne State University, Detroit, MI, USA

Correspondence should be addressed to N. Imran; nimran@med.wayne.edu

Academic Editor: Ricardo Oliveira

Ethylene glycol is found in many household products and is a common toxic ingestion. Acute ingestions present with altered sensorium and an osmolal gap. The true toxicity of ethylene glycol is mediated by its metabolites, which are responsible for the increased anion gap metabolic acidosis, renal tubular damage, and crystalluria seen later in ingestions. Early intervention is key; however, diagnosis is often delayed, especially in elderly patients presenting with altered mental status. There are several laboratory tests which can be exploited for the diagnosis, quantification of ingestion, and monitoring of treatment, including the lactate and osmolal gaps. As methods of direct measurement of ethylene glycol are often not readily available, it is important to have a high degree of suspicion based on these indirect laboratory findings. Mainstay of treatment is bicarbonate, fomepizole or ethanol, and, often, hemodialysis. A validated equation can be used to estimate necessary duration of hemodialysis, and even if direct measurements of ethylene glycol are not available, monitoring for the closure of the anion, lactate, and osmolal gaps can guide treatment. We present the case of an elderly male with altered mental status, acute kidney injury, elevated anion gap metabolic acidosis, and profound lactate and osmolal gaps.

1. Introduction

Ethylene glycol is an alcohol found in many household products such as antifreeze, deicing solutions and windshield wiper fluids [1]. Odorless, colorless, and sweet in taste, it is most commonly ingested by children, animals, and those seeking a substitute for ethanol but has also been reported in cases of homicide [2] and suicide. With oral LD_{LO} of 786 mg/kg for humans, which is about 50 milliliters or 1.7 ounces of ethylene glycol for a 70-kilogram patient, even the ingestion of a small volume can prove lethal [3]. The toxicity of ethylene glycol is mediated by its metabolites, mainly glycolic acid and oxalate [4]. These metabolites are responsible for the pathogenesis of the symptoms with which patients present, which are classically those of profound acidosis (altered sensorium and Kussmaul breathing) and crystalluria (consumptive hypocalcemia, oliguria, hematuria, and flank pain) [5].

Diagnosis is made based on known or suspected ingestion in the appropriate clinical setting, with laboratory evaluation playing a key role. While there are tests to specifically identify ethylene glycol in the serum, they may not be readily available and are not without their limitations. As such, clinicians often rely on clinical presentation and findings on blood tests, such as a severe and unexplained anion gap metabolic acidosis with an osmolar gap, to make the diagnosis.

Prevention of sequelae of ethylene glycol intoxication is dependent upon early identification and intervention in order to minimize the production of its toxic metabolites [6]. Early therapeutic intervention is important as most of the ethylene glycol is absorbed through the gastrointestinal tract within one hour of ingestion. The mainstay of treatment is sodium bicarbonate to treat the acute acidosis, fomepizole or ethanol to block conversion of ethylene glycol to its metabolites, and emergent hemodialysis if the ethylene glycol level is more than 50 mg/dL. It should be noted that initial treatment with sodium bicarbonate, though necessary for correction of severe acidosis, may raise the urine pH and increase the likelihood of the precipitation of calcium oxalate crystals, furthering kidney injury and hypocalcemia. This

Table 1: Lactic acid and ethylene glycol levels at approximate times in case report.

Measurement	18:00	23:00	02:00	07:00[d]	10:00	12:00[e]
Lactic acid from arterial blood gas, mMol/L	6.4[a]	27[b]	24			3.2
Lactic acid from plasma, mMol/L	1.6[c]			1.3		1.6
Ethylene glycol from plasma, mg/dL			54	30	10	6

[a]Point-of-care ABG run in the emergency department using Radiometer ABL 800 analyzer.
[b]Point-of-care ABG run in the ICU using Radiometer ABL 800 analyzer. All subsequent ABG run with this analyzer.
[c]Laboratory lactic acid measured in venous blood using Siemens Dimension EXL analyzer.
[d]Hemodialysis initiated.
[e]Hemodialysis terminated (note closure of lactate gap).

highlights again the importance of early identification and effective intervention. As patients are often critically ill, they frequently require monitoring in an intensive care unit to watch for secondary complications of altered mental status and cardiac arrhythmias. We herein present a case of an accidental ingestion of ethylene glycol in an elderly male that necessitated the above-mentioned therapeutic interventions.

2. Case Presentation

A 78-year-old male with a medical history significant for hypertension, dementia, and prior transient ischemic attack was brought into the hospital by his daughter for altered sensorium and gait disturbance. At baseline, the patient was capable of ambulating without assistance. He was last known well around 23:00 one day prior to his emergency visit. According to the daughter, around 11:00 on the day of his admission, the patient was noted to have difficulty in standing and sitting upright unassisted. His speech was garbled and nearly unintelligible. Earlier, he reported to his daughter that he "felt drunk" and was unable to focus on her face. Subsequently, the daughter brought the patient to the emergency room five hours later at around 16:00.

On presentation, the patient was afebrile, normotensive, tachycardic, and tachypneic. Pulse oximetry showed a hemoglobin saturation of 98% on room air. Physical exam findings were normal except for lethargy, disorientation, and response to deep pain by moving all extremities. His blood profile showed an acute kidney injury with creatinine of 1.24 mg/dL, up from a baseline of 1.0 mg/dL (equivalent to drop in glomerular filtration rate from 95 to 68 mL/min/1.73 m^2), and an elevated anion gap metabolic acidosis with pH of 7.090, $PaCO_2$ of 10.0 mmHg, serum bicarbonate of 8 mMol/L, and an anion gap of 29 mMol/L. Lactic acid was 1.6 mMol/L on a venous sample sent to the laboratory; however, a point-of-care arterial blood gas revealed a lactic acid of 27.0 mMol/L (Table 1).

The venous lactic acid level was initially attributed to a laboratory error given the consistently profound low pH on repeated arterial blood gases. A thorough investigation into the cause of this perceived severe lactic acidosis was undertaken and no clear etiology was identified. There was no evidence of sepsis or postictal symptoms, head CT was negative for stroke, and glucose and beta hydroxybutyrate were within normal limits. Furthermore, there were no signs of gangrenous tissue and surgical and radiological evaluations were negative for ischemic bowel or incarcerated hernia. Additionally, the patient was hemodynamically stable with normal liver enzymes, making systemic hypoperfusion or decreased clearance of lactic acid highly unlikely.

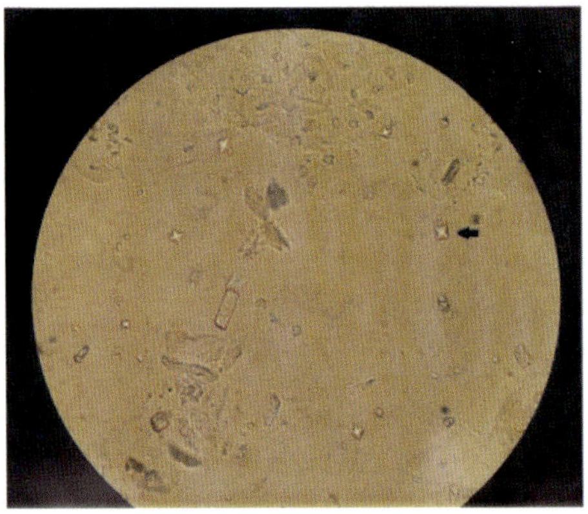

Figure 1: Urine sediment showing envelope-shaped calcium oxalate crystals (arrow).

Despite several fluid boluses and sodium bicarbonate administration, the acidosis and lactate levels did not improve. Further investigation revealed an osmolar gap of 53 mOsm/kg, an undetectable methanol level, and a serum ethylene glycol level of 54 mg/dL. At this time, repeat lactic acid levels were sent from both venous blood and an arterial blood gas and demonstrated the same significant discrepancy (1.3 versus 22 mMol/L, resp.). Subsequently, the patient was admitted to the intensive care unit and continued on intravenous sodium bicarbonate to correct the underlying acidosis and fomepizole to block conversion of ethylene glycol by alcohol dehydrogenase to toxic metabolites and initiated on emergent hemodialysis. Thiamine and pyridoxine were also given to facilitate conversion of glycolate to less toxic metabolites. Serial labs were drawn to monitor acidosis and ethylene glycol levels. When pH normalized and ethylene glycol levels remained <20 mg/dL, hemodialysis and fomepizole were discontinued.

Initially, renal function was stable, with the patient making nearly 2 liters of urine in 24 hours; however, within 48 hours, the patient became oliguric and his renal function deteriorated. Corrected serum calcium dropped from 9.7 to 7.9 mg/dL, which was attributable to precipitation of calcium oxalate crystals, as examination of urine sediment now revealed the typical envelope-shaped calcium oxalate crystals (Figure 1). Though the patient's mental status improved to his

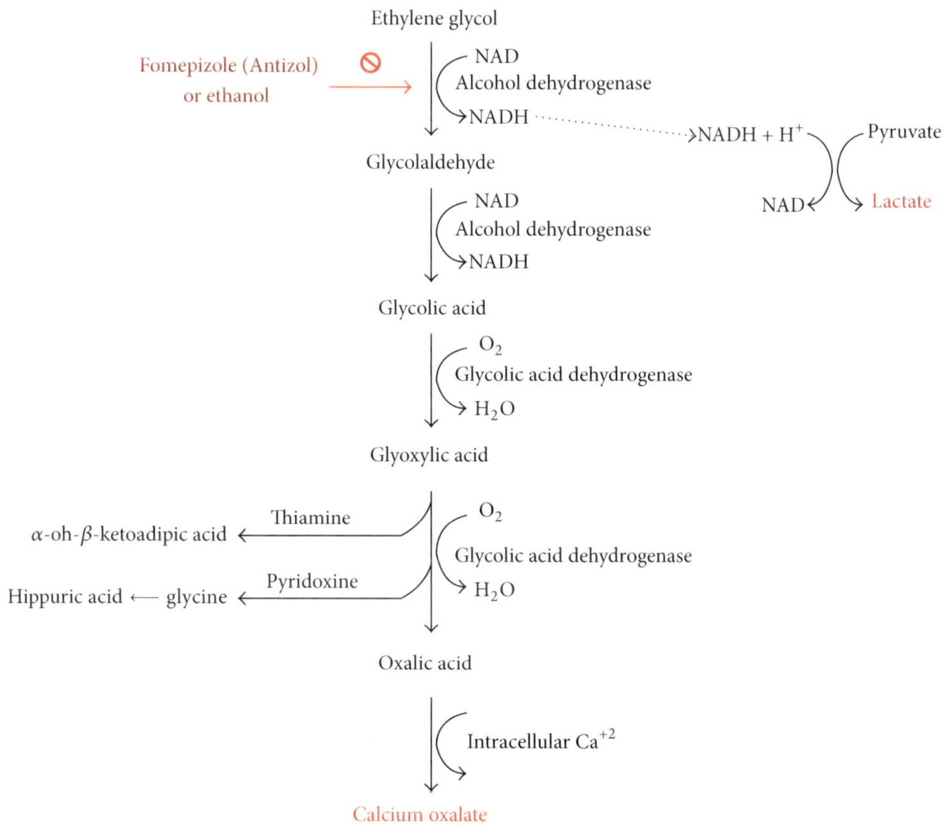

Figure 2: Ethylene glycol metabolism in the human body.

prior baseline, renal function continued to worsen and he became dialysis-dependent. He was discharged on long-term intermittent hemodialysis with uncertain potential for renal recovery.

3. Discussion

When patients present to the emergency room with altered mental status, the differential diagnosis is generally broad. While intoxication is always a consideration, ethylene glycol ingestion is often low on the treating physician's radar, especially in a septuagenarian patient. However, ethylene glycol intoxication is not uncommon. In their annual report, the American Association of Poison Control Centers reported a total of 6600 cases of ethylene glycol poisoning during 2013 alone, a steadily rising number over the years. In 2014, this number rose to a total of 6809 cases. In the report, ethylene glycol was the third most common chemical responsible for deaths by nonpharmaceutical poisoning, following ethanol and carbon monoxide [7]. It should be noted though that reporting of these cases to poison control depends solely on the discretion and initiative of the treating physician and, hence, the true number of cases is likely underestimated. In the UK, the National Poisons Information Service reported a total of 91 cases of ethylene glycol poisoning ranking as the fourth most common after acetaminophen, drugs of misuse, and substance abuse. This number only rose to 92 in the following year [8]. This number is significantly smaller than that in the USA but authors will not speculate on the reason and there were no references exploring the differences.

3.1. Absorption and Toxicity. Ethylene glycol is rapidly absorbed in the gastrointestinal tract within the first hour of ingestion. There have been no reported cases of toxicity after dermal or respiratory exposure [9]. Ingestion of ethylene glycol itself results in an inebriated state and central nervous system depression not unlike that seen in ethanol intoxication. The toxicity of ethylene glycol is mediated by its metabolites (Figure 2) [4]. Ethylene glycol, like other alcohols, is metabolized in the liver. Hepatic oxidation via alcohol dehydrogenase and aldehyde dehydrogenase generates glycolaldehyde and then glycolic acid, respectively. Further metabolism leads to glyoxylate, which may be converted to less toxic metabolites if thiamine and pyridoxine are available, and the final end product, oxalic acid.

Circulating glycolic acid in the blood leads to an elevated anion gap metabolic acidosis with resultant Kussmaul breathing and profound obtundation [4]. Direct renal tubular damage was traditionally attributed to glycolic acid, but there is evidence that glycolaldehyde and glyoxylate may be the principle ethylene glycol metabolites responsible for this mechanism of nephrotoxicity and the ensuing acute renal failure, oliguria, and hematuria (Figure 2). This particular damage was found to be independent of the calcium oxalate crystals formation [10]. As oxalate joins with calcium to form calcium oxalate, the resultant hypocalcemia may lead to nerve palsies and tetany. Seizures and arrhythmias may also develop. Calcium oxalate precipitates in urine and leads to further renal injury via crystal induced nephropathy with occasional flank pain [11]. Because ethylene glycol levels peak at one to four hours after oral ingestion and ethylene glycol's half-life is three to nine hours [11], prompt recognition and intervention are imperative to minimize the production of toxic metabolites.

3.2. Measuring Ethylene Glycol. Unfortunately, even if a clinician suspects ethylene glycol intoxication, definitive methods of detecting ethylene glycol in the serum have limitations which may significantly delay diagnosis and treatment in a situation where time is of the essence. Gas chromatography is the most common method of detecting serum ethylene glycol, but it is not widely available and is often a "send out" test. In a study by Church and Witting, none of the hospitals surveyed had on-site gas chromatography columns for ethylene glycol testing, and the "send out" turn-around time was greater than one hour [12]. Solvent screens for alcohols may not include ethylene glycol and lead the clinician to incorrectly conclude that no ethylene glycol is present, while enzymatic assays have been known to give false positives in patients with elevated levels of lactate or lactate dehydrogenase [13]. Additionally, patients presenting late may have normal ethylene glycol levels but may be critically ill, having already metabolized ethylene glycol to its toxic metabolites. Therefore, recognition of key findings in more readily available laboratory evaluations in the right clinical setting is of utmost importance. Regarding our patient, quantification of ethylene glycol was performed using the Agilent™ 7890A Gas Chromatography per our center (Detroit Medical Center, DMC) Toxicology University Laboratory protocol. The patient's serum was collected in a red top vacutainer and transported at room temperature. The serum was stored in refrigerator temperatures ranging from 2 to 8°C. Working standards were prepared by mixing the combined standard of 25 mg/dL ethylene glycol and 25 mg/dL propylene glycol with an internal standard containing 1000 mg/dL 1,2-butanediol. BioRad™ drug-free serum and serum volatiles containing ethylene glycol were also used. Controls and patient samples were placed into tubes. A set amount of standard was added to each tube. Controls and patient samples were then transferred to an Amicon™ Filter and the protein-free filtrate was transferred to an injection vial with a micro sample insert. The samples, standards, and controls were run in the Agilent 7890A with Autosampler 6850 per DMC toxicology protocol.

An in-depth evaluation of findings and discrepancies in routine laboratory tests plays a key role in raising clinical suspicion of and diagnosing ethylene glycol intoxication. The profound high anion gap metabolic acidosis seen with ethylene glycol and/or methanol intoxication is seen in few other conditions, and, of those conditions, most also present with severely elevated lactic acid levels, such as bowel ischemia or status epilepticus. Ethylene glycol intoxication may lead to a slight elevation in lactic acid, but it is typically not enough to account for the degree of acidosis [11, 14].

3.3. Lactate Gap. One phenomenon which is of great clinical significance and utility is the lactic acid gap. In several studies, it has been noted that lactic acid measurements may be severely but falsely elevated in ethylene glycol intoxication depending on the type of analyzer used. In particular, some point-of-care whole blood analyzers which use L-lactate oxidase may cross-react with glycolate or glyoxylate, leading to massive false-positive lactate elevations [15, 16]. These analyzers are typically used in emergency departments and STAT labs to run arterial blood gases. In contrast, laboratory serum analyzers, which are used for routine analysis of venous blood samples, have less cross-reaction and show very minimal lactate elevation. This lactate gap between an arterial blood gas and venous blood sample is representative then of the presence of toxic ethylene glycol metabolites which are cross-reacting with the point-of-care analyzer. This lactate gap, if present, can be exploited for diagnosis of ethylene glycol intoxication, even in late presentations, as well as for monitoring for clearance of metabolites [16]. In our case, there was a significant lactic acid gap present, which in part prompted investigation into possible ethylene glycol intoxication, and after hemodialysis was initiated, this gap diminished (Table 1).

3.4. Osmolal Gap. Alcohol ingestion often also presents with elevated serum osmolal gaps. Although osmolal gaps up to 15 mOsm may be normal based on the method of calculation [17], significantly elevated and unexplained plasma osmolal gaps greater than 20 to 25 mOsm in the right clinical scenario should raise suspicion of the recent ingestion of an alcohol such as ethanol, methanol, ethylene glycol, or isopropyl alcohol. Because the contribution of an alcohol to the osmolal gap is a direct function of that alcohol's molar mass, if the osmolal gap and type of alcohol are known, the amount of that alcohol in the serum can be determined. For example, an osmolal gap of 10 mOsm is equal to 62 mg/dL of ethylene glycol. Our patient had an osmolal gap of 51 mOsm, which suggests an initial level around 316 mg/dL of ethylene glycol. The parent alcohol contributes initially to both the osmolal and anion gaps. However, after ethylene glycol has been metabolized, there will only be an anion gap without the osmolal gap. This phenomenon can help treating physicians trace back to the approximate time of ingestion.

3.5. Urine Crystals. Finally, another clue in favor of ethylene glycol ingestion is the appearance of calcium oxalate crystals in the urine and concurrent development of hypocalcemia, presumed to be due to the precipitation of calcium oxalate. However, the finding of crystalluria may not be initially present and may take different forms. The classic dihydrate envelope-shaped crystals are only present at high concentrations of calcium oxalate, with the monohydrate needle-shaped crystals being more common and easily confused with hippurate [11]. It is therefore a late and nonspecific finding.

4. Management

Management of ethylene glycol ingestion involves, first and foremost, securing the patient's airway, breathing, and circulation. Severe acidosis and altered sensorium may necessitate endotracheal intubation and hyperventilation. Sodium bicarbonate administration in these patients has two roles, to correct acidosis and to deprotonate glycolic acid and oxalic acid to glycolate and oxalate, making them less likely to penetrate end-organ tissues. However, the delay in hemodialysis initiation to remove oxalate and the continuous bicarbonate infusion may lead to both worsening of hypocalcemia and increasing the risk of calcium oxalate crystal precipitation by raising the urine pH. The next step is to inhibit alcohol dehydrogenase with fomepizole or ethanol. As per current clinical guidelines, fomepizole or ethanol should be given in cases of serum ethylene glycol concentration > 20 mg/dL, known recent ingestion with osmolal gap > 10 mMol, or strong clinical suspicion with three of the following: arterial pH <7.3, serum bicarbonate <20 mMol/L, osmolal gap >10 mMol, or urinary oxalate crystals [18]. Criteria for the initiation of antidotal therapy for known or suspected ethylene glycol intoxication [18] are as follows:

> Serum ethylene glycol of > 20 mg/dL (3.2 mMol/L), or
>
> Documented recent history of ingestion of toxic amounts of ethylene glycol and an osmolal gap >10 mOsm/L, or
>
> Suspected ethylene glycol ingestion and at least two of the following:
>
> (1) Arterial pH <7.3
> (2) Serum bicarbonate <20 mMol/L (mEq/L)
> (3) Osmolal gap >10 mOsm/L
> (4) Oxalate crystalluria.

It should be noted that these guidelines are based on expert opinions not on clinical studies. Hemodialysis is indicated if there is severe acidosis, ethylene glycol levels >50 mg/dL, or evidence of end-organ damage, that is, renal failure. Fomepizole is preferred due to easier dosing and decreased side effects [19]. Thiamine, magnesium, and pyridoxine act as cofactors in different reactions that facilitate the conversion of glyoxylic acid to less toxic metabolites such as glycine (and later hippuric acid) and α-Hydroxy-β-Ketoadipic acid. However, their role is minor and clinicians should not solely rely on them in treating the acute toxicity (Figure 2) [11].

4.1. Role of Hemodialysis. As stated above, in patients with severe poisoning, hemodialysis may be life-saving. The consensus is to start hemodialysis if the level of ethylene glycol is more than 50 mg/dL. Having a normal glomerular filtration rate is not a deterrent to initiate hemodialysis. Intravenous fluid should be switched to normal saline to avoid excessive bicarbonate load and to decrease the risk of calcium oxalate crystals precipitation by raising the urine pH. The calcium level will be maintained during the entire hemodialysis session as calcium concentration in the dialysate is at physiological level. If the patient is receiving fomepizole, then it is crucial to increase the dosing frequency from every 12 hours to four hours as fomepizole is significantly dialyzable. Hemodialysis should be continued until the level of ethylene glycol is consistently < 20 mg/dL with successful resolution of metabolic acidosis [5]. The duration of hemodialysis depends on the level of ethylene glycol upon initiation. A validated equation can be used to estimate the time needed in hours: $-V\ [\ln(5/A)]/[0.06k]$, where V is total body water in liters, ln is the natural logarithm, A is the initial ethylene glycol concentration in mMol/L, and k is 80 percent of the dialyzer urea clearance in mL/min, which is manufacturer-specific and can be easily found using internet search engines [20]. In our patient, weight was 90 kg (45 kg of water), ethylene glycol level upon initiation of dialysis was 54 mg/dL (equal to 8.7 mMol/L), and the dialyzer urea clearance of the filter we used was 266 mL/min at a blood flow of 300 mL/min. We estimated the required duration of hemodialysis to be two hours. Had hemodialysis been started when his presumed ethylene glycol level was 316 mg/dL, he would have required more than 8 hours of hemodialysis.

4.2. Predictors of Renal Recovery. There are not many dedicated studies about predictors of renal recovery after ethylene glycol poisoning. In a retrospective study by Lung et al., patients who had lower chances of recovery were more likely to present with coma or seizures, have profound acidosis, or receive therapy (fomepizole or dialysis) more than 6 hours of presentation [21]. It should be noted that most of cases in the literature involve young patients, and so the recovery likelihood may be higher in this population. Unfortunately, our patient was elderly, had other comorbidities, and presented late with a severe acidosis, giving him a lower chance for recovery.

5. Conclusion

Diagnosing an elderly and demented patient with ethylene glycol toxicity is very challenging. This patient population can present with metabolic acidosis and confusion due to many etiologies and is at risk of decompensating rapidly. Hence, following the well-established algorithms in assessing patients with metabolic acidosis remains the most effective tool to prevent missing any future cases of ethylene glycol ingestion. Given the vague circumstances around our patient's ingestion incidence, we felt the need to alert adult protective services in order to rule out any malicious intent by the caregiver. The patient is still dialysis-dependent and no recovery is expected soon as he remains anuric.

Competing Interests

The authors declare that they have no competing interests.

References

[1] http://www.cdc.gov/niosh/ershdb/emergencyresponsecard_29750031.html.

[2] http://www.cnn.com/2007/LAW/01/05/black.widow/index.html.

[3] Safety Officer in Physical Chemistry, *Safety (MSDS) Data for Ethylene Glycol*, Oxford University, Oxford, UK, 2009.

[4] A. D. Fraser, "Clinical toxicologic implications of ethylene glycol and glycolic acid poisoning," *Therapeutic Drug Monitoring*, vol. 24, no. 2, pp. 232–238, 2002.

[5] J. Brent, K. McMartin, S. Phillips et al., "Fomepizole for the treatment of ethylene glycol poisoning," *The New England Journal of Medicine*, vol. 340, no. 11, pp. 832–838, 1999.

[6] D. Jacobsen, "New treatment for ethylene glycol poisoning," *The New England Journal of Medicine*, vol. 340, no. 11, pp. 879–881, 1999.

[7] https://aapcc.s3.amazonaws.com/pdfs/annual_reports/2013_NPDS_Annual_Report.pdf.

[8] http://www.npis.org/NPISAnnualReport2013-14.pdf.

[9] J. A. Kruse, "Methanol and ethylene glycol intoxication," *Critical Care Clinics*, vol. 28, no. 4, pp. 661–711, 2012.

[10] V. Poldelski, A. Johnson, S. Wright, V. D. Rosa, and R. A. Zager, "Ethylene glycol-mediated tubular injury: identification of critical metabolites and injury pathways," *American Journal of Kidney Diseases*, vol. 38, no. 2, pp. 339–348, 2001.

[11] D. Jacobsen, T. P. Hewlett, R. Webb, S. T. Brown, A. T. Ordinario, and K. E. McMartin, "Ethylene glycol intoxication: evaluation of kinetics and crystalluria," *The American Journal of Medicine*, vol. 84, no. 1, pp. 145–152, 1988.

[12] A. S. Church and M. D. Witting, "Laboratory testing in ethanol, methanol, ethylene glycol, and isopropanol toxicities," *Journal of Emergency Medicine*, vol. 15, no. 5, pp. 687–692, 1997.

[13] A. F. Eder, Y. G. Dowdy, J. A. M. Gardiner, B. A. Wolf, and L. M. Shaw, "Serum lactate and lactate dehydrogenase in high concentrations interfere in enzymatic assay of ethylene glycol," *Clinical Chemistry*, vol. 42, no. 9, pp. 1489–1491, 1996.

[14] P. A. Gabow, K. Clay, J. B. Sullivan, and R. Lepoff, "Organic acids in ethylene glycol intoxication," *Annals of Internal Medicine*, vol. 105, no. 1, pp. 16–20, 1986.

[15] T. J. Morgan, C. Clark, and A. Clague, "Artifactual elevation of measured plasma L-lactate concentration in the presence of glycolate," *Critical Care Medicine*, vol. 27, no. 10, pp. 2177–2179, 1999.

[16] P. G. Brindley, M. S. Butler, G. Cembrowski, and D. N. Brindley, "Falsely elevated point-of-care lactate measurement after ingestion of ethylene glycol," *Canadian Medical Association Journal*, vol. 176, no. 8, pp. 1097–1099, 2007.

[17] R. S. Hoffman, M. J. Smilkstein, M. A. Rowland, and L. R. Goldfrank, "Osmol gaps revisited: normal values and limitations," *Journal of Toxicology: Clinical Toxicology*, vol. 31, no. 1, pp. 81–93, 1993.

[18] D. G. Barceloux, E. P. Krenzelok, K. Olson, W. Watson, and H. Miller, "American academy of clinical toxicology practice guidelines on the treatment of ethylene glycol poisoning," *Journal of Toxicology—Clinical Toxicology*, vol. 37, no. 5, article 537, 1999.

[19] K. J. Lepik, A. R. Levy, B. G. Sobolev et al., "Adverse drug events associated with the antidotes for methanol and ethylene glycol poisoning: a comparison of ethanol and fomepizole," *Annals of Emergency Medicine*, vol. 53, no. 4, pp. 439.e10–450.e10, 2009.

[20] G. M. Youssef and D. J. Hirsch, "Validation of a method to predict required dialysis time for cases of methanol and ethylene glycol poisoning," *American Journal of Kidney Diseases*, vol. 46, no. 3, pp. 509–511, 2005.

[21] D. D. Lung, T. E. Kearney, J. A. Brasiel, and K. R. Olson, "Predictors of death and prolonged renal insufficiency in ethylene glycol poisoning," *Journal of Intensive Care Medicine*, vol. 30, no. 5, pp. 270–277, 2015.

Pancreaticopericardial Fistula: A Case Report and Literature Review

Muhammad S. Khan,[1] Najmi Shahbaz,[2] Hassaan A. Zia,[3] Muhammad Hamza,[2] Henna Iqbal,[2] and Ahmed Awab[1]

[1]*Section of Pulmonary & Critical Care Medicine, University of Oklahoma Health Sciences Center, No. WP1310, 920 Stanton L Young Boulevard, Oklahoma City, OK 73117, USA*
[2]*Dow University of Health Sciences, Mission Road, Karachi 74200, Pakistan*
[3]*Department of Internal Medicine, University of Oklahoma Health Sciences Center, No. WP1310, 920 Stanton L Young Boulevard, Oklahoma City, OK 73117, USA*

Correspondence should be addressed to Muhammad S. Khan; muhammad-khan@ouhsc.edu

Academic Editor: Kurt Lenz

Purpose. Pancreaticopericardial fistula (PPF) is an extremely rare complication of acute or chronic pancreatitis. This paper presents a rare case of PPF and provides systematic review of existing cases from 1970 to 2014. *Methods.* A PubMed search using key words was performed for all the cases of PPF from January 1970 to December 2014. Fourteen cases were included in the study. The cases were reviewed for demographic characteristics, diagnostic modalities, and treatment. Descriptive analysis of these variables was performed. *Results.* Median age was 43 years. 78% were known alcoholics and 73.3% had chronic pancreatitis. Dyspnea was present in 78%. Cardiac tamponade was present in 53%; 75% of patients had known chronic pancreatitis (RR = 0.74). Surgery was associated with best treatment outcomes and 50% of patients who underwent endoscopic treatment survived. *Conclusion.* PPF is a rare disease. This paper indicates that acute cardiac tamponade in patients with history of alcoholism and chronic pancreatitis could be a sign of an existing pancreaticopericardial fistula and early surgical intervention could be life-saving.

1. Introduction

Pancreatic pseudocyst is a known complication of pancreatitis. Persistent leakage of pancreatic secretions can result in development of internal fistula due to spontaneous erosion into neighboring hollow viscus and cavities. Leakage from pancreatic secretions can cause significant morbidity due to malnutrition and infections. A fistula from pancreatic pseudocyst to pericardium is a rare complication and can present with cardiac tamponade. In this paper we describe a case of pancreaticopericardial fistula and review similar cases from 1970 to 2014.

2. Case

A middle-aged African American male presented to hospital with complaints of shortness of breath and feeling of dizziness for 3 days. Patient had known history of alcoholism and was admitted at a rehabilitation center 3 weeks before presentation for an elective detoxification. His initial course at rehabilitation center was uneventful; however, 3 days before presentation he started feeling dizzy and had gradual onset dyspnea on exertion that progressed to resting dyspnea. This was associated with sharp 3/10 epigastric pain radiating to his chest and back, which was aggravated by deep breaths. His past medical history was also significant for hypertension and episodes of delirium tremens. On admission his temperature was 37 degrees Celsius and blood pressure (BP) was 96/48 mmHg after 2-liter fluid bolus in emergency department, with pulse of 110/min, respiratory rate of 20/min, and oxygen saturation of 96% on 2 L nasal cannula. Examination was significant for decreased breath sounds in lung bases, increased vocal fremitus in left lower lobe, and dullness to percussion at lung bases bilaterally.

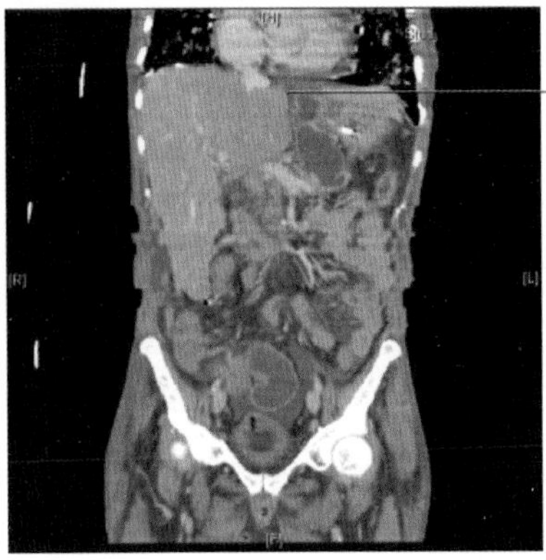

FIGURE 1: Abdominal CT showing cyst extension into mediastinum.

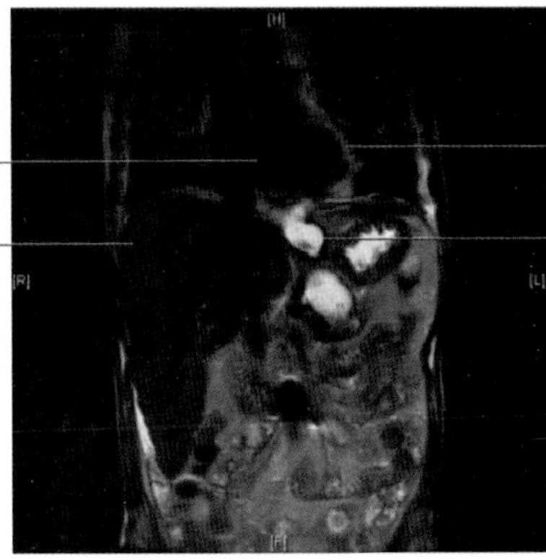

FIGURE 2: MRCP showing cyst extension into the mediastinum.

Jugular venous distension of 7 cm when sitting and pulsus paradoxus of 15 mmHg were also noted. His white blood cell (WBC) count was 18.5 K/mm^3 (normal range 4–11 K/cc^3) and hemoglobin (Hb) was 10.5 g/dL (normal range Hb 13–18 g/dL), with normal electrolytes, liver function tests, cardiac enzymes, and amylase. Due to concern for cardiac tamponade, urgent transthoracic echocardiography was performed that demonstrated a large pericardial effusion with early tamponade physiology. Computed tomography (CT) scan of chest done on admission showed large pericardial effusion and reticular ground glass opacities within the lungs bilaterally. The patient was started on broad spectrum antibiotics and underwent urgent pericardiocentesis and pericardial drain placement, with 280 mL of serosanguineous fluid obtained. The fluid analysis showed 59500 red blood cells, 3750 white blood cells, lipase of 196 IU, and amylase of 101 IU. Pericardial fluid cultures and blood cultures remained negative. On day 2 of admission the pericardial drainage decreased, and the drain was removed. However, after removal the patient acutely became short of breath with oxygen saturation in low 80s despite a 15 L nonrebreather mask. He was moved to the medical intensive care unit and intubated. Repeat transthoracic echocardiography showed reaccumulation of pericardial effusion. Due to concern for pulmonary embolism, a CT angiogram of the chest was done, which was negative for pulmonary embolism but showed an abdominal pseudocyst extending from the esophageal hiatus into the mediastinum. This was subsequently followed by a CT of the abdomen, showing necrotizing pancreatitis with multiloculated pseudocyst formation. The largest fluid collection was 4.1 cm × 3.6 cm traversing the mediastinal plane concerning for pancreaticopleural-pericardial fistula (Figure 1).

To further elaborate the pancreatic cyst and fistula, magnetic resonance cholangiopancreatography (MRCP) was also done which confirmed the findings of a large pseudocyst extending into the mediastinum (Figure 2).

The patient was subsequently extubated and moved to the medicine floor. Endoscopic retrograde cholangiopancreatography (ERCP) was performed to visualize the fistulous tract but was limited due to presence of a calculus in ventral pancreatic duct. Endoscopic ultrasound for cystgastrostomy was attempted and showed a fistulous tract towards the left pleural space. A 4 cm 7 French double-pigtail Zimmon stent was successfully placed into the pseudocyst cavity for decompression. The patient's symptoms improved after this procedure and he was discharged from the hospital on day 14. Unfortunately the patient was lost to follow-up in our clinic.

3. Materials and Methods

An extensive PubMed search was performed for all the cases of pancreaticopericardial fistula (PPF) using the key words "pancreatic fistula", "pericardial tamponade", and "chronic pancreatitis" from January 1970 to December 2014. A total of 15 cases were found. Fourteen cases were included in the study; one case was excluded as the pericardial effusion was not from fistulous tract. The cases were reviewed for age; sex; alcohol abuse; past history of chronic pancreatitis; acute pancreatitis on admission; presenting symptoms; associated symptoms of fever, abdominal pain, and chest pain; and hypotension, serum amylase levels, tamponade physiology on echocardiography, pericardiocentesis performed, pericardial amylase levels, diagnostic modality used for confirming the fistula, type of treatment offered, and patient outcomes of recovery versus death. Missing variables were marked as "unknown." Finally a descriptive analysis of the variables was done.

4. Results

A total of 15 cases of PPF were found from 1971 to 2014 including our case (Table 1). All reported cases were of male gender. Median age was found to be 43 years. Seventy-eight percent of patients had history of alcoholism; 73.3% cases had a known diagnosis of chronic pancreatitis. Dyspnea was the chief presenting symptom (78%) followed by hypotension (53%), chest pain (50%), fever (43%), abdominal pain (26.6%), syncope (6.6%), weight loss (6.6%), and ascites (6.6%). Acute pancreatitis was present in 42% of cases. Cardiac tamponade was present in a total of eight cases, was negative in five cases, and was unknown in two cases. Of the patients presenting with cardiac tamponade, 75% had a past medical history of chronic pancreatitis (relative risk = 0.74,

TABLE 1: Pancreaticopericardial fistula cases from 1971 to 2014 with patient demographics, symptoms, diagnostic test, and treatments.

Author	Year	Sex	Age	Alcohol	Chronic pancreatitis	Acute pancreatitis	Presenting symptoms	Dyspnea	Abdominal pain	Fever	Hypotension	Chest pain	Tamponade physiology	Pericardial drain	Diagnostic modality	Serum amylase	Pericardial amylase	Treatment	Patient outcomes
Lipson and Stephenson [1]	1971	M	40	N	Y	N	Ascites	N	N	N	N	N	N/A	N	Surgical exploration	613	N/A	Surgical	Recovered
Davidson et al. [2]	1979	M	39	Y	Y	N	Chest pain	Y	N	Y	N/A	Y	N	Pericardiocentesis	Surgical exploration	2000	12700	Surgical	Recovered
Imai et al. [3]	1993	M	42	Y	Y	Y	Dyspnea	Y	N	N	N	N	Y	Pericardiocentesis	ERCP	1681	6094	Surgical	Recovered
Schoonjans et al. [4]	1996	M	42	Y	Y	Y	Impending tamponade	Y	N	Y	N	N	N	N	ERCP	1413	N/A	Conservative management	Recovered
Tan et al. [5]	2002	M	28	Y	Y	N	Weight loss	Y	N	Y	N	N	Y	Pericardial drain	CT scan	N/A	5900	Surgical	Recovered
Oláh et al. [6]	2002	M	41	Y	Y	N	Dyspnea	Y	N	Y	Y	Y	Y	Pericardiocentesis	CT scan	748	226	Ultrasound guided drain placed transhepatically	Recovered
Balasubramanian et al. [7]	2004	M	16	N	Y	N	Dyspnea	Y					N	Pericardiocentesis	CT scan			Surgical	Recovered
François et al. [8]	2005	M	60	N/A	Pancreatic abscess	N/A	Back pain and dyspnea	Y	N	N/A	N/A	N/A	N/A	Pericardiocentesis	ERCP	20	328	Pericardial window	Recovered
Komtong et al. [9]	2006	M	43	Y	N	Y	Epigastric pain, dysphagia, orthopnea		Y	N	N	Y	N	N	ERCP and CT scan	285	N/A	ERCP stenting	Recovered
Ching et al. [10]	2007	M	45	Y	Y	N	Hemoptysis	Y	N	Y	Y	Y	N	N	CTA and MRCP	Normal	N/A	Surgical	Recovered
Bhatt et al. [11]	2011	M	47	Y	N	Y	Epigastric pain	Y	Y	N	Y	N	Y	Pericardial window		1830	N/A	Pericardial window	Death
Lamparter and Sundermann [12]	2013	M	57	Y	N	Y	Abdominal pain	N	Y	N	Y	N/A	Y	Y	ERCP	130	21560	ERCP stenting	Recovered
Parekh et al. [13]	2013	M	67	N	Y	Y	Chest pain	Y	N	N	Y	Y	Y	Pericardiocentesis	Surgical exploration	N/A	24000	ERCP stenting	Death
Sommer and Wilcox [14]	2014	M	58	Y	Y	N	Syncope	Y	N	N	N	N	Y	Y	ERCP	386	633	ERCP stenting	Death
Khan et al. (above reported case)	2014	M	45	Y	Y	N	Dyspnea	Y	N	N	y	Y	Y	Pericardiocentesis	CTA and MRCP	Normal	101	Endoscopic ultrasound & cystgastrostomy	Recovered

M = male, Y = yes, N = no, and N/A = not available.

95% confidence interval: 0.32 to 1.67, and p value = 0.46). Of the patients presenting with cardiac tamponade, 50% had acute pancreatitis on admission (RR = 1.25, 95% CI: 0.34 to 4.48, and p value = 0.73). Pericardiocentesis was done in a total of 11 patients (73.3%). Of the patients who underwent pericardiocentesis, eight patients recovered (72.7% recovery). Endoscopic retrograde cholangiopancreatography (ERCP) was used in 40% of the patients to diagnose PPF. Computed tomography (CT) abdomen was used to make the diagnosis in 26.6% of patients. Two patients had CT angiogram of the chest to rule out pulmonary embolism that revealed suspected pancreaticopericardial fistula, which was later confirmed by MRCP. Three cases were diagnosed by direct surgical exploration of the pancreatic duct. For definitive treatment, six patients underwent surgery (40%) with complete recovery in all six patients. Endoscopic retrograde cholangiopancreatography (ERCP) was done for four patients (26.6% cases) of which two patients recovered completely and two patients died. Two patients underwent pericardial window only (13.3%) of which only one patient recovered. One patient was managed conservatively without any invasive intervention. An external transhepatic drain was placed in one patient. Endoscopic ultrasound guided cystgastrostomy was done in one patient. All three patients had a complete recovery.

5. Discussion

A pancreatic fistula (PF) is defined as an abnormal connection between the pancreas and adjacent or distant organs, structures, and spaces [15]. PFs are classified as "internal" if the pancreatic duct communicates with the peritoneal or pleural cavity or any other hollow viscus and "external" if the pancreatic duct communicates with the skin [1]. The pathogenic mechanism of both internal and external PFs consists of disruption of the pancreatic duct secondary to pancreatitis or trauma [16, 17]. Persistent leakage of pancreatic secretions can result in development of internal pancreatic fistulas to neighboring hollow viscus (colon, duodenum, stomach, and esophagus), body cavities (peritoneal, pleural, and mediastinal), and vasculature (splenic vein, portal vein, and aorta). If the communication occurs anteriorly into the peritoneal cavity, it results in pancreatic ascites. A posterior communication may track into the pleural cavity or mediastinum [18]. A mediastinal pseudocyst occurs if the secretions are confined to mediastinum [18]. However, penetration of the secretion through pleura into pleural cavities, pericardium, or bronchial tree results in pancreaticopleural, pancreaticopericardial, or pancreaticobronchial fistula, respectively.

5.1. Incidence. The incidence of PFs after pancreatic resection ranges from 10 to 29% depending upon the type of surgery and underlying pancreatic pathology [15, 16]. The exact incidence of thoracopancreatic fistula and especially pancreaticopericardial fistula (PPF) is unknown. A review of English medical literature extending from 1965 to 1990 showed only 89 cases of thoracopancreatic fistulas [19]. The incidence of pancreaticopleural fistula has been reported in roughly 0.4% of patients with pancreatitis and 2.3–4.5% of patients presenting with pancreatic pseudocyst [20]. Our report indicates an increased incidence of pancreaticopericardial fistula in patients with existing history of chronic pancreatitis (73.3%). Acute pancreatitis was present in 42% of patients with PPF on admission. It is interesting to note that, of the patients with acute pancreatitis, 66% did not have any history of chronic pancreatitis. This association could be due to an undetected chronic subclinical pancreatitis in this patient population. However, we cannot exclude the possibility of acute pancreatitis resulting in fistula to pericardium based on the available information.

5.1.1. Clinical Presentation. The clinical symptoms of thoracopancreatic fistula include cough, shortness of breath, chest pain, wheezing, palpitations, and dysphagia [21]. Patients with pancreaticopleural fistula can have unilateral and bilateral pleural effusions with dullness to percussion over the thorax and diminished breath sounds on physical examination. Our study indicates that patients with PPF are predominately male with median age of 43 years and a strong history of alcoholism (78%). Dyspnea is the most common clinical symptom (78%) followed by hypotension (53%), chest pain (50%), fever (43%), abdominal pain (26.6%), syncope (6.6%), weight loss (6.6%), and ascites (6.6%). Cardiac tamponade was present in 53% of patients, and of all the patients with cardiac tamponade 75% had history of chronic pancreatitis (RR = 0.74, 95% CI: 0.32 to 1.67, and p value = 0.46). Because of small sample size and the fact that PPF is a rare disease, the relative risk and confidence interval cannot be interpreted inaccurately. However, given that majority of patients with PPF had past medical history of chronic pancreatitis, a PPF should be suspected in patients with chronic pancreatitis presenting with cardiac tamponade.

5.1.2. Diagnosis. The diagnosis of thoracopancreatic fistula should be suspected in patients with history of pancreatitis, pancreatic trauma, or surgery who present with a combination of abdominal and chest symptoms (dyspnea, orthopnea, chest pain, wheezing, etc.). The diagnosis is established by the finding of high levels of amylase in extravasated pancreatic fluid and evidence of duct disruption on imaging. For pancreaticopleural fistulas, the pleural effusions are exudative and amylase-rich with pleural fluid amylase greater than the upper limit of normal for serum amylase or a pleural fluid to serum amylase ratio greater than 1.0 [22]. To date there is no published data regarding the cardiac fluid analysis in patients with pancreaticopericardial fistula. Our study indicates that the cardiac fluid in such patients is exudative and amylase-rich in nature with pericardial fluid amylase to serum amylase ratio greater than 1.0. Our case and three more cases found an increased level of pericardial fluid lipase levels in patients with PPF.

5.2. Imaging. A number of imaging studies have been proposed to diagnose internal pancreatic fistulas. A CT scan of abdomen may demonstrate free fluid and walled-off collections in abdominal and thoracic cavities and changes of acute and chronic pancreatitis. However, a CT scan is diagnostic of pancreatic fistula only if performed immediately after an ERCP when it may demonstrate a fistulous tract [23]. MRCP is also another noninvasive method of diagnosing fistulas and should be performed if there is concern for adjacent complications (example is a pseudoaneurysm on CT) or if an ERCP is not performed. MRCP has advantage of guiding the clinical management by delineating the pancreatic duct injuries including those upstream of a complete duct disruption that would not be visualized on ERCP [24, 25]. ERCP provides direct evidence of a pancreatic fistula and is the test of choice if therapeutic pancreatic stenting is planned [26]. Unlike abdominal CT or MRCP, ERCP has the ability to demonstrate contrast filling the pancreatic ducts and extravasation in real time. ERCP has higher sensitivity and specificity for pancreatic duct leak as compared to CT scan [27]. Our report indicates that 40% of patients with pancreaticopericardial fistula were diagnosed by ERCP. CT abdomen was used to make the diagnosis in 26.6% of patients. Two patients had CT angiogram of the chest to rule out pulmonary embolism which revealed suspected pancreaticopericardial fistula which was later confirmed by MRCP. Three cases were diagnosed by direct surgical exploration of the pancreatic duct. In the above-mentioned patient the CT scan of chest on admission was done without contrast and failed to demonstrate the fistula. However CT angiogram of chest done in later hospital course demonstrated the fistula, indicating that contrast enhancement is required for visualization of fistulous tract.

5.3. Management. The management of pancreatic fistula is based on case reports and small observational studies [28]. The initial care depends on the presence of symptoms of abdominal pain, fever, and hypotension; presence of pancreatic necrosis on imaging and associated complications of infection; septic shock; and so forth. Reducing pancreatic stimulation by maintaining nil-by-mouth (NPO) status is part of initial management. Nasojejunal feeding to correct malnutrition is essential, and enteral nutrition is associated with lower incidence of infection, higher 30-day fistula closure rates, and shorter time to closure of postoperative pancreatic fistula as compared to total parenteral nutrition [29–31]. Octreotide 100 mcg three times daily in patients with high output fistula has been reported to be effective in reducing the fistula output, but it does not affect rate of fistula closure [29]. Fifty to sixty-five percent of internal fistulas close with supportive care [32]. In patients with persistent symptomatic fistula, additional interventions are required. Endoscopic treatment is preferred approach for management of most pancreatic fistulas. The goal of endoscopic therapy is internal drainage of pancreatic secretions, which thereby reduces flow through the fistula tract via placement of a pancreatic stent and/or pancreatic sphincterotomy [33, 34]. In a case series, endoscopic therapy for pancreatic fistulas has been associated with success rates of 85–100% [32]. Surgery for pancreatic fistula is indicated when endoscopic management fails or is technically difficult and is associated with a success rate of 90% with an associated mortality of 6–9% [32]. In case of pericardial tamponade, pericardiocentesis and pericardial drain placement becomes essential for initial stabilization of the patient followed by definitive treatment. All patients in our study who presented with acute tamponade had pericardial effusion drained. Four patients underwent ERCP guided stenting (26.6%) of which two patients recovered while two patients died. Six patients underwent surgical treatment (40%) with complete recovery in all six patients. Our patient underwent endoscopic ultrasound guided cystgastrostomy with complete recovery. Pericardial window was done as primary treatment in two patients (13.3%) of which one patient survived. Two patients were managed conservatively and one patient eventually had a transhepatic drain placed. Both these patients recovered without any complications.

6. Conclusion

PPF is a rare complication of pancreatitis. To our knowledge this is the first paper on this subject discussing the patient demographics, clinical picture, diagnostic modalities, and treatment options. The data is limited owing to rarity of the disease and no randomized trials are available that guide the diagnosis and treatment options. Identification and reporting of cases are required to have a better understanding of the disease process, which can affect treatment modes and patient outcomes.

Competing Interests

The authors declare that they have no competing interests.

References

[1] J. D. Lipson and H. E. Stephenson Jr., "Pancreatitis complicated by pericardial effusion and cardiac tamponade. Recovery after prolonged cerebral anoxia," *Archives of Surgery*, vol. 103, no. 3, pp. 414–416, 1971.

[2] E. D. Davidson, J. T. Horney, and P. P. Salter III, "Internal pancreatic fistula to the pericardium and pleura," *Surgery*, vol. 85, no. 4, pp. 478–480, 1979.

[3] Y. Imai, M. Taniguchi, K. Tagawa et al., "A case of chronic pancreatitis complicated by massive pericardial and right pleural effusion," *Gastroenterologia Japonica*, vol. 28, no. 5, pp. 734–738, 1993.

[4] R. Schoonjans, K. Vandewoude, E. Cesmeli et al., "Recurrent pericardial effusion as a result of chronic pancreatitis. Successful treatment with somatostatin," *Journal of Clinical Gastroenterology*, vol. 23, no. 3, pp. 224–227, 1996.

[5] M. H. Tan, G. Kirk, P. Archibold, P. Kennedy, and M. C. Regan, "Cardiac compromise due to a pancreatic mediastinal pseudocyst," *European Journal of Gastroenterology and Hepatology*, vol. 14, no. 11, pp. 1279–1282, 2002.

[6] A. Oláh, A. S. Nagy, I. Rácz, and M. E. Gamal, "Cardiac tamponade as complication of pseudocyst in chronic pancreatitis," *Hepato-Gastroenterology*, vol. 49, no. 44, pp. 564–566, 2002.

[7] P. Balasubramanian, R. Jeyamani, S. Govil et al., "Pancreaticopericardial fistula: a rare complication of chronic pancreatitis," *Indian Journal of Gastroenterology*, vol. 23, no. 1, pp. 31–32, 2004.

[8] C. J. François, T. C. Demos, and N. Iqbal, "Pancreaticothoracic fistulas: imaging findings in five patients," *Abdominal Imaging*, vol. 30, no. 6, pp. 761–767, 2005.

[9] S. Komtong, R. Chanatrirattanapan, P. Kongkam, R. Rerknimitr, and P. Kullavanijaya, "Mediastinal pseudocyst with pericardial effusion and dysphagia treated by endoscopic drainage," *Journal of the Pancreas*, vol. 7, no. 4, pp. 405–410, 2006.

[10] S.-S. Ching, M. M. Rao, A. Ali, S. Yeluri, A. G. Chalmers, and M. J. McMahon, "Chronic pancreatitis complicated by pancreaticopericardial fistula," *Surgical Practice*, vol. 11, no. 3, pp. 130–133, 2007.

[11] V. R. Bhatt, A. Koirala, R. V. Wetz, S. Kedia, P. Ghimire, and R. Bartaula, "Cardiac tamponade in acute pancreatitis," *BMJ Case Reports*, vol. 2011, 2011.

[12] S. Lamparter and H. Sundermann, "Swinging heart in acute pancreatitis," *American Journal of the Medical Sciences*, vol. 346, no. 2, pp. 160–161, 2013.

[13] P. Parekh, D. Howerton, and D. Johnson, "Not your everyday case of acute pancreatitis: a rare complication of a common diagnosis," *ACG Case Reports Journal*, vol. 1, no. 1, pp. 40–43, 2013.

[14] C. A. Sommer and C. M. Wilcox, "Pancreatico-pericardial fistula as a complication of chronic pancreatitis," *F1000Research*, vol. 3, article 31, 2014.

[15] C. Bassi, G. Butturini, E. Molinari et al., "Pancreatic fistula rate after pancreatic resection: the importance of definitions," *Digestive Surgery*, vol. 21, no. 1, pp. 54–59, 2004.

[16] G. G. Tsiotos, C. D. Smith, and M. G. Sarr, "Incidence and management of pancreatic and enteric fistulas after surgical management of severe necrotizing pancreatitis," *Archives of Surgery*, vol. 130, no. 1, pp. 48–52, 1995.

[17] J. L. Cameron, R. S. Kieffer, W. J. Anderson, and G. D. Zuidema, "Internal pancreatic fistulas: pancreatic ascites and pleural effusions," *Annals of Surgery*, vol. 184, no. 5, pp. 587–593, 1976.

[18] L. Kaman, A. Behera, R. Singh, and R. N. Katariya, "Internal pancreatic fistulas with pancreatic ascites and pancreatic pleural effusions: recognition and management," *ANZ Journal of Surgery*, vol. 71, no. 4, pp. 221–225, 2001.

[19] P. A. Lipsett and J. L. Cameron, "Internal pancreatic fistula," *The American Journal of Surgery*, vol. 163, no. 2, pp. 216–220, 1992.

[20] D. Semba, Y. Wada, Y. Ishihara, T. Kaji, A. Kuroda, and Y. Morioka, "Massive pancreatic pleural effusion: pathogenesis of pancreatic duct disruption," *Gastroenterology*, vol. 99, no. 2, pp. 528–532, 1990.

[21] D. C. Rockey and J. P. Cello, "Pancreaticopleural fistula: report of 7 patients and review of the literature," *Medicine*, vol. 69, no. 6, pp. 332–344, 1990.

[22] A. S. Fulcher, G. W. Capps, and M. A. Turner, "Thoracopancreatic fistula: clinical and imaging findings," *Journal of Computer Assisted Tomography*, vol. 23, no. 2, pp. 181–187, 1999.

[23] J. Joseph, S. Viney, P. Beck, C. Strange, S. A. Sahn, and G. S. Basran, "A prospective study of amylase-rich pleural effusions with special reference to amylase isoenzyme analysis," *Chest*, vol. 102, no. 5, pp. 1455–1459, 1992.

[24] J. S. Barkin, R. M. Ferstenberg, W. Panullo, H. D. Manten, and R. C. Davis Jr., "Endoscopic retrograde cholangiopancreatography in pancreatic trauma," *Gastrointestinal Endoscopy*, vol. 34, no. 2, pp. 102–105, 1988.

[25] A. S. Fulcher, M. A. Turner, J. A. Yelon et al., "Magnetic resonance cholangiopancreatography (MRCP) in the assessment of pancreatic duct trauma and its sequelae: preliminary findings," *Journal of Trauma—Injury, Infection and Critical Care*, vol. 48, no. 6, pp. 1001–1007, 2000.

[26] J. A. Soto, O. Alvarez, F. Múnera, N. L. Yepes, M. E. Sepúlveda, and J. M. Pérez, "Traumatic disruption of the pancreatic duct: diagnosis with MR pancreatography," *American Journal of Roentgenology*, vol. 176, no. 1, pp. 175–178, 2001.

[27] J. Devière, H. Bueso, M. Baize et al., "Complete disruption of the main pancreatic duct: endoscopic management," *Gastrointestinal Endoscopy*, vol. 42, no. 5, pp. 445–451, 1995.

[28] J. A. Blatnik and J. M. Hardacre, "Management of Pancreatic fistulas," *Surgical Clinics of North America*, vol. 93, no. 3, pp. 611–617, 2013.

[29] S. L. Gans, H. L. van Westreenen, J. J. S. Kiewiet, E. A. J. Rauws, D. J. Gouma, and M. A. Boermeester, "Systematic review and meta-analysis of somatostatin analogues for the treatment of pancreatic fistula," *British Journal of Surgery*, vol. 99, no. 6, pp. 754–760, 2012.

[30] S. Klek, M. Sierzega, L. Turczynowski, P. Szybinski, K. Szczepanek, and J. Kulig, "Enteral and parenteral nutrition in the conservative treatment of pancreatic fistula: a randomized clinical trial," *Gastroenterology*, vol. 141, no. 1, pp. 157–163.e1, 2011.

[31] D. K. Heyland, R. Dhaliwal, J. W. Drover, L. Gramlich, and P. Dodek, "Canadian clinical practice guidelines for nutrition support in mechanically ventilated, critically ill adult patients," *Journal of Parenteral and Enteral Nutrition*, vol. 27, no. 5, pp. 355–373, 2003.

[32] N. Alexakis, R. Sutton, and J. P. Neoptolemos, "Surgical treatment of pancreatic fistula," *Digestive Surgery*, vol. 21, no. 4, pp. 262–274, 2004.

[33] J. J. Telford, J. J. Farrell, J. R. Saltzman et al., "Pancreatic stent placement for duct disruption," *Gastrointestinal Endoscopy*, vol. 56, no. 1, pp. 18–24, 2002.

[34] R. A. Kozarek, T. J. Ball, D. J. Patterson, P. C. Freeny, J. A. Ryan, and L. William Traverso, "Endoscopic transpapillary therapy for disrupted pancreatic duct and peripancreatic fluid collections," *Gastroenterology*, vol. 100, no. 5, part 1, pp. 1362–1370, 1991.

A Case of Invasive Pneumococcal Infection with Septic Shock and Rare Complications

John R. Woytanowski,[1] Nausheen Hakim,[1] Caytlin Deering,[2] and Sara Schultz[2]

[1]Department of Internal Medicine, Drexel University College of Medicine, Philadelphia, PA, USA
[2]Department of Infectious Disease and HIV Medicine, Drexel University College of Medicine, Philadelphia, PA, USA

Correspondence should be addressed to John R. Woytanowski; john.woytanowski@tenethealth.com

Academic Editor: Mehmet Doganay

Invasive pneumococcus is a serious illness with potentially devastating outcomes. A 64-year-old female with a medical history of psoriatic arthritis and diabetes was transferred from an outside hospital for ventilator dependent respiratory failure and altered mental status. She initially presented with worsening back pain and was found to have leukocytosis with bandemia and acute renal failure but she was in septic shock upon arrival to our tertiary care center. Her blood cultures grew *Streptococcus pneumoniae* and MRI of the brain revealed pus within the posterior lateral ventricles and multiple infarcts. MRI of the spine revealed a psoas abscess. Transesophageal echocardiogram revealed mitral valve vegetation and her right eye developed endogenous endophthalmitis. She was treated with intravenous and intravitreal antibiotics and underwent drainage of the abscess with no improvement in mental status. Repeat imaging revealed multiple new thalamic, basal ganglia, and parietal lobe infarcts likely from septic emboli. After a protracted ICU stay, the patient's family opted for comfort care. The incidence of invasive pneumococcal infections has declined rapidly since the advent of antibiotics and vaccines. With the growing incidence of antibiotic resistance as well as the emergence of new immunomodulating drugs for various pathologies, there is a concern that invasive infections will reemerge. Ventriculitis and endogenous endophthalmitis are very rare complications of pneumococcal bacteremia.

1. Introduction

The incidence of invasive pneumococcal infections has declined rapidly since the advent of both antibiotics and vaccines [1–4]. More likely to occur at the extremes of age or in immunocompromised individuals, invasive pneumococcus is a serious illness with potentially devastating outcomes. Although the most commonly associated pneumococcal infections are sinusitis, otitis media, and meningitis, a variety of case reports have demonstrated highly atypical pneumococcal infections including those of the central nervous system, gastrointestinal tract, genitourinary tract, ocular system, and integumentary system [1]. As antibiotic resistance becomes more prevalent, there is an increased concern for reemergence of invasive infections.

2. Case Report

A 64-year-old female with a medical history of psoriatic arthritis (not currently on immunosuppressive agents) and type 2 diabetes mellitus presented to an outside community hospital with worsening lower back pain. Three weeks prior to admission, it was noted that the patient had a severe sinus infection and also had a molar implantation around the same time. One week later, she developed pain in her lumbar spine and was prescribed tizanidine and prednisone by her primary care physician with no relief. At the time of presentation to the hospital, she was found to have creatinine of 2.95 (baseline normal renal function) and leukocytosis of 14 ($\times 10^3$) with 57% bands. She was admitted and within hours she acutely decompensated and was intubated for airway protection. A lumbar puncture was attempted unsuccessfully by interventional radiology. MRI of the brain showed restricted diffusion in the supratentorial region consistent with small infarctions or encephalitis. She was started on broad-spectrum antibiotic coverage for meningitis/encephalitis and was transferred to our tertiary care center.

Upon arrival to our facility, she was febrile and hypotensive. Neurologically, she was unresponsive, but flexion of

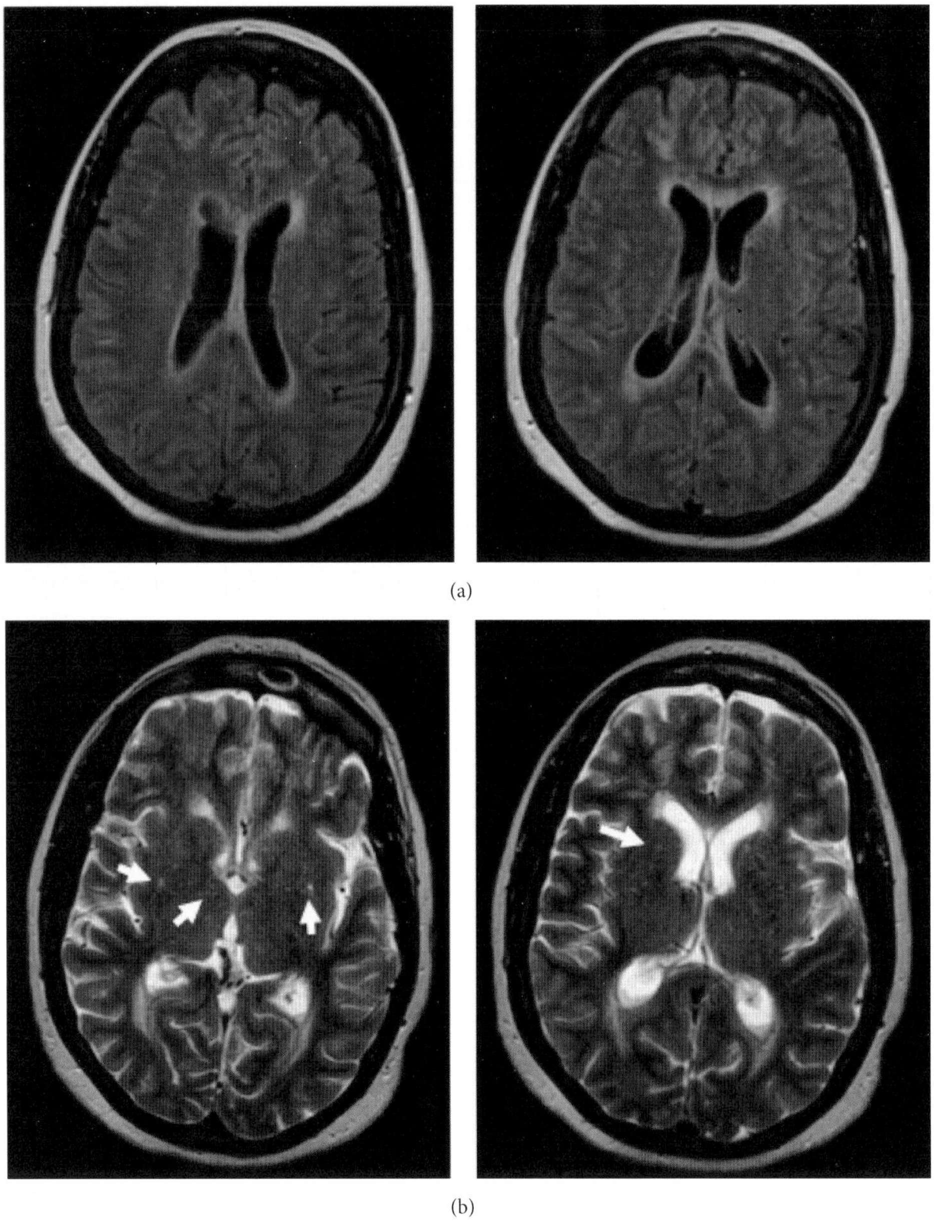

Figure 1: MRI brain taken on hospital day 3. (a) FLAIR enhancement of the ventricles and fluid levels within the posterior lateral ventricles, consistent with ventriculitis. (b) T2 enhanced images showing acute infarcts in the periventricular areas (arrows).

her neck caused her to wince. Her extremities had good tone and reflexes. She was started on norepinephrine to maintain her mean arterial pressure and continuous venovenous hemodialysis (CVVHD) for fluid overload. A lumbar puncture was performed which showed 3,000,000 RBCs and 722 WBCs (likely a traumatic tap) and cultures were positive for methicillin-resistant *Staphylococcus epidermidis*—likely a contaminant, as it grew in broth only several days after the initial sample with no organisms on Gram stain. On the following day, we received word that 4 out of 4 bottles of blood cultures from the initial hospital grew *Streptococcus pneumoniae* that was sensitive to penicillin.

After two days of antibiotic treatment, the decision was made to repeat MRI of the brain and spine as there was no improvement in her condition. FLAIR enhancement showed enhancement of the ventricles and pooling of purulent material into the posterior lateral ventricles, consistent with ventriculitis (Figure 1). T2 enhancement showed acute infarcts in the periventricular areas, likely from septic emboli (Figure 1). Spine imaging showed a fluid collection in the left psoas muscle (Figure 2). Neurosurgery was consulted who recommended medical management only. Interventional radiology performed CT guided drainage of the psoas fluid collection, which produced 10 cc of reddish-brown material consistent with an abscess; subsequently, Gram stain and cultures were negative. A transesophageal echo showed 0.5 × 0.3 cm vegetation on the mitral valve; it was unclear whether

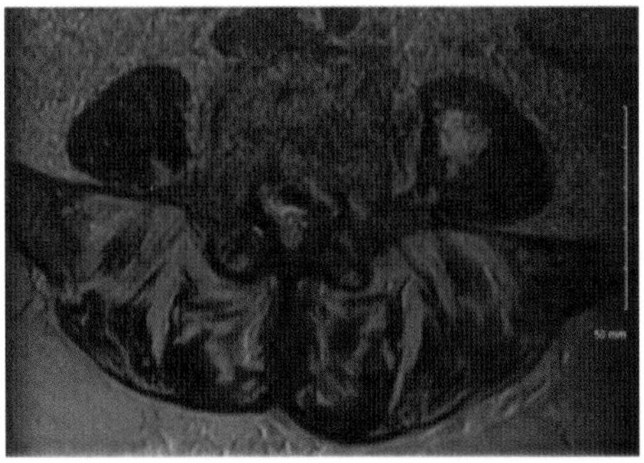

Figure 2: MRI of the lumbar spine on hospital day 3. This MRI shows a fluid collection within the left psoas muscle. The collection was aspirated and revealed purulent brown material, consistent with an abscess.

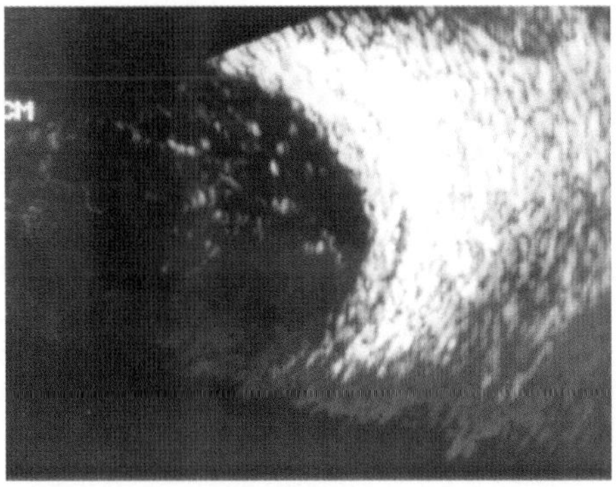

Figure 3: Ultrasound of the right eye. Ultrasound of the right eye shows a thickened retina and debris within the vitreous humor. These findings are consistent with inflammation and purulent material within the eye.

this was the source of emboli given its size and unlikely appearance on the echocardiogram.

A few days later, physical examination revealed a fluid level and debris in the anterior chamber of her right eye. Ophthalmological ultrasound revealed a thickened retina and debris within the vitreous fluid (Figure 3). She was diagnosed with endogenous bacterial endophthalmitis. A vitreous tap was performed and she was given intravitreal doses of vancomycin, amphotericin, and ceftazidime. Cultures of the vitreous fluid were subsequently negative. Because of the patient's altered mental status, a visual acuity assessment was unable to be performed prior to and following treatment. The gross appearance of the external eye did not seemingly improve in the following days.

The patient's fevers, blood pressure, leukocytosis, and kidney function improved over several days—she was weaned off pressors and her renal function returned to normal with adequate urine output. Her mental status, however, seemed to worsen as her extremities became flaccid. All cultures (except for the initial outside hospital blood cultures) remained negative. MRI of the brain and lumbar spine was repeated on day 10. FLAIR enhancement showed improvement in the ventriculitis (Figure 4); T2 enhancement showed additional infarcts now within the bilateral thalami, basal ganglia, and right parietal lobe (Figure 4). Lumbar spine showed an increase in size of the fluid collection within the psoas muscle (Figure 5). Several days later, the patient developed intracranial hemorrhage. The family ultimately opted for comfort care.

3. Discussion

In the preantibiotic and prevaccine eras, invasive pneumococcal infections were far more common than in current day [1–4]. With the growing incidence of antibiotic resistance, there is a concern that invasive infections similar to our case will become, again, increasingly prevalent. In this section, we will discuss two of the less common complications that our patient presented with.

Pyogenic ventriculitis is an inflammation of the ciliated ependymal lining of the brain's ventricles, leading to an accumulation of pus within the ventricles themselves [5]. Ventriculitis most commonly occurs in situations where infectious agents (most commonly *Staphylococcus*, approximately 90% of cases) have a route to enter the brain ventricles, that is, neurosurgical procedures such as external drains and intracranial stents. Many cases are also seen concomitantly with meningitis via contiguous spread. While incidence has increased recently given the rise in drug-resistant nosocomial infections, ventriculitis is still a rare but potentially lethal infection. Clinical presentation often overlaps with a meningitis-type picture; patients typically present with severe headache, fever, nuchal rigidity, photophobia, and changes in mental status [5–8]. CSF analysis generally reveals low glucose and elevated protein as well as a high neutrophil count, but subsequent neuroimaging is essential for diagnosis. CT scan of the head can show fluid levels and hyperdensities along the ependymal lining of the dilated ventricles. MRI of the brain can show dilated ventricles with fluid levels as well [7, 9]. Intravenous antibiotic therapy is the mainstay of treatment; it is initiated broadly and subsequently tailored to results of the CSF cultures. Intrathecal antibiotics can be considered if the ventriculitis is refractory to IV antibiotics. Progress of treatment can be monitored both by clinical picture and by serial imaging. Serial imaging can also be used to monitor complications of the disease, most commonly hydrocephalus or brain abscess. There are no particular guidelines for neurosurgical intervention in purulent ventriculitis, and surgical intervention is often deferred as the risk of further infection and other surgical complications is too high. There are a few case reports, especially in pediatric patients, of endoscopic ventricular washouts and drainage in refractory cases, as well as septostomy to restore CSF flow in cases complicated by unilateral hydrocephalus [10, 11]. Tabuchi and Kadowaki (2015) proposed that neurosurgical intervention be considered after two weeks of antibiotic therapy with no improvement [11]. In patients with simultaneously infected shunts, the shunt is often removed and a new shunt is reimplanted once antibiotic therapy is complete [10]. Our patient did not have any history of intracranial procedures. She likely developed ventriculitis after first developing meningitis. Consideration of both surgical intervention and

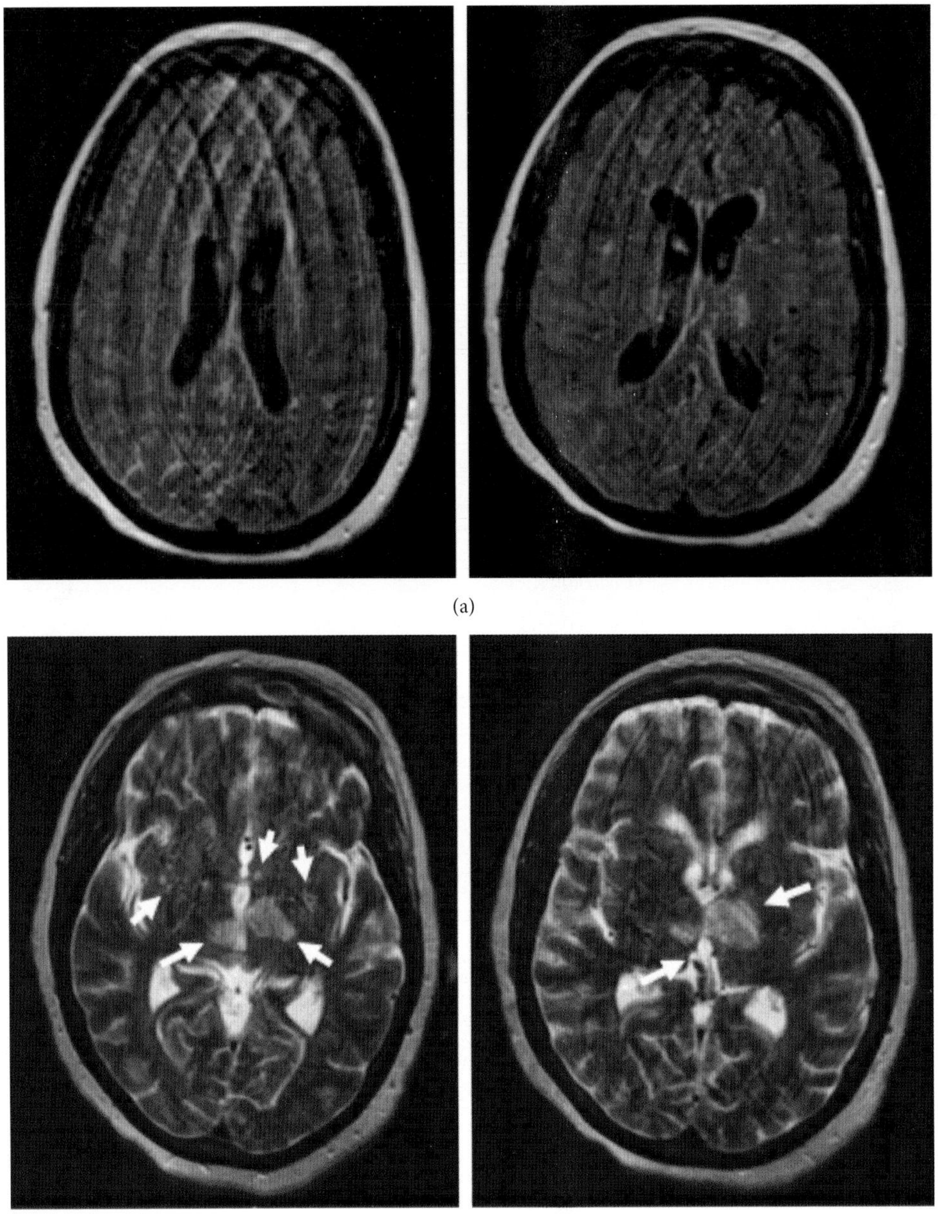

(a)

(b)

Figure 4: Repeat MRI of the brain on hospital day 10. (a) There is much less FLAIR enhancement of the ventricles, consistent with improving infection. (b) T2 weighted images showing several new infarcts within the bilateral thalami, basal ganglia, and right parietal lobe (arrows). Also visible are older, evolving infarcts.

intrathecal antibiotics was deferred in our patient's case as her repeat imaging showed improvement in the purulent material within her ventricles.

Endogenous bacterial endophthalmitis is a rare subset of endophthalmitis; it is an ophthalmologic emergency that often leads to poor visual outcomes [12, 13]. Endogenous endophthalmitis with meningitis is an extraordinarily rare combination of complications from invasive *Strep. pneumoniae* infections, having only been described in isolated case reports [14]. Endogenous endophthalmitis occurs when bacteria reach the eye via bloodstream infection or through central nervous infection spread via the optic nerve [15, 16]. It is often associated with chronic predisposing conditions such as those that cause a baseline immunodeficient state (i.e., diabetes mellitus, HIV, and ESRD). Symptoms are nonspecific and include decreased vision, seeing floaters, headache, redness, and discharge. Previously, it was mainly caused by pneumococcal infections; however, more recent literature describes other streptococcal species, such as *Streptococcus bovis* (GI procedures such as endoscopy and colonoscopy have had high associations with endogenous endophthalmitis). Fungal infections have also been implicated quite often. The right eye is more often affected than the left due to a more direct route through the right carotid artery [12, 16].

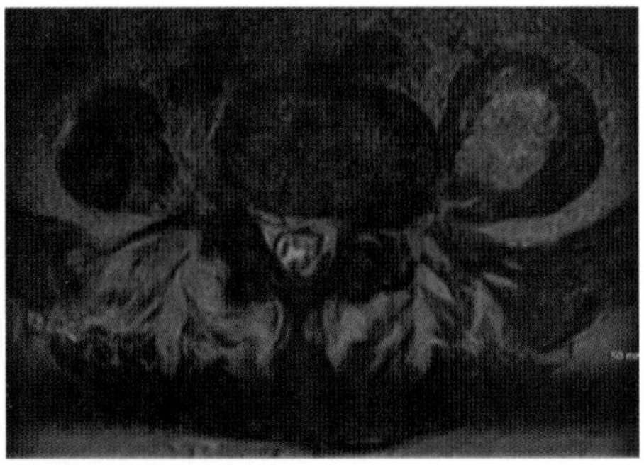

FIGURE 5: Repeat MRI of the lumbar spine on hospital day 10. Visible here is a persistent fluid collection within the left psoas muscle that has increased in size from previous MRI (Figure 2) despite CT guided aspiration.

Diagnosis is made with high clinical suspicion in the setting of other risk factors such as systemic infection and imaging concerning for intraocular infection. Clinical signs include uveal tissue abscesses, vitreous exudates, panophthalmitis, intraretinal hemorrhages, conjunctival injection, and scleritis. Vitreous aspiration and cultures, as well as RT-PCR of vitreous fluid, can identify a specific organism. Diagnostic vitrectomy has a higher rate of positive cultures than does aspiration, but it is not required for diagnosis [16]. According to Okada et al. (1994), diagnosis is correctly made only 50% of the time and is delayed up to four days in 29% of patients [12]. Treatment includes intravenous antibiotics for the underlying source of infection as well as intravitreal antibiotics to treat the endophthalmitis directly. There are conflicting studies on the use of steroids; however, the current literature does recommend corticosteroid use. Vitrectomy should be considered in treatment refractory cases. Evisceration of the eye is often performed in cases refractory to both antibiotics and vitrectomy [17].

Both the visual and the overall prognosis of endogenous endophthalmitis are dismal. Most cases result in a complete vision loss, and the risk of this increases with delay in diagnosis [12, 13, 15, 16]. Miller et al. (2004) completed a large retrospective analysis of patients with endophthalmitis caused by *Streptococcus pneumoniae* between the years of 1989 and 2003. Of the 27 cases examined, only 2 patients developed the infection endogenously. Both patients had poor outcomes; the first patient had 20/30 vision before infection, was unable to perceive light during infection, and ultimately required evisceration of the affected eye. The second patient was able to perceive light prior to and during infection but was left unable to perceive light despite receiving systemic and intravitreal antibiotics [18]. Sekiguchi and Inaba (2015) reported a case of endogenous endophthalmitis following *Streptococcus pneumoniae* meningitis. This patient was also left unable to perceive light, despite both systemic and intravitreal antibiotics and full recovery from his meningitis. Because our patient did not recover mental status, it is unclear what her visual outcome would have been. Furthermore, she was transferred to us in an altered state and thus we are unsure whether she had been experiencing any visual symptoms prior to presentation, making it difficult to assess whether we made the diagnosis early enough to save her vision.

We presented a case of a 64-year-old female, whose only risk factor for immunocompromise was diabetes, who developed a highly atypical invasive pneumococcal infection with numerous complications. Although it is not entirely clear what started this patient's disease process, we believe that her dental procedure led to hematological seeding of the bacteria and subsequent endocarditis of her mitral valve, an abscess in her psoas muscle, endophthalmitis in her right eye, and seeding into the cerebrospinal fluid (CSF) through a compromised blood-brain barrier. She developed meningitis which spread contiguously to the ventricles causing a pyogenic ventriculitis. Finally, the endocarditis released septic emboli which caused infarcts in regions of the brain as above. Initially, her rapid decline in mental status can likely be attributed to the CNS infections. Because her mental status did not improve with antibiotic therapy, her permanent decline in mental status is likely a result of the infarcts.

References

[1] S. N. Taylor and C. V. Sanders, "Unusual manifestations of invasive pneumococcal infection," *American Journal of Medicine*, vol. 107, no. 1, pp. 12–27, 1999.

[2] "Direct and indirect effects of routine vaccination of children With 7-valent pneumococcal conjugate vaccine on incidence of invasive pneumococcal disease-United States, 1998-2003," *Journal of the American Medical Association*, vol. 294, no. 16, pp. 2022–2026, 2005.

[3] S. S. Shah and A. J. Ratner, "Trends in invasive pneumococcal disease-associated hospitalizations," *Clinical Infectious Diseases*, vol. 42, no. 1, 2006.

[4] C. A. Lexau, R. Lynfield, R. Danila et al., "Changing epidemiology of invasive pneumococcal disease among older adults in the era of pediatric pneumococcal conjugate vaccine," *Journal of the American Medical Association*, vol. 294, no. 16, pp. 2043–2051, 2005.

[5] A. Agrawal, "Pyogenic ventriculitis in an immunocompetent adult female," *Narayana Medical Journal*, vol. 4, no. 1, pp. 43–46, 2015.

[6] A. Yuen and F. Mok, "Ventriculitis, an unusual cause of sepsis in an elderly patient who presented with persistent fever," *Asian Journal of Gerontology Geriatrics*, pp. 49–52, 2006.

[7] R. A. Hirst, B. Gosai, A. Rutman, P. W. Andrew, and C. O'Callaghan, "Streptococcus pneumoniae damages the ciliated ependyma of the brain during meningitis," *Infection and Immunity*, vol. 71, no. 10, pp. 6095–6100, 2003.

[8] R. Beer, B. Pfausler, and E. Schmutzhard, "Management of nosocomial external ventricular drain-related ventriculomeningitis," *Neurocritical Care*, vol. 10, no. 3, pp. 363–367, 2009.

[9] M. B. Fukui, R. L. Williams, and S. Mudigonda, "CT and MR imaging features of pyogenic ventriculitis," *American Journal of Neuroradiology*, vol. 22, no. 8, pp. 1510–1516, 2001.

[10] A. Agrawal, R. Cincu, and J. Timothy, "Current concepts and approach to ventriculitis," *Infectious Diseases in Clinical Practice*, vol. 16, no. 2, pp. 100–104, 2008.

[11] S. Tabuchi and M. Kadowaki, "Neuroendoscopic surgery for ventriculitis and hydrocephalus after shunt infection and malfunction: Preliminary report of a new strategy," *Asian Journal of Endoscopic Surgery*, vol. 8, no. 2, pp. 180–184, 2015.

[12] A. A. Okada, R. P. Johnson, W. C. Liles, D. J. D'Amico, and A. S. Baker, "Endogenous bacterial endophthalmitis: report of a ten-year retrospective study," *Ophthalmology*, vol. 101, no. 5, pp. 832–838, 1994.

[13] S.-P. Chee and A. Jap, "Endogenous endophthalmitis," *Current Opinion in Ophthalmology*, vol. 12, no. 6, pp. 464–470, 2001.

[14] T. Sekiguchi and A. Inaba, "Endogenous endophthalmitis following streptococcus pneumoniae meningitis," *Internal Medicine*, vol. 54, no. 18, pp. 2401–2404, 2015.

[15] M. Cubillas, A. Sampedro, B. Domınguez, I. Carrio, V. Bango, and J. Barbón, "Endogenous bacterial endophthalmitis. A report of 2 cases," *Archivos de la Sociedad Española de Oftalmología (English Edition)*, vol. 92, no. 6, pp. 280–282, 2017.

[16] M. A. Sadiq, M. Hassan, A. Agarwal et al., "Endogenous endophthalmitis: diagnosis, management, and prognosis," *Journal of Ophthalmic Inflammation and Infection*, vol. 5, no. 1, article no. 32, pp. 1–11, 2015.

[17] F. Soriano, E. Pérez-Trallero, R. Pallarés et al., "Streptococcus pneumoniae endophthalmitis: A study of 36 cases with special reference to antibiotic resistance and treatment options," *Clinical Microbiology and Infection*, vol. 12, no. 6, pp. 519–526, 2006.

[18] J. J. Miller, I. U. Scott, H. W. Flynn Jr., W. E. Smiddy, R. P. Corey, and D. Miller, "Endophthalmitis caused by streptococcus pneumoniae," *American Journal of Ophthalmology*, vol. 138, no. 2, pp. 231–236, 2004.

40

Abnormal Breathing Patterns Predict Extubation Failure in Neurocritically Ill Patients

Pragya Punj,[1] Premkumar Nattanmai,[1] Pravin George,[2] and Christopher R. Newey[1]

[1]*Department of Neurology, University of Missouri, 5 Hospital Drive, CE 540, Columbia, MO 65211, USA*
[2]*Cleveland Clinic, Cerebrovascular Center, Neurological Institute, 9500 Euclid Avenue, Cleveland, OH 44195-5245, USA*

Correspondence should be addressed to Christopher R. Newey; neweyc@health.missouri.edu

Academic Editor: Kurt Lenz

In neurologically injured patients, predictors for extubation success are not well defined. Abnormal breathing patterns may result from the underlying neurological injury. We present three patients with abnormal breathing patterns highlighting failure of successful extubation as a result of these neurologically driven breathing patterns. Recognizing abnormal breathing patterns may be predictive of extubation failure and thus need to be considered as part of extubation readiness.

1. Introduction

Extubation in neurologically injured patients can be challenging. Typical factors considered for extubation readiness are stable cardiorespiratory status along with decreased risk for aspiration [1, 2]. Common predictors of extubation failure are longer duration on mechanical ventilation, poor cough reflex, upper airway obstruction, low hemoglobin concentration, continued intravenous sedation, and comorbid medical conditions such as left ventricular failure [1, 2]. Despite optimizing these components, extubation failure still occurs in 2 to 25% of cases in the intensive care unit (ICU) likely from a disparity between work of breathing (WOB) and capacity of respiratory muscles [1, 2]. A trial of spontaneous breathing (SBT) is typically performed prior to extubation as a predictor of success [1, 3]. If a patient breathes shallow and rapidly during the trial, the patient may not tolerate spontaneous breathing [1, 3]. However, neurologically injured patients have abnormal breathing patterns as a result of their injury. These patients may breathe rapid and/or irregularly as a result of their injury. Thus, SBTs are less reliable. Predictors of extubation success in these patients are less clear. This article describes three cases of extubation failure who had an associated abnormal breathing pattern as a result of their underlying neurological injury.

2. Case Report

2.1. Case 1. An 80-year-male presented to the emergency department (ED) with acute onset of right sided facial droop, right sided hemiplegia, numbness, swallowing difficulty, and dysphonia. He had a past history of hypertension, diabetes, gout, prior ischemic stroke without any residual neurological deficit, and peripheral vascular disease. On examination, he was noted to have nystagmus on upward gaze and weakness with loss of sensation in the right upper and lower extremities. He was unable to coordinate the control of secretions. He was intubated for airway protection given his poor orolingual control. A magnetic resonance imaging (MRI) of the brain was obtained which showed left lateral and medial medullary acute ischemia (Figures 1(a)-1(b)).

His hospital stay was complicated by aspiration pneumonia. He was treated with antibiotics. Subsequently, his chest X-ray and neurological examination improved. However, the waveform on the ventilator showed a cluster breathing pattern (Figure 1(c)). He was eventually extubated. However, he did not tolerate secondary breathing irregularity and was subsequently reintubated. A tracheostomy and percutaneous gastrostomy were performed.

2.2. Case 2. A 60-year-male presented to the ED with headache, frequent falls, and dizziness for prior 3 months. He

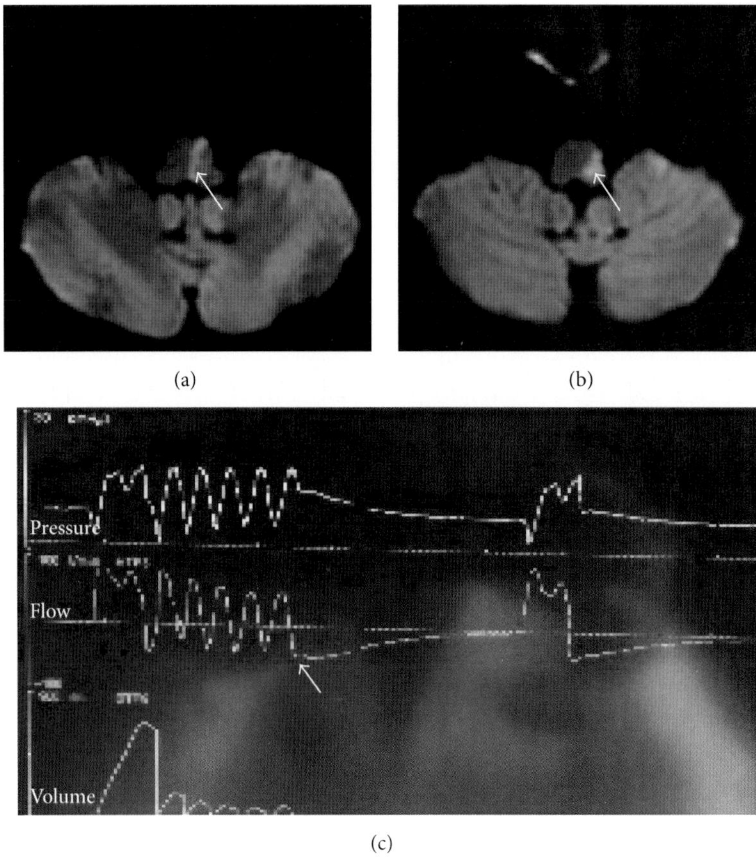

FIGURE 1: Magnetic resonance imaging of the brain. Diffusion weighted imaging (DWI) showing left medial (a, arrow) and lateral (b, arrow) medullary acute ischemia. (c) Ventilator picture showing cluster breathing pattern (arrow).

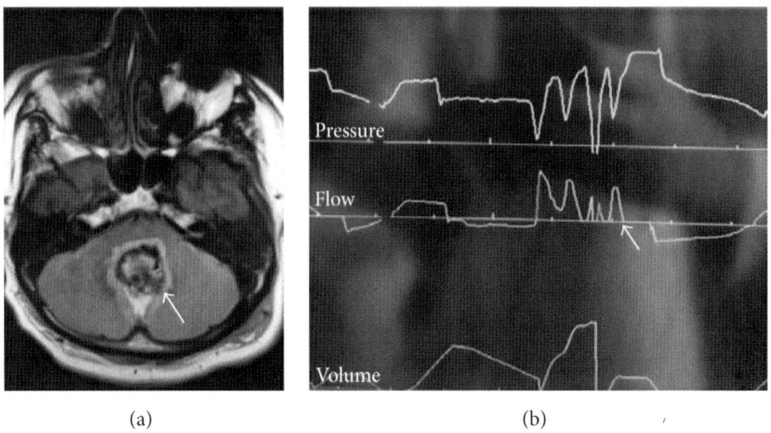

FIGURE 2: Magnetic resonance imaging of the brain. (a) T2 fluid attenuated inversion recovery (FLAIR) sequence showing medulloblastoma status after resection causing effacement of the fourth ventricle (arrow). (b) Ventilator picture showing cluster breathing pattern (arrow).

had a past medical history of glaucoma and hypothyroidism. Computed tomography (CT) head showed a large medial cerebellar mass with compression of the brainstem and effacement of the fourth ventricle. The mass was resected (Figure 2(a), arrow). Postoperatively, he remained intubated for stuporous mental state.

His hospital course was complicated by aspiration pneumonia and development of acute respiratory distress syndrome (ARDS). He made remarkable recovery from the lung injury. His level of consciousness remained lethargic. The ventilator waveform consistently showed cluster breathing pattern preventing extubation (Figure 2(b), arrow).

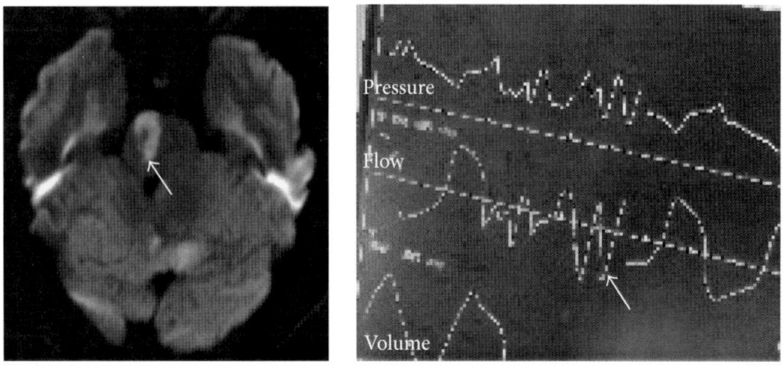

(a) (b)

FIGURE 3: Magnetic resonance imaging of the brain. (a) Diffusion weighted imaging (DWI) showing right acute pontine ischemia (arrow). (b) Ventilator picture showing ataxic breathing pattern (arrow).

A tracheostomy and percutaneous gastrostomy were then performed.

2.3. Case 3. A 43-year-old male presented to the ED with altered mental status, slurred speech, and left sided hemiplegia. He had a past medical history of diabetes, hypertension, and hypertriglyceridemia. Neurological examination confirmed the left sided hemiplegia and decreased arousal. CT head showed moderate sized left medial posterior inferior cerebellar artery (PICA) infarct with obstructive hydrocephalus. MRI confirmed the CT scan findings (Figure 3(a), arrow). CT-angiography (CTA) demonstrated right vertebral artery dissection. His examination acutely worsened. He was intubated and required a decompressive suboccipital craniectomy. He slowly improved and eventually was extubated. He failed extubation and was reintubated. The ventilator waveform on reintubation showed an ataxic breathing pattern (Figure 3(b), arrow). He eventually required tracheostomy and percutaneous gastrostomy.

2.4. Weaning. Prior to extubation, a standard checklist was reviewed. The patients' respiratory statuses were PaO2 > 60 mmHg with FiO2 < 50% and positive end expiratory pressure (PEEP) of <8. The patients were hemodynamically stable. Arterial blood gasses showed a pH range of 7.44–7.46, PaO2 68–98 mmHg, PaCO2 of 33–35 mmHg, and bicarbonate of 23-24 mEq/L. Spontaneous breathing trials were performed in all three patients. This breathing trial consisted of a 30-minute trial on 0 pressure support and 0 PEEP. All three patients passed this breathing trial. Patient 2 was not extubated given his lethargic mental status and cluster breathing pattern. The other two patients' levels of consciousness were awake and following commands. All three patients had a cough reflex.

3. Discussion

We presented three cases of neurologically injured patients who were otherwise ready for extubation. However, they each had a neurologically driven breathing pattern. All required tracheostomy and percutaneous gastrostomy. These cases highlight that the finding of a breathing abnormality attributed to the underlying brain injury should be considered when predicting extubation success.

The patients of these three cases were unable to be extubated secondary to abnormal neurogenic breathing patterns. Cluster breathing pattern, as observed in cases 1 and 2, has been characterized as "respiratory pattern characterized by periods or clusters of rapid respirations of near equal depth or tidal volume followed by regular periods of apnea" [4]. It classically results from injury to pons due to stroke, trauma, or increased pressure on medulla from tumor or herniation [4]. Ataxic breathing as seen in case 3 is classically seen in medullary ischemia [4, 5]. However, as we demonstrate here, the breathing patterns may be seen in injuries elsewhere in the brainstem. For example, cluster breathing, as in case 1, associated with medullary ischemia, and ataxic breathing, as in case 3, associated with pontine ischemia.

The respiratory system functions to maintain adequate oxygenation for energy production and ventilation to maintain physiological acid base balance [6]. The primitive respiratory control centers are located within the pons and medulla of the brainstem [6]. It receives afferent signals from peripheral and central chemoreceptors, stretch receptors in lung, and higher cortical centers [6]. These afferent inputs are analyzed and efferent signals are sent to respiratory muscle groups to maintain a stable tidal volume as well as respiratory rate and rhythm [6]. Damage to any of these areas can create classic respiratory patterns [5, 6]. These include Cheyne Stokes (bilateral cerebral hemisphere injury), hyperventilation (midbrain injury), apneustic (cephalad pons injury), cluster (caudal pons/cephalad medulla injury), and ataxic (medullary injury) breathing patterns [5, 6]. These breathing patterns are summarized in Table 1.

The decision to perform tracheostomy in the neurocritical care patient is individualized. Predictors for tracheostomy in patients with intracerebral hemorrhage have been proposed to be hematoma volume (≥30 cc), intraventricular hemorrhage, obstructive hydrocephalus, Glasgow Coma Scale (GCS; <8), prolonged intubation (≥14 days), and pneumonia [7]. The timing of when to perform tracheostomy

TABLE 1: Neurologically driven breathing patterns and anatomic correlation.

Respiratory control centers	Function	Abnormal breathing pattern associated with injury
Cerebral hemisphere	Regulates respiratory center located in pons and medulla	Cheyne stokes breathing pattern
Midbrain	Rate of inspiration	Hyperventilation
Pons		
Pneumotaxic center	Intensity of respiration	Cluster breathing pattern
Apneustic center	Rate of inspiration	Apneustic breathing pattern
Medulla oblongata		
Ventral breathing center Dorsal breathing center	Responsible for expiratory movement	Ataxic breathing pattern

(early or late) in intracerebral hemorrhage patients has been proposed with the TRACH score [8]. Significant predictors from the TRACH score indicating need for early tracheostomy included GCS score and radiological findings of obstructive hydrocephalus, septum pellucidum shift, and thalamic hemorrhage [8]. Early tracheostomy may be beneficial in the neurocritical care patient. In subarachnoid hemorrhage patients, performing early (days 1–7) versus later (days 8–20) tracheostomy resulted in less pneumonia, less respiratory adverse events, shorter duration of mechanical ventilation, and ultimately earlier decannulation [9]. In an analysis of 10 trials in acute brain injured patients, early tracheostomy was found to reduce long-term mortality, duration of mechanical ventilation, and ICU length of stay; however delaying tracheostomy resulted in an increased probability of not needing a tracheostomy [10]. Assessing need for tracheostomy at day 7 has been recommended [11]. However, in general critical care, early tracheostomy only reduced the duration of ventilator but not the incidence of pneumonia, length of stay, or long-term mortality [12]. Another study in critically ill patients only found early tracheostomy useful in reducing duration of sedation [13]. It was not found to change mortality, pneumonia incidence, duration of mechanical ventilation, or length of stay [13]. In general, we assess the need for tracheostomy around day 7. Unfortunately, algorithms for determining who would benefit from tracheostomy and timing of tracheostomy are largely lacking and do not include neurologically driven breathing patterns.

In conclusion, the finding of neurologically driven breathing patterns should be considered in predicting extubation failure.

Competing Interests

The authors have no financial disclosure or conflict of interests to report.

Authors' Contributions

Pragya Punj, Premkumar Nattanmai, Pravin George, and Christopher R. Newey contributed equally to the writing of the case and formatting of the images.

References

[1] A. Kulkarni and V. Agarwal, "Extubation failure in intensive care unit: predictors and management," *Indian Journal of Critical Care Medicine*, vol. 12, no. 1, pp. 1–9, 2008.

[2] R. C. Rothaar and S. K. Epstein, "Extubation failure: magnitude of the problem, impact on outcomes, and prevention," *Current Opinion in Critical Care*, vol. 9, no. 1, pp. 59–66, 2003.

[3] M. El-Khatib, G. Jamaleddine, R. Soubra, and M. Muallem, "Pattern of spontaneous breathing: potential marker for weaning outcome," *Intensive Care Medicine*, vol. 27, no. 1, pp. 52–58, 2001.

[4] http://www.breathsounds.org/docs/Breathing%20Patterns.pdf.

[5] R. M. Youngson, *Collins. Dictionary of Medicine*, Collins, 2004-2005.

[6] H. K. Walker, W. D. Hall, and J. W. Hurst, Eds., *Clinical Methods: The History, Physical, and Laboratory Examinations*, Butterworths, Boston, Mass, USA, 3rd edition, 1990.

[7] S. Yaghi, P. Moore, B. Ray, and S. G. Keyrouz, "Predictors of tracheostomy in patients with spontaneous intracerebral hemorrhage," *Clinical Neurology and Neurosurgery*, vol. 115, no. 6, pp. 695–698, 2013.

[8] V. Szeder, S. Ortega-Gutierrez, W. Ziai, and M. T. Torbey, "The TRACH score: clinical and radiological predictors of tracheostomy in supratentorial spontaneous intracerebral hemorrhage," *Neurocritical Care*, vol. 13, no. 1, pp. 40–46, 2010.

[9] F. Gessler, H. Mutlak, S. Lamb et al., "The impact of tracheostomy timing on clinical outcome and adverse events in poor-grade subarachnoid hemorrhage," *Critical Care Medicine*, vol. 43, no. 11, pp. 2429–2438, 2015.

[10] V. A. McCredie, A. S. Alali, D. C. Scales et al., "Effect of early versus late tracheostomy or prolonged intubation in critically ill patients with acute brain injury: a systematic review and meta-analysis," *Neurocritical Care*, vol. 26, no. 1, pp. 14–25, 2017.

[11] J. Bösel, "Tracheostomy in stroke patients," *Current Treatment Options in Neurology*, vol. 16, article 274, 2014.

[12] N. Raimondi, M. R. Vial, J. Calleja et al., "Evidence-based guidelines for the use of tracheostomy in critically ill patients," *Journal of Critical Care*, vol. 20, pp. 304–318, 2016.

[13] L. Meng, C. Wang, J. Li, and J. Zhang, "Early vs late tracheostomy in critically ill patients: a systematic review and meta-analysis," *Clinical Respiratory Journal*, vol. 10, pp. 684–692, 2016.

41

Use of Continuous Renal Replacement Therapy for Removal of Dabigatran in a Patient in Need of Emergent Surgery

Sara E. Parli,[1,2] Melissa L. Thompson Bastin,[1,2] and Daniel A. Lewis[3]

[1]*Department of Pharmacy Services, University of Kentucky HealthCare, Lexington, KY 40536, USA*
[2]*Department of Pharmacy Practice and Science, University of Kentucky College of Pharmacy, Lexington, KY 40536, USA*
[3]*Department of Pharmacy Services, South Pointe Hospital, Cleveland Clinic, Cleveland, OH 44195, USA*

Correspondence should be addressed to Sara E. Parli; sara.parli@uky.edu

Academic Editor: Petros Kopterides

Purpose. To report the ability to remove serum dabigatran using continuous renal replacement therapy (CRRT) in a patient with life-threatening bleeding. *Summary.* A 77-year-old female with history of atrial fibrillation who takes dabigatran for stroke prevention presented with abdominal pain. Patient was found to have bleeding and possible mesenteric ischemia and was taken to the operating room and had continued bleeding postoperatively. CRRT was initiated for the removal of any remaining dabigatran, with serum dabigatran levels collected to evaluate removal of dabigatran with CRRT. This patient had an increased dabigatran level prior to intervention, which decreased to an undetectable level after use of CRRT. Greater than 80% of the drug was removed due to 4 hours of CRRT and residual kidney function. Reversal of dabigatran is an area of current research with recent FDA approval of idarucizumab for use. *Conclusion.* Bleeding may occur as a result of the use of dabigatran and change in patient's clinical condition. Use of CRRT may be an option in removing serum dabigatran in the case of a life-threatening bleed.

1. Introduction

Dabigatran etexilate is an oral reversible direct thrombin inhibitor, approved for anticoagulation for prevention of stroke and systemic embolism in nonvalvular atrial fibrillation, as well as the treatment and reduction in risk of recurrence of pulmonary embolism and deep vein thrombosis (DVT). It offers a predictable anticoagulation response without the need for routine coagulation test monitoring and therefore is becoming a viable alternative to vitamin K antagonists, such as warfarin [1]. The pharmacokinetics have previously been described in detail [1, 2]. Dabigatran etexilate is rapidly absorbed from the gastrointestinal tract and quickly hydrolyzed to its active form (dabigatran) and follows first-order kinetics with a two-compartment distribution model. Effects of food and drug interactions are negligible, as the anticoagulant effect is immediate and predictable. Metabolism occurs by way of liver conjugation with glucuronic acid, with 80% of unchanged drug recovered in the urine; therefore, dabigatran must be dose-adjusted for renal insufficiency. Steady state concentrations are reached within three days of oral dosing, and the average half-life is 12–17 hours. Although dabigatran exhibits an ideal pharmacokinetic profile, a potential pitfall to its use is the difficulty in accurately assessing the degree of anticoagulation in a supratherapeutic dosing situation [2]. In this report, we describe a case of utilizing continuous renal replacement therapy (CRRT) for the removal of dabigatran from the serum of a patient with an ischemic bowel requiring emergent surgery. The report of this case did not require Institutional Review Board review by the investigators institution.

2. Case

A 77-year-old Caucasian female presented to an outside hospital via Emergency Medical Services with complaints of abdominal pain, bright red blood in her stools, and an episode of melena. She was found to be hypotensive and tachycardic and have coagulation lab abnormalities. The international normalized ratio (INR) was elevated at 9 and guaiac test was positive. The patient was given two liters of intravenous fluids, which stabilized her blood pressure before she was transferred to our institution for further evaluation and treatment.

The patient's past medical history included paroxysmal atrial fibrillation, chronic obstructive pulmonary disease, and depression, with past surgical history of hip repair and left above-knee amputation. Pertinent oral home medications included dabigatran etexilate 150 mg twice daily, duloxetine HCl 30 mg every morning and 60 mg at bedtime, carvedilol 6.25 mg daily, lisinopril 2.5 mg daily, furosemide 40 mg daily, and diltiazem 120 mg daily. The last known dose of dabigatran was taken the morning prior to transfer.

Upon admission, the patient was volume-resuscitated with crystalloid fluids, which improved the blood pressure and heart rate. Lab abnormalities on presentation to our facility included hemoglobin and hematocrit (H/H) of 7.2 and 20.6, an increased serum creatinine (SCr) of 1.54 mg/dL (estimated creatinine clearance of 38 mL/min using Cockcroft Gault (CG) formula [weight 80.6 kg]), activated partial thromboplastin time (aPTT) of >160 seconds, INR of 6.2, prothrombin time (PT) of 58.2 seconds, and lactate of 3.5 mmol/L, which decreased to INR of 3.2, prothrombin time of 31.5 seconds, and lactate of 2.4 mmol/L after 2 units of packed red blood cells and 3 units of fresh frozen plasma. Her H/H improved to 9.8 and 27.7, respectively. A physical examination found the patient to have mild abdominal distention with positive bowel sounds and a left lower quadrant implanted pain pump.

An additional 2 units of packed red blood cells and 3 units of fresh frozen plasma were given due to elevated INR, and the patient was started on a pantoprazole drip for further management of a gastrointestinal bleed as well as antibiotics for possible infection. A computed tomography scan of her abdomen/pelvis was obtained which revealed some thickening of the colon, pneumatosis, and portal venous air, following which she was seen by general surgery and taken emergently to the operating room for an exploratory laparotomy. Ischemia of the hepatic flexure was found and resected. The patient was noted to have a small tear in the liver capsule, which was sprayed with thrombin and Surgicel, covered with laparotomy pads and a wound vacuum assisted closure device was placed. Her labs at this time included H/H of 9.3 and 26.8, INR of 2.8, and aPTT of 80 seconds. Patient had an estimated blood loss of 2 liters in the operating room and continued to have oozing from her wound postoperatively. A nephrology consult was then obtained to initiate dialysis in an attempt to remove any remaining dabigatran from the serum that may be contributing to her current bleeding. Access was obtained, and since the patient remained hypotensive postoperatively despite volume resuscitation with colloids, crystalloids, and norepinephrine infusion, the decision was made to initiate CRRT for treatment of the acute nonoliguric renal failure as well as to augment dabigatran removal from the serum. Serum dabigatran levels were determined using high performance liquid chromatography (HPLC); margin of error was not reported. Samples were collected prior to initiation of CRRT, as well as approximately 8, 12, and 24 hours after initiation of CRRT (Figure 1). Serum drug levels were send-out tests performed at National Medical Services, Willow Grove, PA.

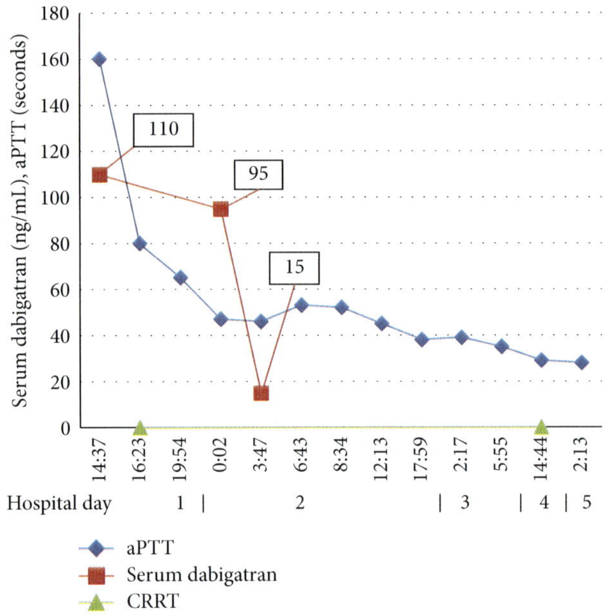

FIGURE 1: Serum dabigatran levels and aPTT trend over time.

CRRT was initiated as continuous venovenous hemodiafiltration (CVVHD/F). The dialysis set utilized the Prismasate® system, with the HF1400 polyarylethersulfone filter (Gambro®). CVVHD/F hemofiltration was prescribed at a total hemofiltration dose of 2500 ml/hr (32 ml/kg/hr) with a blood flow rate of 250 ml/min, dialysate flow rate of 1500 ml/hr, and replacement flow rate of 1000 mL/hr, with infused 100% post-filter; the preceding settings are common rates used at our institution. Circuit anticoagulation was not initiated as the patient was actively bleeding, requiring transfusions, and extent of liver injury previously described was not yet known. A hemofiltration fluid consisting of bicarbonate 22 mEq/L, calcium 0 mEq/L, chloride 120.5 mEq/L, lactate 3 mEq/L, magnesium 1.5 mEq/L, sodium 140 mEq/L, and potassium 4 mEq/L was utilized for both dialysate and replacement.

The initial dabigatran level, collected approximately 2 hours prior to start of CVVHD/F, was 110 ng/mL. This decreased to 95 ng/mL and 15 ng/mL, 7.5 h (after 5.5 h of CVVHD/F) and 11.5 h (after 9.5 h of CVVHD/F) after initial level, respectively. The final serum level was obtained approximately 24 h after the first level and returned undetectable (after 22 h of CVVHD/F). Dialysis was no longer necessary at this point for the indication of drug toxicity and rather was continued for volume status and hemodynamic instability. In relation to the last known time of ingestion (which was approximately 0900 the morning of transfer), the levels were drawn at the following intervals: 31.5 h, 39 h, 43 h, and 55 h after the dose. The calculated estimated creatinine clearance just prior to initiation of CVVHD/F had improved to 58 mL/min (CG), with adequate urine output of 1 mL/kg/hour which was maintained throughout the first 48 hours of CRRT therapy, as renal function improved daily upon admission. CVVHD/F was continued overnight for approximately 18 hours until the patient was taken back to the operating room on hospital day 2 for relaparotomy and removal of packing and evaluation for ongoing bleeding. She received another unit of packed red blood cells prior to operation, with hemoglobin and hematocrit of 7.4 g/dL and 20.3%, respectively, which was decreased from previous value, as well as INR of 1.6 and aPTT of 53 seconds at the time. Hemorrhage was noted to be controlled, blood and coagulation products were no longer necessary, and the patient underwent resection of nonviable cecum and ileostomy creation. The patient returned to the intensive care unit where CVVHD/F was restarted and continued through hospital day 4 for management of volume status (3 days total of CRRT), at which time she returned to the operating room for removal of packing with fascia and abdominal wall closure. The patient was transferred to a progressive care unit and discharged to a nursing and rehabilitation facility on hospital day 21, a prolonged stay which was not deemed to be related to bleeding complications. She did return to the hospital 4 days after discharge for possible infection requiring an 18-day hospital stay until she was discharged alive.

Pharmacokinetic calculations were done utilizing linear noncompartmental pharmacokinetic methods [3]. The elimination rate constant (k_e) was calculated using the only 2 detectable levels which were drawn during the treatment with CRRT (level 2 = 95 ng/mL and level 3 = 15 ng/mL). The final level drawn 22 h after CRRT commencement was not able to be used as it is below the limit of detection of the laboratory. The k_e calculation includes elimination on CRRT plus renal elimination from a calculated GFR of 58 mL/min. Pharmacokinetic parameters are as follows: [k_e = 0.461 hours^{-1}] and [elimination half-life = 1.5 hours]. $C_{\max}$ and V_d were not calculated, as the elimination prior to starting CRRT is not known. Based on calculated clearance, the dabigatran level would be expected to fall below 1 ng/mL approximately 6 hours after the last measured serum concentration. Compared to published pharmacokinetic information, the half-life exhibited during the treatment with CRRT was significantly shorter compared to healthy elderly female volunteers with normal renal function (1.5 hours versus 13 hours) [2] although our patient did have adequate renal function during the treatment with CRRT, and this seems to be a significant decrease in the half-life of this drug. It is not possible to determine exactly how much clearance is due to the effects of the CRRT, as effluent levels were not measured; however, our observed elimination half-life was approximately 8 times faster than expected [2]. Limitations to the pharmacokinetic calculations include assumption of steady state dosing, consistent renal elimination over the time course of serum sampling, compliance with home medication regimen, and inability to calculate V_d. Regardless of the inherent limitations of the calculations and serum measurements, we believe that the enhanced clearance seen with CRRT as well as residual renal function is worth noting. While it is impossible to predict the exact elimination from the CRRT circuit without measuring drug effluent levels, the total dabigatran clearance was observed to be significantly higher in our patient, as compared to expected clearance seen in previous pharmacokinetic studies in a similar patient population.

3. Discussion

We describe a case of dabigatran induced life-threatening bleeding, a unique case in which the primary treatment modality used for reversal was CRRT. Other cases utilizing CRRT to remove dabigatran from the serum of bleeding patients have been reported [4, 5], yet data are still lacking for removal constants and dosage adjustments during CRRT. Dosing adjustment recommendations exist for patients with moderate renal dysfunction; however, patients with severe renal dysfunction were excluded from phase III clinical trials. A group of patients with end-stage renal disease requiring intermittent hemodialysis were included in a pharmacokinetic study of dabigatran and it was determined that approximately 68% of the 50 mg dose was removed after the 4-hour dialysis session, with 62% removed at 2 hours [6]. Chang et al. describe a case of intermittent hemodialysis for emergent dabigatran removal which resulted in a serum decrease in serum dabigatran concentration of about 10 ng/mL per hour during the time of monitoring. After hemodialysis was completed, further serum monitoring showed a rebound of drug levels possibly due to the large volume of distribution of dabigatran [7]. A well designed pharmacokinetic study by Khadzhynov et al. reports the results of phase I study of dabigatran elimination by hemodialysis [8]. Serum levels of dabigatran were reduced by 59.3% after a four-hour session of hemodialysis at a blood flow rate of 400 mL/min. At a lower blood flow rate of 200 mL/min, they observed a 48.8% removal of serum dabigatran. This study is unique in that the investigators were able to observe greater extent of extracorporeal removal of dabigatran with a higher blood flow rate, although the authors state that this effect was not linear. The investigators of this study did not detect a significant rebound effect of dabigatran after the dialysis session, although clinically significant bleeding due to rebound drug levels has been described in a setting of extracorporeal drug removal [5]. In our case, we did not collect serum dabigatran levels after the termination of CRRT in order to measure a rebound effect. The patient required CRRT for 3 days total to treat the acute nonoliguric renal failure and dabigatran toxicity; it was assumed at that time that the dabigatran had been adequately removed from the serum, renal function had recovered, and the clinically significant bleeding had since stopped.

Reversal of dabigatran is difficult due to its specific action on thrombin generation. Vitamin K and protamine will have little to no effect on reversal [9]. Use of recombinant factors has been investigated as potential reversal agents, including recombinant factor VIIa which has been used to study the reversal effects of direct thrombin inhibitors with conflicting results [7, 10]. Rat models of bleeding have shown that activated factor products (PCC), such as FEIBA® (Factor Eight Inhibitor Bypassing Activity), have significantly slowed bleeding times following dabigatran overdose [11]. In contrast, nonactivated PCCs, such as Cofact®, have not had the same reversal effects on anticoagulation due to dabigatran [11]. Additional limitations include the lack of routinely available four-factor PCCs in the United States at some institutions due to cost constraints. In an ex vivo model of dabigatran therapy, Khoo and colleagues examined the effects of FEIBA on coagulation abnormalities induced by dabigatran at therapeutic doses (serum concentration range 96–286 ng/mL). The authors found that a 50 u/kg dose was efficacious in reversing the effects of dabigatran [12]. A case presented by Dager et al. reported successful reversal of a life-threatening bleed caused by dabigatran utilizing FEIBA [13]. A dose of 26 u/kg actual body weight was used to treat the bleeding caused by a transseptal perforation in the presence of anticoagulation with dabigatran. The aPTT values did not correlate well with clinical bleeding or doses of FEIBA; however, the bleeding time decreased in a linear manner after administration of the FEIBA [12, 13]. Idarucizumab, a monoclonal antibody fragment, binds to both free and thrombin-bound dabigatran to inhibit its activity and recently gained fast track FDA approval. The RE-VERSE AD trial showed 100% median maximum percentage reversal in patients taking dabigatran who had serious bleeding or required a procedure within 8 hours [14]. Given the lack of clinical experience of the product, safety concerns exist. The RE-VERSE AD trial lists several early and late adverse events of concern including DVT and ischemic stroke; however, none of these patients were receiving antithrombotic therapy in a patient population with known risk (hence taking dabigatran prior to admission). In addition, cost may be an issue as hospitals predict use and inventory management. Critical access hospitals should attempt to carry this product if possible. CRRT may be considered in a patient who is not able to receive this reversal agent given drug acquisition due to unavailability or cost constraints. Additional postmarketing surveillance data will help determine the role of CRRT in these cases.

Dabigatran was developed as an alternative to warfarin with less need for routine laboratory monitoring. There are times when monitoring of the coagulation levels may become necessary, as in the example above during a life-threatening bleeding event, although consensus on a readily available test to define coagulation status in these patients is lacking. Previous studies have shown that the aPTT is prolonged with increasing doses of dabigatran, although the result becomes less accurate with larger doses of the drug [2]. PT and INR are not significantly altered by therapeutic doses of dabigatran (although they can be elevated with supratherapeutic concentrations). The ecarin clotting time (ECT) and thrombin clotting time (TT) have the strongest correlation with increasing serum drug concentrations, although they are not widely available as a point-of-care test in most hospitals [2, 15].

4. Conclusion

The case above reports a successful treatment utilizing CRRT to remove dabigatran from the serum of a patient with a life-threatening bleed. The use of CRRT along with residual kidney function removed 84 percent of the drug serum level over approximately 4 hours, enhancing the elimination of the drug 8-fold compared to healthy volunteers. Although a 4-hour intermittent hemodialysis session may be a more efficient modality to dialyze toxic dabigatran levels [5, 8], our reported case enhances the body of literature suggesting that CRRT is a safe and efficacious therapy to employ in the treatment of a dabigatran induced life-threatening bleed in a hemodynamically unstable patient.

Competing Interests

All authors report no conflict of interests, including pharmaceutical or industry support, regarding any of the information contained in this report.

References

[1] B. E. Baetz and S. A. Spinler, "Dabigatran etexilate: an oral direct thrombin inhibitor for prophylaxis and treatment of thromboembolic diseases," *Pharmacotherapy*, vol. 28, no. 11, pp. 1354–1373, 2008.

[2] J. Stangier, "Clinical pharmacokinetics and pharmacodynamics of the oral direct thrombin inhibitor dabigatran etexilate," *Clinical Pharmacokinetics*, vol. 47, no. 5, pp. 285–295, 2008.

[3] M. E. Winter, *Basic Clinical Pharmacokinetics*, Lippincott Williams & Wilkins, Philadelphia, Pa, USA, 4th edition, 2004.

[4] J. Bouchard, M. Ghannoum, A. Bernier-Jean et al., "Comparison of intermittent and continuous extracorporeal treatments for the enhanced elimination of dabigatran," *Clinical Toxicology*, vol. 53, no. 3, pp. 156–163, 2015.

[5] T. Singh, T. T. Maw, B. L. Henry et al., "Extracorporeal therapy for dabigatran removal in the treatment of acute bleeding: a single center experience," *Clinical Journal of the American Society of Nephrology*, vol. 8, no. 9, pp. 1533–1539, 2013.

[6] J. Stangier, K. Rathgen, H. Sthle, and D. Mazur, "Influence of renal impairment on the pharmacokinetics and pharmacodynamics of oral dabigatran etexilate: an open-label, parallel-group, single-centre study," *Clinical Pharmacokinetics*, vol. 49, no. 4, pp. 259–268, 2010.

[7] D. N. Chang, W. E. Dager, and A. I. Chin, "Removal of dabigatran by hemodialysis," *American Journal of Kidney Diseases*, vol. 61, no. 3, pp. 487–489, 2013.

[8] D. Khadzhynov, F. Wagner, S. Formella et al., "Effective elimination of dabigatran by haemodialysis: a phase I single-centre study in patients with end-stage renal disease," *Thrombosis and Haemostasis*, vol. 109, no. 4, pp. 596–605, 2013.

[9] *Idarucizumab*, Boehringr Ingelheim Pharmaceuticals, Ridgefield, Conn, USA, 2015.

[10] T. E. Warkentin, P. Margetts, S. J. Connolly, A. Lamy, C. Ricci, and J. W. Eikelboom, "Recombinant factor VIIa (rFVIIa) and hemodialysis to manage massive dabigatran-associated postcardiac surgery bleeding," *Blood*, vol. 119, no. 9, pp. 2172–2174, 2012.

[11] M. Wolzt, M. Levi, T. C. Sarich et al., "Effect of recombinant factor VIIa on melagatran-induced inhibition of thrombin generation and platelet activation in healthy volunteers," *Thrombosis and Haemostasis*, vol. 91, no. 6, pp. 1090–1096, 2004.

[12] E. S. Eerenberg, P. W. Kamphuisen, M. K. Sijpkens, J. C. Meijers, H. R. Buller, and M. Levi, "Reversal of rivaroxaban and dabigatran by prothrombin complex concentrate: a randomized, placebo-controlled, crossover study in healthy subjects," *Circulation*, vol. 124, no. 14, pp. 1573–1579, 2011.

[13] T.-L. Khoo, C. Weatherburn, G. Kershaw, C. J. Reddel, J. Curnow, and S. Dunkley, "The use of FEIBA[5] in the correction of coagulation abnormalities induced by dabigatran," *International Journal of Laboratory Hematology*, vol. 35, no. 2, pp. 222–224, 2013.

[14] W. E. Dager, R. C. Gosselin, and A. J. Roberts, "Reversing dabigatran in life-threatening bleeding occurring during cardiac ablation with factor eight inhibitor bypassing activity," *Critical Care Medicine*, vol. 41, no. 5, pp. e42–e46, 2013.

[15] C. V. Pollack, P. A. Reilly, J. Eikelboom et al., "Idarucizumab for dabigatran reversal," *The New England Journal of Medicine*, vol. 373, no. 6, pp. 511–520, 2015.

42

Diffuse Alveolar Hemorrhage Associated with Edoxaban Therapy

Kenichi Nitta, Hiroshi Imamura, Akihiro Yashio, Satoko Kashima, and Katsunori Mochizuki

Department of Emergency and Critical Care Medicine, Shinshu University School of Medicine, Nagano, Japan

Correspondence should be addressed to Kenichi Nitta; nittaken@shinshu-u.ac.jp

Academic Editor: Kenneth S. Waxman

Introduction. The main adverse effect of anticoagulant therapy is bleeding, and major bleeding, including intracranial, gastrointestinal, and retroperitoneal bleeding, has been reported as an adverse effect of edoxaban, a direct oral anticoagulant (DOAC). Bleeding during systemic anticoagulation with edoxaban presents a therapeutic conundrum, because there is currently no safe or efficacious reversal agent to stop major bleeding. *Case Report.* A 51-year-old woman had multiple traumatic injuries, including lower limb fractures. On day 8, she developed deep venous thrombosis, and edoxaban was administered orally. On day 38, she developed fungemia, which was treated with an antifungal drug. On day 43, she presented with dyspnea. Chest computed tomography scan showed bilateral diffuse ground-glass opacities in the whole lung fields. The results of the subsequent workup (i.e., serum levels of the antineutrophil cytoplasmic antibody, antinuclear antibody, and antiglomerular basement membrane antibody) and microbiological study were unremarkable. Based on these findings, her condition was diagnosed as diffuse alveolar hemorrhage (DAH) associated with edoxaban therapy. The lung opacities disappeared spontaneously after edoxaban therapy was discontinued. *Conclusion.* DAH is a dangerous complication associated with edoxaban therapy. DOACs, including edoxaban, should be prescribed with caution, especially for patients in a critical condition.

1. Introduction

Venous thromboembolism is the third most common cardiovascular disorder after coronary heart disease and stroke [1]. Treatment of the venous and arterial thrombotic phenomena is a main medical challenge, and the development of anticoagulant drugs is a revolution in medicine. Edoxaban, a direct oral anticoagulant (DOAC), was approved by the United States Food and Drug Administration in January 2015 to prevent stroke in patients with nonvalvular atrial fibrillation and treat deep venous thrombosis (DVT) and pulmonary embolism after 5 to 10 days of parenteral anticoagulation. The main adverse effect of anticoagulant therapy is bleeding, and major bleeding, including intracranial, gastrointestinal, and retroperitoneal bleeding, has been reported to be an adverse effect of edoxaban [2]. Bleeding during systemic anticoagulation with edoxaban presents a therapeutic conundrum, because there is currently no safe or efficacious reversal agent to stop major bleeding [3].

Diffuse alveolar hemorrhage (DAH) has not been previously reported to be a complication of edoxaban therapy. Herein, we describe a case of DAH associated with edoxaban therapy in a woman who suffered multiple traumatic injuries accompanied by DVT and a fungal infection.

2. Case Presentation

A 51-year-old woman with no relevant medical history was admitted to the emergency department with shock due to multiple traumatic injuries caused by a traffic crash. An occlusion balloon catheter was introduced temporarily from the femoral artery to the descending aorta. The patient simultaneously received blood transfusion, and the patient's cardiorespiratory condition gradually stabilized. Whole-body computed tomography (CT) scan showed injuries to the wall of the small and large intestines. Radiographic imaging demonstrated a right femoral shaft fracture and a left open tibial fracture. Consequently, the patient underwent resection

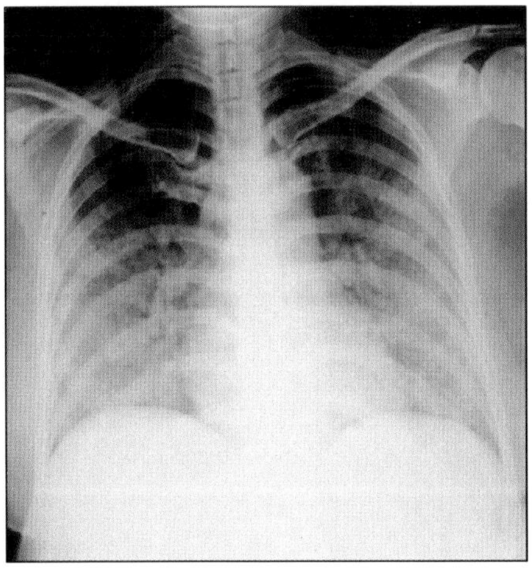

Figure 1: Chest radiograph showing infiltrates bilaterally.

of the small and large intestines, two colostomies, and osteosynthesis, after which the patient was admitted to the intensive care unit.

On the fourth day after admission (postoperative day 2), anticoagulant therapy with heparin was initiated to prevent DVT. On the eighth day after admission, the patient's D-dimer level increased, and contrast-enhanced CT scan showed DVT in the right femoral vein. Therefore, edoxaban (30 mg/day) was administered orally. Ordinarily, 60 mg edoxaban is administered once daily, but since the patient weighed 51 kg and had normal renal function, the dose was reduced.

On day 36, the patient developed a fever with nausea and vomiting. Blood cultures were performed, and a course of antibiotics was initiated for a possible intraperitoneal infection. On day 38, the patient's condition was diagnosed as sepsis due to *Candida guilliermondii*, and treatment with micafungin was initiated. On day 43, coagulation tests showed a prothrombin time (PT) of 16.2 s, prothrombin time-international normalized ratio (PT-INR) of 1.44, and activated partial thromboplastin time of 35.6 s. The patient had already received a dose of edoxaban (30 mg) that day. That night, the patient demonstrated dyspnea with tachypnea and had blood in her sputum along with an abrupt decrease in oxygen saturation. Chest radiography scan showed lung opacities bilaterally (Figure 1). The patient was intubated and underwent mechanical ventilation with positive end-expiratory pressure (PEEP) because of worsening hypoxemia. The arterial partial pressure of oxygen to fraction of inspired oxygen (PaO_2/FiO_2) ratio was 113 mmHg on PEEP with 6 cm H_2O. Chest CT scans showed diffuse ground-glass opacities bilaterally (Figures 2(a) and 2(b)). At this point, the PT was 18.7 s and PT-INR was 1.66. Echocardiography results showed normal left ventricular function and no valvular disease. Serum levels of the antineutrophil cytoplasmic antibody, perinuclear antineutrophil cytoplasmic antibody, antinuclear antibody, anti-dsDNA antibody, and antiglomerular basement membrane antibody were negative. Bronchoscopy results showed bloody discharge around the bifurcation of the trachea and no malignant tumor (Figure 2(c)), and subsequent bronchoalveolar lavage (BAL) findings showed a bloody gross appearance. All results of the sputum cultures and BAL fluid did not indicate any causative pathogen. The patient had a pure DAH confined to the lungs with no evidence of disseminated intravascular coagulation or hemorrhagic events occurring elsewhere in the body. In addition, the patient did not receive any concomitant therapy with specific P-glycoprotein inhibitors (i.e., verapamil; quinidine; or short-term use of azithromycin, clarithromycin, erythromycin, oral itraconazole, or oral ketoconazole), which may increase the serum concentration of edoxaban. Finally, we diagnosed this case as DAH associated with edoxaban therapy, which was triggered by fungemia.

Conservative therapy with PEEP was continued, and the lung opacities disappeared spontaneously following the discontinuation of edoxaban therapy. The bloody sputum gradually diminished, and the patient's respiratory status recovered over time.

The patient was extubated on day 50, and the patient showed gradual improvement without DVT recurrence. Additionally, the patient could walk using a crutch. On day 84, chest radiography scan showed almost normal findings, and the patient was transferred to another hospital for leg rehabilitation.

3. Discussion

To the best of our knowledge, this is the first reported case of DAH associated with edoxaban therapy. DAH is a clinical syndrome resulting from extensive bleeding in the acinar portion of the lung [4], and it is caused by diseases that damage the alveolar capillary barrier or by coagulation disorders. Generally, DAH may develop in several pathologic conditions, including vasculitis, autoimmune diseases, acute poststreptococcal glomerulonephritis, and any pneumorenal syndrome. However, the incidence of DAH in patients receiving anticoagulant therapy is low [5]. DAH secondary to warfarin therapy has been rarely reported [6, 7], but DAH is a serious adverse effect of dabigatran [8] and apixaban [9]. However, DAH associated with edoxaban has not been reported in the literature. In our patient, the BAL fluid became progressively more hemorrhagic, with no evidence of massive bleeding or endobronchial pathology. In addition, tests for specific antibodies were negative, and although the patient had a fungal infection, all sputum and BAL fluid cultures were negative for any causative pathogen. Moreover, the patient's lung opacities disappeared spontaneously after edoxaban therapy was discontinued. On the basis of these findings, the patient's condition was diagnosed as DAH associated with edoxaban therapy, which was triggered by fungemia.

Routine coagulation tests are not conducted to determine the anticoagulation status of patients receiving DOACs. However, edoxaban and other factor Xa inhibitors prolong the clotting time tests, including the PT, PT-INR, and activated partial thromboplastin time (aPTT). Additionally, these clotting time tests are not indicative of bleeding risks, because there is no dose-response relationship that correlates the changes between PT and aPTT to a specific dose of

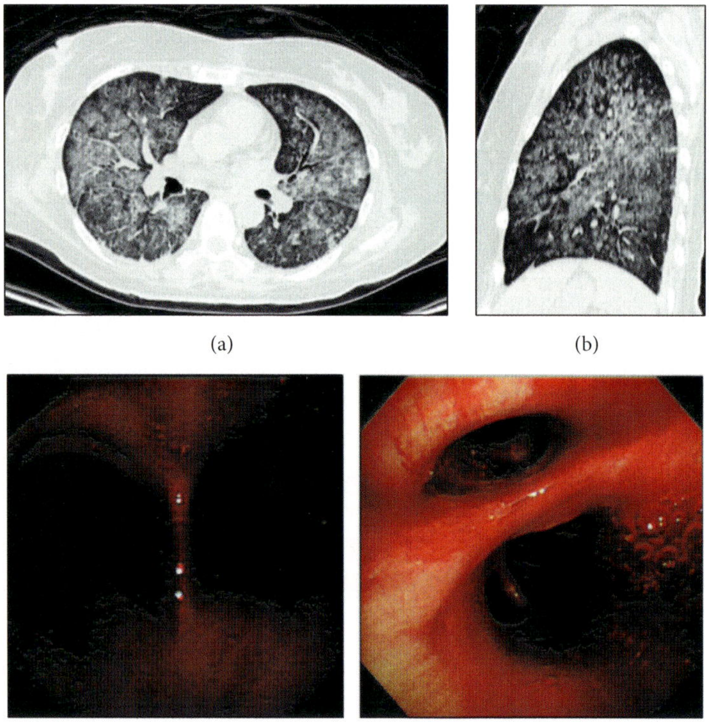

(a) (b)

(c)

Figure 2: Imaging studies. Axial (a) and sagittal (b) chest computed tomography scans showing diffuse ground-glass opacities bilaterally. Bronchoscopy images (c) showing bloody discharge around the bifurcation of the trachea and the right intermediate and inferior bronchi.

DOACs [10]. As traditional coagulation assays do not reliably measure the anticoagulant effects of DOACs, viscoelastic assays may be a useful tool for assessing coagulation function in the presence of DOACs [11]. In the present case, although we monitored the patient's PT-INR daily after fungemia was diagnosed, we could not prevent DAH. One of the disadvantages of DOACs is physicians' limited experience with these drugs in cases of abnormal coagulation. Accordingly, DOACs should be used cautiously in patients who require invasive procedures [12] and intensive care.

Warfarin anticoagulation can be reversed. A recent study suggested that andexanet alfa can reverse the anticoagulant activity of apixaban and rivaroxaban in older healthy participants without clinical toxic effects [3]. However, there is still no safe or efficacious reversal agent to stop factor Xa inhibitor-associated acute major bleeding. The peak plasma concentration of edoxaban occurs 1 to 2 h after oral administration, and the usual plasma half-life is 8 to 10 h [13]. As DOACs have short elimination half-lives, time is the most important antidote. In many cases, a bleeding event can be managed effectively by simply providing supportive therapy and withholding the DOAC in question at least temporarily [14]. Fatal bleeding associated with edoxaban is particularly challenging, because there is limited experience with the expected clinical course. Fortunately, our patient's respiratory status improved spontaneously with the discontinuation of edoxaban therapy. Moreover, recent data from human studies have indicated that prothrombin complex concentrate (PCC) products may be viable agents for correcting coagulation changes associated with dabigatran, rivaroxaban, and apixaban [15, 16]. However, the use of PCCs may increase the risk for thrombosis; therefore, it is important to monitor signs and symptoms of thrombotic events in patients at high risk of thrombosis [11]. Therefore, reversal by a specific antidote (as yet unavailable) is unlikely to change the priority given to conservative therapy, which was used successfully in this case.

The present case is the first reported case of DAH associated with edoxaban. DOACs, including edoxaban, should be prescribed with caution, especially for patients in a critical condition, as there is still no safe or efficacious reversal agent to stop factor Xa inhibitor-associated acute major bleeding.

Competing Interests

The authors declare that there is no conflict of interests regarding the publication of this paper.

References

[1] S. Z. Goldhaber and H. Bounameaux, "Pulmonary embolism and deep vein thrombosis," *The Lancet*, vol. 379, no. 9828, pp. 1835–1846, 2012.

[2] H. R. Büller, H. Décousus, M. A. Grosso et al., "Edoxaban versus warfarin for the treatment of symptomatic venous thromboembolism," *The New England Journal of Medicine*, vol. 369, no. 15, pp. 1406–1415, 2013.

[3] D. M. Siegal, J. T. Curnutte, S. J. Connolly et al., "Andexanet alfa for the reversal of factor Xa inhibitor activity," *New England Journal of Medicine*, vol. 373, no. 25, pp. 2413–2424, 2015.

[4] A. R. Lara and M. I. Schwarz, "Diffuse alveolar hemorrhage," *Chest*, vol. 137, no. 5, pp. 1164–1171, 2010.

[5] M. Santalo, P. Domingo, J. Fontcuberta, M. Franco, and J. Nolla, "Diffuse pulmonary hemorrhage associated with anticoagulant therapy," *European Journal of Respiratory Disease*, vol. 69, no. 2, pp. 114–119, 1986.

[6] A. Waness, T. Aldabbagh, and M. Harakati, "Diffuse alveolar haemorrhage secondary to warfarin therapy for atrial fibrillation: a case report and literature review," *BMJ Case Reports*, 2009.

[7] E. Uysal, E. Çevik, S. Solak, Y. A. Acar, and M. Yalimol, "A life-threatening complication of warfarin therapy in ED: diffuse alveolar hemorrhage," *The American Journal of Emergency Medicine*, vol. 32, no. 6, pp. 690.e3–690.e4, 2014.

[8] K. Yokoi, K. Isoda, T. Kimura, and T. Adachi, "Diffuse alveolar hemorrhage associated with dabigatran," *Internal Medicine*, vol. 51, no. 18, pp. 2667–2668, 2012.

[9] M. I. Gabrilovich, D. E. Buxton, D. M. Lykins, S. M. McMillen, and O. O. A. Onadeko, "Diffuse alveolar hemorrhage secondary to apixaban administration," *Chest*, vol. 146, no. 3, pp. e115–e116, 2014.

[10] A. Cuker, D. M. Siegal, M. A. Crowther, and D. A. Garcia, "Laboratory measurement of the anticoagulant activity of the non-vitamin K oral anticoagulants," *Journal of the American College of Cardiology*, vol. 64, no. 11, pp. 1128–1139, 2014.

[11] D. R. Rinehart, N. R. Lockhart, L. A. Hamilton, J. R. Langdon, and A. S. Rowe, "Management of apixaban-associated subdural hematoma: a case report on the use of factor eight inhibitor bypassing activity," *Critical Care Medicine*, vol. 43, no. 6, pp. e203–e207, 2015.

[12] P. Prandoni, "The treatment of venous thromboembolism with novel oral anticoagulants: warnings and limitations," *Blood Transfusion*, vol. 13, no. 2, pp. 178–180, 2015.

[13] C. Minor, K. B. Tellor, and A. L. Armbruster, "Edoxaban, a novel oral factor Xa inhibitor," *The Annals of Pharmacotherapy*, vol. 49, no. 7, pp. 843–850, 2015.

[14] C. V. Pollack Jr., "Coagulation assessment with the new generation of oral anticoagulants," *Emergency Medicine Journal*, vol. 33, no. 6, pp. 423–430, 2016.

[15] E. S. Eerenberg, P. W. Kamphuisen, M. K. Sijpkens, J. C. Meijers, H. R. Buller, and M. Levi, "Reversal of rivaroxaban and dabigatran by prothrombin complex concentrate: a randomized, placebo-controlled, crossover study in healthy subjects," *Circulation*, vol. 124, no. 14, pp. 1573–1579, 2011.

[16] R. Marlu, E. Hodaj, A. Paris, P. Albaladejo, J. L. Crackowski, and G. Pernod, "Effect of non-specific reversal agents on anticoagulant activity of dabigatran and rivaroxaban: a randomised crossover ex vivo study in healthy volunteers," *Thrombosis and Haemostasis*, vol. 108, no. 2, pp. 217–224, 2012.

43

Hemadsorption with Adult CytoSorb® in a Low Weight Pediatric Case

Catalin Gabriel Cirstoveanu,[1,2] Ileana Barascu,[2] and Samantha Mc Kenzie Stancu[1]

[1] *"Carol Davila" University of Medicine & Pharmacy Bucharest, 37 Dionisie Lupu Street, District 1, 020021 Bucharest, Romania*
[2] *"Marie S. Curie Children's Emergency Hospital" Bucharest, Neonatal Intensive Care Unit, 20 Constantin Brancoveanu Street, District 4, 041451 Bucharest, Romania*

Correspondence should be addressed to Catalin Gabriel Cirstoveanu; cirstoveanu@yahoo.com

Academic Editor: Zsolt Molnár

Cytokine adsorber (CytoSorb) has been used successfully as adjunctive treatment for adult patients with elevated cytokine levels in the setting with severe sepsis and septic shock and to reduce blood myoglobin, unconjugated bilirubin, and conjugated bilirubin. In this article we present the case of a nine-month-old male infant who was admitted to the NICU due to sepsis after cardiac surgery, Fallot tetralogy, and multisystem organ failure (MSOF) including liver failure and renal failure which was successfully treated by a combination of continuous hemodiafiltration (HDF) and hemadsorption with CytoSorb. HDF was safe and effective from the first day for urea removal, but the patient's bilirubin levels kept increasing gradually, culminating on the 9th day with a maximum value of 54 mg/dL of total bilirubin and 31.67 mg/dL of direct bilirubin when we performed hemadsorption with CytoSorb. Over the 49-hour period of hemadsorption, the total bilirubin value decreased from 54 to 14 mg/dL, and the patient's general status improved considerably accompanied by a rapid drop of aminotransferases. Hemodynamic status has been improved as well and inotropes dropped rapidly. The patient's ventilation settings improved during CytoSorb treatment permitting weaning the patient from mechanical ventilation after five days of hemadsorption. The patient was discharged home after 34 days of hospitalization, in a good general status.

1. Introduction

Hemadsorption is a means of artificial extracorporeal liver support designed to remove toxins accumulating in patients suffering from acute liver failure (ALF). First developed in the 1950s, although scarcely employed, hemadsorption gained its reputation as an efficacious modality of bridging to liver transplant [1].

In 1996, Bhaduri and Mieli-Vergani proposed the definition of ALF as "a rare multisystem disorder in which severe impairment of liver function, with or without encephalopathy, occurs in association with hepatocellular necrosis in a patient with nonrecognized underlying chronic liver disease" [2].

Although it is a rare entity encountered in neonates, without liver transplantation it is a highly fatal condition, with mortality of 70%. The main parameter used to establish the need for transplantation is an INR $\geq$ 4, representing a mortality of 90% [3]. The causes of ALF are diverse ranging from perinatal infections and inborn errors of metabolism to septicemia and shock [4, 5]. Due to its markedly high mortality rate, neonates suffering from ALF should be admitted to the Neonatal Intensive Care Unit (NICU) and managed by a highly skilled, multidisciplinary team comprising neonatologists, hepatologists, and transplant surgeons until either hepatic transplantation or liver regeneration takes place [3].

As a result of the detrimental clinical course and prognosis of ALF, liver support devices have been advocated [6] in order to act as bridge to transplantation [3]. Bridging therapy is in even higher demand in cases where transplantation is contraindicated, for example, in patients with consequences of ALF such as uncontrolled sepsis. Liver support devices are promising in ALF due to their inherent capacity of removing accumulated metabolites secondary to deficient hepatic clearance [6].

Extracorporeal liver support (ELS) devices can be divided into bioartificial systems, which use human or animal hepatocytes, and artificial, cell-free systems, as hemadsorption. Currently, there are three types of artificial extracorporeal liver support devices available: Single Pass Albumin Dialysis (SPAD), Molecular Adsorbent Recirculating System (MARS®), and the Fractionated Plasma Separation and Absorption (FPSA), called the "Prometheus System" [7].

Scientific data on ELS concerning the pediatric population is scarce in literature [8, 9]. Although MARS dialysis is the most extensively studied type of ELS, it is limited to case reports and small case series [10].

In the last years, hemadsorption using CytoSorb initially intended as adjunctive treatment for patients with elevated cytokine levels in the setting of SIRS, severe sepsis, and septic shock has gained attention as a potential tool to also reduce various other endogenous and exogenous compounds from blood such as myoglobin, bilirubin, and others. Several publications have shown excellent removal of unconjugated bilirubin (0.6 kDa) and conjugated bilirubin (0.8 kDa) by CytoSorb, with binding confirmed by the beads turning yellow [11, 12]. The CytoSorb polymer is both highly adsorptive and biocompatible, facilitating a concentration-dependent but size-selective removal of molecules with middle molecular weight (approx. 10–50 kDa). Of note, standard high-flux dialysis or CRRT is only capable of removing substances with a molecular weight below 15 kDa.

Herein we present the case of a nine-month-old male infant who was admitted to the NICU due to sepsis after cardiac surgery, Fallot tetralogy and multisystem organ failure (MSOF), respiratory failure, cardiac failure, liver failure, and renal failure which was successfully treated by a combination of continuous hemodiafiltration (HDF) and hemadsorption with a cytokine adsorber (CytoSorb) even despite the lack of an indication and limited information on the use of CytoSorb in children.

2. Case Presentation

A nine-month-old male infant, weighing 9 kilograms, was admitted to the NICU of "Marie Curie" Children's Hospital in Bucharest. The patient was admitted from the Pediatric Cardiovascular Surgery Unit, on his fourth postoperative day after the correction of tetralogy of Fallot. The patient was extubated on the first postoperative day, only to be reintubated on the second following the diagnosis of pleural and peritoneal effusions. On the third postoperative day the patient became febrile; therefore a complete blood count (CBC), biochemistry, and a blood culture were performed. The infant entered the NICU in a seriously degraded general status, intubated, and mechanically ventilated (CMV), presenting unilaterally diminished breath sounds, hypoxemia (oxygen saturation: 90%), oliguria, tachycardia (137 beats per minute), hypotension (74/44/59 mmHg), and abdominal distention with anasarca and fever (39-40°C). Physical examination revealed hepatosplenomegaly.

Upon admission, the CBC was reviewed showing hemoconcentration (Hb: 14.2 g/dL, Ht: 45%), thrombocytopenia (27,000/mm^3), and leukocytosis (17,800/mm^3) with neutrophilia (66.6%). Coagulation tests revealed a grossly elevated INR (4.66), hypofibrinogenemia (113 mg/dL), and a prolonged aPPT time (63 seconds). From the biochemical tests a severe inflammatory response was noticed (CRP: 47.76 U/L, procalcitonin: 10 ng/L). Furthermore, liver function tests (LFTs) were greatly abnormal (ALT: 1883.1 U/L, AST: 4214.5 U/L, GGT 72 U/L, total bilirubin: 10.05 mg/dL, and direct bilirubin: 7.59 mg/dL), consistent with hepatocellular necrosis. Renal impairment was also evident with creatinine of 1.15 mg/dL and urea of 55 mg/dL. Creatinine kinase and creatine kinase-MB were also elevated with values of 1619 U/L and 159.6 U/L, respectively. Acid-base balance was deranged, revealing metabolic acidosis. Blood culture was sterile and the culture from tracheal aspirate revealed *Escherichia coli* colonies.

Antibiotic and antifungal therapies with Meropenem, Vancomycin, and Fluconazole were initiated. Multiple episodes of severe hypotension and bradycardia were treated with Adrenaline, Noradrenaline, and Dopamine. A central venous catheter was inserted into the left subclavian vein and kept for 34 days. Due to persistence of the systemic inflammatory response syndrome (SIRS) at increasing CRP values from 47.76 to 54.76, Meropenem and Vancomycin were replaced by Tienam (Imipenem and Cilastin) and Amikacin (the dose was adjusted for renal failure) for the duration of 9 days. The metabolic acidosis was managed with sodium bicarbonate. Thrombocytopenia with values as low as 15,000/mm^3 was treated with multiple transfusions of thrombocyte mass and fresh frozen plasma (FFP). The anasarca was managed with a continuous Furosemide and Aminophylline perfusion and repeated albumin transfusions.

Two days after NICU admission oliguria rapidly evolving to anuria was noticed, and peritoneal dialysis was initiated. While the patient's fluid intake continued to exceed the output the decision was made to start hemodiafiltration (Prismaflex, Baxer) and to insert a double lumen Gambro 6.5 Fr venovenous catheter into the right femoral vein as the access route for HDF. Throughout HDF, the patient continued to be hypotensive and bradycardic necessitating an increased dose of inotropic agents. Metabolic acidosis was also persistent requiring repeated sodium bicarbonate administration. The patient continued to be thrombocytopenic needing multiple thrombocyte mass transfusions. In addition, the infant developed macrocytic, hyperchromic anemia. After initiation of HDF the patient continued to be oliguric presenting intensely hyperchromic hematuria.

The patient's fever did not subside, as a result of which antibiotic therapy was modified once again—this time Tienam and Amikacin were replaced by Meropenem and Ciprofloxacin for a duration of 16 days. Antibiotic doses were kept constant during. The patient's bilirubin levels kept increasing gradually, culminating in a maximum value of 54 mg/dL of total bilirubin and 31.67 mg/dL of direct bilirubin. Intense scleral and cutaneous jaundice was observed and the patient was diagnosed with cholestatic jaundice.

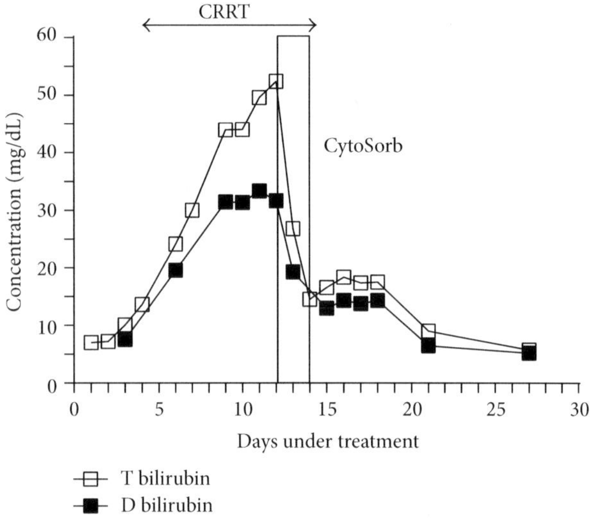

Figure 1: Level of total and direct bilirubin 48 hours before, during, and 48 hours after CytoSorb.

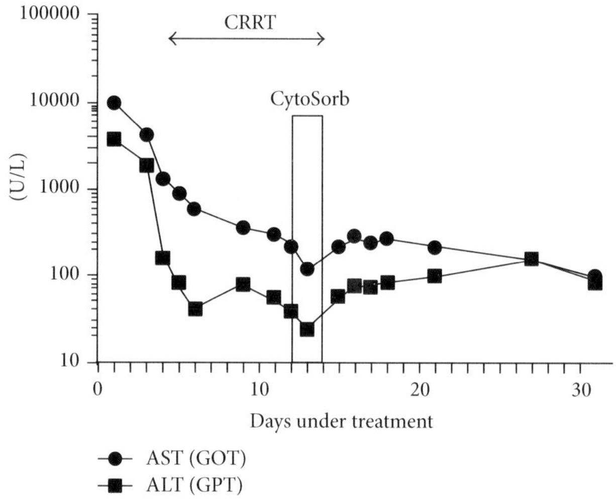

Figure 2: Level of aminotransferases 48 hours before, during, and 48 hours after CytoSorb.

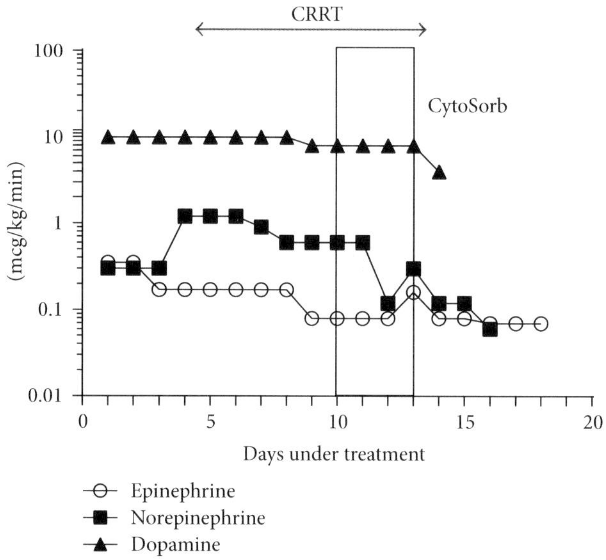

Figure 3: Norepinephrine doses before, during, and 48 hours after CytoSorb.

On the 9th day of HDF the therapeutic decision of commencing hemadsorption with a cytokine adsorber (CytoSorb) was taken. Blood flow was maintained at 40 mL/min and anticoagulation was achieved using heparin. The adsorber was placed in postdialyzer position.

Due to the paucity of recommendations in the literature and the fact that a flow of only 40 mL/min—1/5 of the recommended flow for hemadsorption of 200 mL/min—could be maintained throughout the HDF process, the procedure was maintained for 49 hours, 8 times more than normal (6 hours).

Over the 24-hour period of hemadsorption (during the first half period of the procedure), the total bilirubin value decreased from 54 to 17 mg/dL and the patient's general status improved considerably. Finally, after 49 hours of hemadsorption, the total bilirubin was 14 mg/dL (Figure 1).

During hemadsorption we noticed a rapid drop of the aminotransferases, which rose back to their previous values as soon as CytoSorb was removed. The infant was discharged three weeks later with aminotransferase values of 95 and 87 U/L for AST and ALT, respectively (Figure 2).

Our choice of inotropic drugs included norepinephrine, epinephrine, and Dopamine. We were able to decrease the dose rapidly from 0.8 to 0.18 mcg/kg/min during the first day and to stop norepinephrine administration in less than 48 hours from the initiation of CytoSorb treatment. We also managed to decrease the dose from 8 to 5 mcg/kg/min and to finally withdraw Dopamine administration during liver support (6.67 mcg/kg/min represents the medium dose during the CytoSorb treatment) (Figure 3).

The dose of epinephrine was decreased within 48 hours of CytoSorb treatment and withdrawn after 5 days. We observed a slight increase of the dose during CytoSorb treatment. Forty-eight hours after CytoSorb treatment, epinephrine was stopped.

On May 29, HDF was stopped after 11 days. The patient's cardiovascular status improved, which allowed for the dose of the inotropic agents to be decreased. Furthermore, a major attenuation of the SIRS was noticed in addition to a significant improvement of hepatocellular necrosis.

The patient's ventilation settings also improved during CytoSorb treatment. The fraction of inspired oxygen (FiO_2) dropped from 0.4 to 0.3 in the first day and subsequently to room air on the third day of liver treatment (at 49 hours). The respiratory rate (RR) decreased rapidly from 29 to 22 breaths/minute during the first day and then to 20 breaths/minute and maintained there for five days until extubation. Positive inspiratory pressure (PIP) decreased from 24 to 18 cm/H_2O while positive end expiratory pressure (PEEP) decreased from 7 to 6 cm/H_2O for the last five days on mechanical ventilation until extubation, having totally 27 days of mechanical ventilation (Figure 4).

Diuresis gradually reached normal values and on the same day enteral nutrition was initiated.

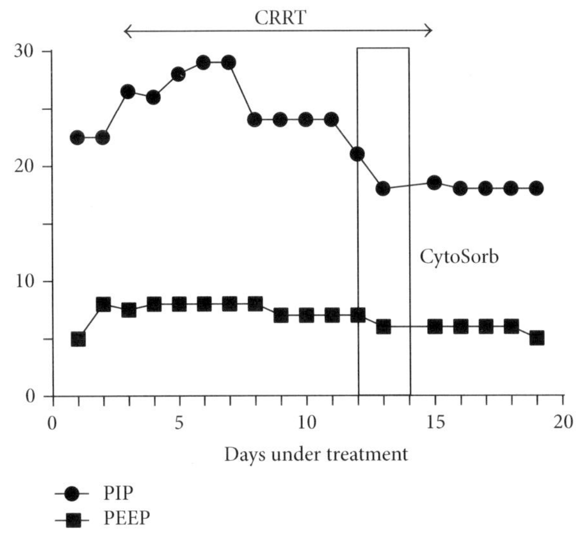

FIGURE 4: PIP and PEEP settings before, during, and after CytoSorb treatment.

Antibiotic doses could also be kept constant during the entire hemadsorption procedure using CytoSorb.

Renal function returned to normal with normochromic urine in a normal quantity while renal function tests showed normalization of the values of serum creatinine and urea.

The patient was discharged home on June 18, after 34 days of hospitalization, in a good general status, hemodynamically stable, afebrile, and weighing 9.6 kilograms. The patient's blood tests upon discharge were as follows: CBC within normal limits, mild inflammatory syndrome (slight leukocytosis (11,500/mm^3), CRP 5.27 mg/dL), hyperbilirubinemia (total: 5.89 mg/dL, conjugated: 5.24 mg/dL), increased transaminases (ALT: 87 U/L, AST: 95 U/L), normal serum creatinine, urea, and electrolytes. He was referred as well to pediatric neurologist for follow-up.

3. Discussion

Despite progress in critical care and highly specialized intensive care units, ALF is still a multisystem condition associated with high mortality [3, 13]. Artificial extracorporeal liver support devices were designed to improve the survival of patients with ALF by carrying out the detoxification processes, in the form of bridge therapy, while awaiting transplantation [14].

Hemadsorption has proven to be a safe and efficacious modality of bridging therapy in adults for treating complications of liver failure such as hepatic encephalopathy (HE), hemodynamic instability, and progressive hyperbilirubinemia [6].

The scientific data about ELS regarding the pediatric population is scarce. The largest study on the pediatric population thus far is coming from a hospital with ten years of experience with the MARS method. In the study performed by Lexmond et al., MARS was employed as ELS in 20 pediatric patients suffering from ALF listed for high urgency liver transplantation. The decision to put the children on MARS was made by a multidisciplinary team consisting of pediatricians, hepatologists, nephrologists, neurologists, and transplant surgeons. MARS was applied for eight consecutive hours daily, every day, up until transplantation. All patients were mechanically ventilated and on vasopressors [10], as was the case in our patient. This method decreased serum ammonia and bilirubin [10]. The only encountered adverse effect from the therapy in this study was thrombocytopenia with bleeding requiring blood and platelet mass transfusions in five children, with one case of mortality [10].

The first particularity of this case was the extreme condition of the infant suffering from sepsis with MSOF, with intravascular hemolysis and thrombocytopenia reaching a value of 15.000/mm^3. Next, the etiology of the severe coagulopathy was questionable; it could have been attributable solely to ALF, but also to sepsis, or a combination of both. Also, the jaundice could have been a result of ALF, but also of TPN. Parenteral nutrition-associated cholestasis (PNAC) is one of the most common complications of TPN in neonates and infants. In a study performed by Hsieh et al. in 2009 on 62 infants on TPN, 11 developed PNAC [15]. Furthermore, another particularity that arose was the degree of association between congenital heart disease and ALF. A link between vascular malformations and congenital heart disease with ALF has been described in literature [4, 5]. Another particularity of the case was the advanced degree of hemodynamic instability with hypotension present despite a triple regimen of vasopressors (Adrenaline, Noradrenaline, and Dopamine).

Progressive liver failure can result in death within a few days if no liver is transplanted [16]. We performed hemadsorption on a nine-month-old male infant as a worldwide novel procedure and obtained favorable results. Despite the extreme general status of our intubated patient requiring triple vasopressor therapy, at total bilirubinemia of 54 mg/dL, 24 hours of hemadsorption deemed to be successful. However, since literature regarding hemadsorption in the pediatric population is scarce, large scale prospective studies are needed to determine the exact benefit and possible adverse effects as well as assess survival rates after such a procedure.

Competing Interests

The authors declare no conflict of interests.

References

[1] J. M. Millis and J. E. Losanoff, "Technology insight: liver support systems," *Nature Clinical Practice Gastroenterology and Hepatology*, vol. 2, no. 9, pp. 398–405, 2005.

[2] B. R. Bhaduri and G. Mieli-Vergani, "Fulminant hepatic failure: pediatric aspects," *Seminars in Liver Disease*, vol. 16, no. 4, pp. 349–355, 1996.

[3] A. Dhawan and G. Mieli-Vergani, "Acute liver failure in neonates," *Early Human Development*, vol. 81, no. 12, pp. 1005–1010, 2005.

[4] A. W. Marian, A. Dhawan, A. Baker, and G. Mieli-Vergani, "Neonatal paracetamol overdose—management with N-acetyl cystine," *Archives of Disease in Childhood*, vol. 81, p. F78, 1999.

[5] M. Cheung, S. Bansal, M. M. Aw, C. R. Buchanan, G. Mieli-Vergani, and A. Dhawan, "Liver failure in a neonate with congenital adrenal hyporesponsiveness," *European Journal of Pediatrics*, vol. 162, no. 7-8, p. 558, 2003.

[6] S. R. Mitzner, "Extracorporeal liver support-albumin dialysis with the molecular adsorbent recirculating system (MARS)," *Annals of Hepatology*, vol. 10, no. 1, pp. S21–S28, 2011.

[7] T. J. McKenzie, J. B. Lillegard, and S. L. Nyberg, "Artificial and bioartificial liver support," *Seminars in Liver Disease*, vol. 28, no. 2, pp. 210–217, 2008.

[8] B. Schaefer and C. P. Schmitt, "The role of molecular adsorbent recirculating system dialysis for extracorporeal liver support in children," *Pediatric Nephrology*, vol. 28, no. 9, pp. 1763–1769, 2013.

[9] V. Jain and A. Dhawan, "Quest for life on MARS: mission incomplete," *Journal of Pediatric Gastroenterology and Nutrition*, vol. 58, no. 2, pp. 140–141, 2014.

[10] W. S. Lexmond, C. M. L. Van Dael, R. Scheenstra et al., "Experience with molecular adsorbent recirculating system treatment in 20 children listed for high-urgency liver transplantation," *Liver Transplantation*, vol. 21, no. 3, pp. 369–380, 2015.

[11] B. Hinz, O. Jauch, T. Noky, S. Friesecke, P. Abel, and R. Kaiser, "CytoSorb, a novel therapeutic approach for patients with septic shock: a case report," *International Journal of Artificial Organs*, vol. 38, no. 8, pp. 461–464, 2015.

[12] M. Wiegele and C. G. Krenn, "Cytosorb™ in a patient with *Legionella* pneumonia-associated rhabdomyolysis: a case report," *ASAIO Journal*, vol. 61, no. 3, pp. e14–e16, 2015.

[13] W. M. Lee, "Etiologies of acute liver failure," *Seminars in Liver Disease*, vol. 28, no. 2, pp. 142–152, 2008.

[14] P. Tissières, J. S. Sasbón, and D. Devictor, "Liver support for fulminant hepatic failure: is it time to use the molecular adsorbents recycling system in children?" *Pediatric Critical Care Medicine*, vol. 6, no. 5, pp. 585–591, 2005.

[15] M.-H. Hsieh, W. Pai, H.-I. Tseng, S.-N. Yang, C.-C. Lu, and H.-L. Chen, "Parenteral nutrition-associated cholestasis in premature babies: risk factors and predictors," *Pediatrics and Neonatology*, vol. 50, no. 5, pp. 202–207, 2009.

[16] W. Bernal, G. Auzinger, A. Dhawan, and J. Wendon, "Acute liver failure," *The Lancet*, vol. 376, no. 9736, pp. 190–201, 2010.

Endobronchial One-Way Valve Therapy Facilitates Weaning from Extracorporeal Membrane Oxygenation in a Patient with ARDS and Persistent Air Leak

Alessandro Ghiani,[1] **Matthias Hansen**,[2] **Konstantinos Tsitouras**,[1] **and Claus Neurohr**[1]

[1]*Schillerhoehe Lung Clinic (Robert-Bosch Hospital), Department of Pneumology and Critical Care Medicine, Solitudestr. 18, 70839 Gerlingen, Germany*
[2]*Schillerhoehe Lung Clinic (Robert-Bosch Hospital), Department of Anesthesiology and Critical Care Medicine, Solitudestr. 18, 70839 Gerlingen, Germany*

Correspondence should be addressed to Alessandro Ghiani; alessandro.ghiani@klinik-schillerhoehe.de

Academic Editor: Chiara Lazzeri

Prolonged pulmonary air leak (PAL) is a common clinical problem, associated with significant morbidity and mortality. There are numerous reports of treatment of PAL using endobronchial valves (EBV) in respiratory stable patients, but only few reports on critically ill patients, and there is virtually no practical knowledge in the treatment of PAL in mechanically ventilated patients with acute respiratory distress syndrome (ARDS), treated with veno-venous extracorporeal membrane oxygenation (vvECMO). We describe a case where EBV placement was performed in a patient with ARDS and PAL, treated with mechanical ventilation and vvECMO. Despite a lung protective ventilation strategy, a persistent air leak along with a large left-sided pneumothorax was observed. After bronchoscopic localisation of the fistula, two endobronchial valves were inserted into the left upper lobe, leading to an immediate decrease in the air flow and reexpansion of the left lung. During the following two weeks, the patient was weaned from vvECMO, and after another three weeks, complete liberation from mechanical ventilation was accomplished. EBV placement seems to be a safe method even in the presence of coagulopathy and may facilitate mechanical ventilation and weaning from vvECMO in patients with ARDS and PAL.

1. Introduction

Prolonged pulmonary air leaks (PAL) are common and may cause considerable morbidity, prolonged hospital stay, and increased health-care costs [1]. They occur in about 15% of patients after thoracic surgery [2] or develop spontaneously due to an underlying pulmonary disease such as bullous emphysema, advanced interstitial lung disease, lung cancer, or cavernous tuberculosis. Poor performance status caused by pulmonary disease may limit surgical interventions. Therefore, less invasive therapeutic options have been developed in the past 20 years, such as fibrin sealants [3], metal coils [4], chemical pleurodesis [5], and endobronchial valves (EBV) [6].

There is little practical knowledge in the treatment of PAL in mechanically ventilated patients with acute respiratory distress syndrome (ARDS) [7] and even less experience in patients with ARDS and PAL, treated with veno-venous extracorporeal membrane oxygenation (vvECMO) [8].

We describe a case where bedside EBV placement was performed in a patient with ARDS and PAL, while being on invasive mechanical ventilation and vvECMO.

2. Case Report

A 60-year-old healthy male patient (no comorbidities, never-smoker) with ARDS due to influenza A pneumonia was admitted to our specialised lung clinic for further treatment. Endotracheal intubation due to severe hypoxemic respiratory failure was already performed prior to admission (day 0). Transference of the patient to the hospital occurred on day 6. The first chest X-ray after admission revealed an apical

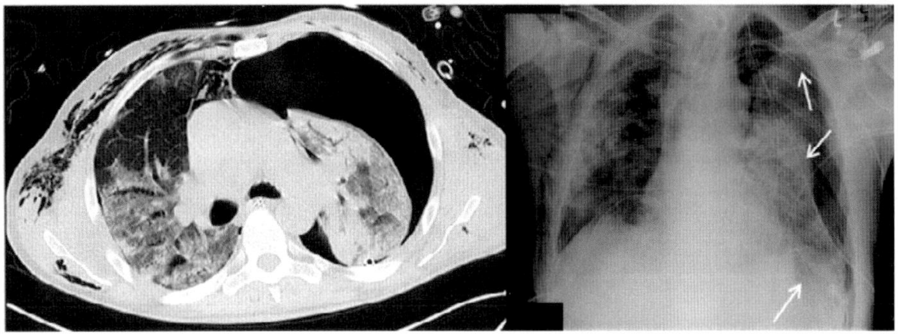

Figure 1: CT-scan (left image) and chest X-ray (right image) on day 16 before endobronchial valve placement: large pneumothorax despite three chest drainages on the left (white arrows).

left-sided pneumothorax of approximately 2 cm, accompanied by a large subcutaneous emphysema. Two chest tubes were inserted, one on each side. After that, the left lung was again fully expanded, the subcutaneous emphysema resolved, and no air leak could be observed. On day 14, the patient developed once again spontaneously a massive and progressive subcutaneous emphysema, accompanied by a large air leak of about 5000 ml per minute on the left side. A second and a third chest tube were inserted on the left, one in Monaldi's position (3rd intercostal space midclavicular) and the other in Bülau's position (5th intercostal space slightly anterior the mid-axillary line). However, the chest X-ray and chest CT-scan on day 16 showed a complete, left-sided pneumothorax (Figure 1). Central venous catheter placement on the left (internal jugular vein) was performed six days before the onset of the air leak. We interpreted the occurrence of the air leak, the pneumothorax, and the subcutaneous emphysema as a result of barotrauma due to invasive mechanical ventilation. Because of progressive hypercapnia and severe respiratory acidosis, a tracheostomy was performed and a vvECMO (PLS Set and ROTAFLOW Console) was established (day 16), using an Avalon Elite™ Bi-Caval Dual Lumen Catheter (Maquet Cardiopulmonary GmbH, Germany). Blood gas analysis immediately before the start of the extracorporeal lung assistance revealed a P_aCO_2 of 88 mmHg with a pH of 7.30, and P_aO_2 was 90 mmHg. At this point, the patient was ventilated in the assist-controlled mode (BIPAP-ASB, Evita 4, Dräger®). F_iO_2 was 0.85, and P_{insp} was set at 28 mBar with a PEEP of 7 mBar. This resulted in a tidal volume of approximately 400 ml and a minute ventilation of 8.4 l/min. After the cannulation of the patient and the commencement of vvECMO support, a lung protective ventilation strategy with low tidal volumes (P_{insp} 20 mBar, PEEP 10 mBar, F_iO_2 0.6, V_T 250 ml) was established. This resulted in acceptable blood gas values (P_aCO_2 49 mmHg, P_aO_2 74 mmHg, pH 7.52) on vvECMO (blood flow 2.5 l/min, $F_iO_{2\text{-vvECMO}}$ 1.0, sweep gas flow 4.0 l/min); however, the air leak persisted (day 17), and in the chest X-rays the left lung remained collapsed. In the further course of treatment, the blood gas analyses revealed persistent hypercapnia with a P_aCO_2 of approximately 60–65 mmHg, and even though the sweep gas flow was increased, a state of normocapnia could not be achieved. Therefore, an interventional closure of the fistula with endobronchial valves was planned.

On the day of the procedure (day 21), F_iO_2 on the ventilator was 0.6, and P_{insp} was set at 17 mBar and PEEP at 5 mBar, resulting in tidal volumes of about 450 ml and minute ventilation of approximately 9.2 l/min. vvECMO blood flow was 2.6 l/min with a sweep gas flow of 5.5 l/min. Valve placement was done bedside on the intensive care unit. The patient was under deep sedation/analgesia with midazolam and sufentanil, respectively. Cis-Atracurium (10 mg) for muscle relaxation was administered immediately before the procedure. Bronchoscopy was performed through the tracheal cannula. The exact bronchoscopic localisation of the fistula was assessed by occlusion of the upper and lower lobe bronchus on the left, using a bronchus blocker while measuring the fistula flow with the Thopaz Digital Chest Drainage System (Medela AG, Switzerland). First of all, as we blocked the left upper lobe bronchus (corresponding to the segment bronchi LB1–5), the air leak was stopped entirely. Then we occluded each segment of the left upper lobe separately, but we did not achieve any significant result. The occlusion of the lingula bronchus (LB4/5) had no significant effect on the air leak as well. Thus, decision was made to close LB1/2 and LB3 with two Zephyr® endobronchial valves (2 × 4.0-LP, Pulmonx®, Redwood City, USA). This initially led to an immediate decrease of the air leak to about 400–700 ml/min, and the left lung was then again fully expanded (Figure 2). After valve placement, P_aCO_2 decreased slowly during the following six days, while there were no major adjustments of the ventilator settings or the vvECMO parameters. Normocapnia was detected for the first time on day 27, so that blood flow and sweep gas flow on vvECMO could be slowly reduced. During the following two weeks, the air leak stopped completely and the patient could be weaned from vvECMO on day 48. The patient was transferred from the intensive care unit to the weaning unit on day 61. Removal of the endobronchial valves occurred on day 62, after which the chest X-rays showed a persistently expanded left lung (Figure 3). As there was no evidence of an air leak once again, the chest tubes were removed one after another, liberation from the ventilator on day 72 and discharge to neurological rehabilitation on day 89.

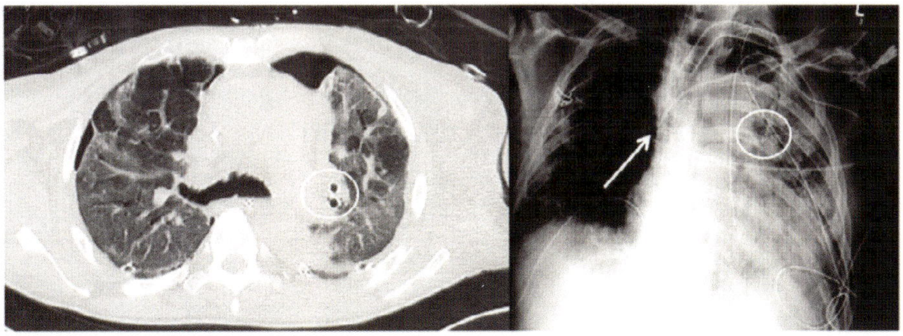

Figure 2: CT-scan (left image) and chest X-ray (right image) after endobronchial valve placement. The left lung is again fully expanded. The circled areas depict the two endobronchial valves within the left upper lobe segmental bronchi (LB1/2 and LB3). The Avalon Elite™ Bi-Caval Dual Lumen Catheter is visible on the chest X-ray (white arrow).

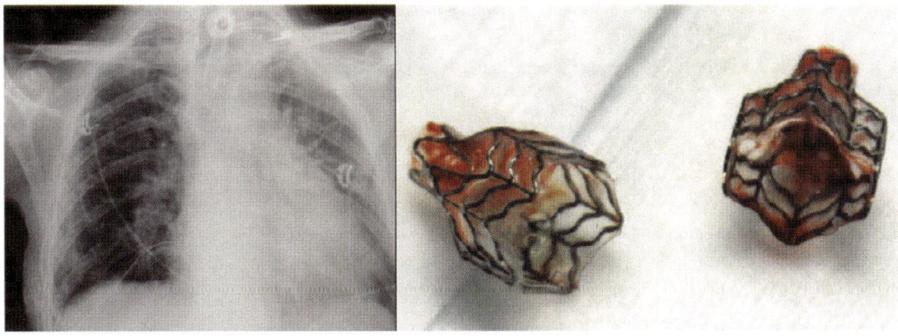

Figure 3: Chest X-ray (left image) after removal of the endobronchial valves (right image).

3. Discussion

Persistent pulmonary air leak is a common clinical problem, associated with significant morbidity and mortality [9]. Large air leaks themselves can lead to respiratory failure, which may necessitate mechanical ventilation or even extracorporeal lung assistance. To date, only a few reports exist on mechanically ventilated, critically ill patients with PAL [10], and there is little practical knowledge in the treatment of PAL in patients with ARDS. Recently, a case series described endobronchial one-way valve placement as a feasible procedure in those patients [7].

In mechanical ventilation due to ARDS, high inspiratory and expiratory airway pressures may delay or even prevent the spontaneous closure of the fistula, because the persistent air flow through this low-resistance pathway averts healing of the affected lung. This effect is even enhanced by spontaneous breathing efforts during controlled mechanical ventilation, referred to as patient-ventilator asynchrony, which may generate highly negative pleural pressure swings and therefore increase the pressure gradient between the airway and the pleural cavity. This is why patients with ARDS have a low likelihood of unprompted resolution of large fistulas, as long as they are mechanically ventilated. We interpreted the observed residual air leak of 400–700 ml/min after placement of the two valves as "intralobar" collateral ventilation between the closed segments 1–3 (localisation of the fistula) and the ventilated segments 4/5 of the left upper lobe. In order to maintain gas exchange through the lingula segments, we decided to leave the lingula bronchus open, because in our experience such a low flow usually stops spontaneously during the following days.

To our knowledge, this is the second report on a patient with EBV treatment while being on vvECMO [8]. Under these circumstances, the risk of bleeding due to heparin anticoagulation is difficult to predict but must be weighed against the expected therapeutic effect. Nevertheless, the longer the air leak persists, the greater the likelihood of complications in the course of treatment will be, such as severe bleeding. Early bronchoscopic intervention in patients with PAL may shorten the duration of extracorporeal lung assistance and mechanical ventilation and, in our opinion, can help to avoid complications due to vvECMO.

4. Conclusion

Endobronchial valve placement seems to be a feasible procedure even in the presence of coagulopathy and may facilitate mechanical ventilation and weaning from vvECMO in patients with ARDS and PAL.

Roche. The remaining authors have no conflicts of interest to disclose.

Authors' Contributions

Alessandro Ghiani serves as the guarantor of the paper and takes responsibility for the integrity and accuracy of the data. All authors had full access to all of the data and contributed to the revision of the manuscript.

References

[1] M. Lois and M. Noppen, "Bronchopleural fistulas: an overview of the problem with special focus on endoscopic management," *Chest*, vol. 128, no. 6, pp. 3955–3965, 2005.

[2] A. Abolhoda, D. Liu, A. Brooks, and M. Burt, "Prolonged air leak following radical upper lobectomy: An analysis of incidence and possible risk factors," *Chest*, vol. 113, no. 6, pp. 1507–1510, 1998.

[3] C. Lopez, F. Facciolo, C. Lequaglie et al., "Efficacy and safety of fibrin sealant patch in the treatment of air leakage in thoracic surgery," *Minerva Chirurgica*, vol. 68, no. 6, pp. 559–567, 2013.

[4] S.-I. Watanabe, T. Watanabe, and H. Urayama, "Endobronchial occlusion method of bronchopleural fistula with metallic coils and glue," *The Thoracic and Cardiovascular Surgeon*, vol. 51, no. 2, pp. 106–108, 2003.

[5] M. Liberman, A. Muzikansky, C. D. Wright et al., "Incidence and Risk Factors of Persistent Air Leak After Major Pulmonary Resection and Use of Chemical Pleurodesis," *The Annals of Thoracic Surgery*, vol. 89, no. 3, pp. 891–898, 2010.

[6] J. M. Travaline, R. J. McKenna Jr., T. De Giacomo et al., "Treatment of persistent pulmonary air leaks using endobronchial valves," *CHEST*, vol. 136, no. 2, pp. 355–360, 2009.

[7] Haris Kalatoudis, Meena Nikhil, Fuad Zeid, and Yousef Shweihat, "Bronchopleural Fistula Resolution with Endobronchial Valve Placement and Liberation from Mechanical Ventilation in Acute Respiratory Distress Syndrome: A Case Series," *Case Reports in Critical Care*, vol. 2017, Article ID 3092457, 4 pages, 2017.

[8] A. M. Hodges, M. J. Gillham, and C. A. Lewis, "Bedside placement of an endobronchial valve to aid invasive ventilation and weaning from extracorporeal membrane oxygenation," *Critical Care and Resuscitation*, vol. 17, no. 3, pp. 219–222, 2015.

[9] M. Ding, Y. Gao, X. Zeng, Y. Guo, and J. Yang, "Endobronchial one-way valves for treatment of persistent air leaks: a systematic review," *Respiratory Research*, vol. 18, no. 1, 2017.

[10] A. K. Mahajan, P. Verhoef, S. B. Patel, G. Carr, and D. K. Hogarth, "Intrabronchial valves: a case series describing a minimally invasive approach to bronchopleural fistulas in medical intensive care unit patients," *Journal of Bronchology & Interventional Pulmonology*, vol. 19, no. 2, pp. 137–141, 2012.

45

Intravenous Vitamin C Administered as Adjunctive Therapy for Recurrent Acute Respiratory Distress Syndrome

Amit Bharara, Catherine Grossman, Daniel Grinnan, Aamer Syed, Bernard Fisher, Christine DeWilde, Ramesh Natarajan, and Alpha A. (Berry) Fowler

Division of Pulmonary Disease and Critical Care Medicine, Department of Internal Medicine, The VCU Johnson Center for Critical Care and Pulmonary Research, Virginia Commonwealth University School of Medicine, Richmond, VA, USA

Correspondence should be addressed to Alpha A. (Berry) Fowler; alpha.fowler@vcuhealth.org

Academic Editor: Kenneth S. Waxman

This case report summarizes the first use of intravenous vitamin C employed as an adjunctive interventional agent in the therapy of *recurrent* acute respiratory distress syndrome (ARDS). The two episodes of ARDS occurred in a young female patient with Cronkhite-Canada syndrome, a rare, sporadically occurring, noninherited disorder that is characterized by extensive gastrointestinal polyposis and malabsorption. Prior to the episodes of sepsis, the patient was receiving nutrition via chronic hyperalimentation administered through a long-standing central venous catheter. The patient became recurrently septic with Gram positive cocci which led to two instances of ARDS. This report describes the broad-based general critical care of a septic patient with acute respiratory failure that includes fluid resuscitation, broad-spectrum antibiotics, and vasopressor support. Intravenous vitamin C infused at 50 mg per kilogram body weight every 6 hours for 96 hours was incorporated as an adjunctive agent in the care of this patient. Vitamin C when used as a parenteral agent in high doses acts "pleiotropically" to attenuate proinflammatory mediator expression, to improve alveolar fluid clearance, and to act as an antioxidant.

1. Introduction

For many years, intensivists have searched for some agent which will attenuate the lung injury induced by the onset of pathological processes which lead to acute respiratory distress syndrome (ARDS). Thus far, following decades of research, utilizing both preclinical research employing animal model systems and clinical trials in human subjects with ARDS, no agent has been identified which attenuates ARDS-induced lung injury. Currently, ARDS continues to be associated with an approximately 25% mortality. Patients who survive ARDS often suffer long-term morbid complications from critical care support as well as posttraumatic stress disorder derived from protracted hospitalization and critical care support. In this case report, we describe the first use of intravenous vitamin C as an agent to attenuate sepsis-induced ARDS.

2. Case Presentation

31-year-old Sudanese female with a medical history of Cronkhite-Canada syndrome, a malabsorptive gastrointestinal genetic disease, who was receiving chronic hyperalimentation through a long-lasting Hickman central venous catheter, presented to the emergency department with fever (101.7 F), myalgia, and tachycardia. The patient was normotensive. Blood cultures were obtained and admission was recommended, but the patient declined admission. PA and lateral chest X-ray film was clear. No antibiotics were administered at this time (Figure 1). Forty-eight hours later, she returned to the emergency department with worsened fever and myalgia. Blood cultures returned positive for Gram positive cocci. The patient was admitted to acute care medicine but soon became hypotensive and tachycardic. She was transferred to the medical intensive care unit after

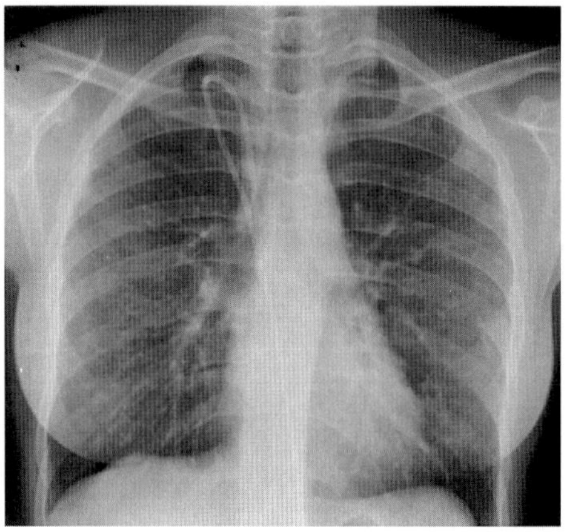

Figure 1

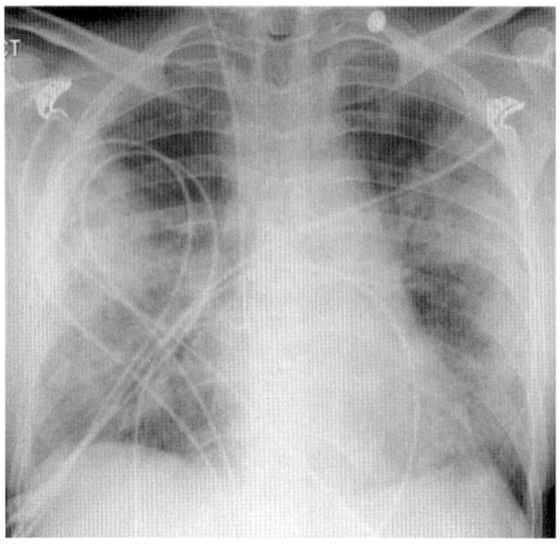

Figure 2

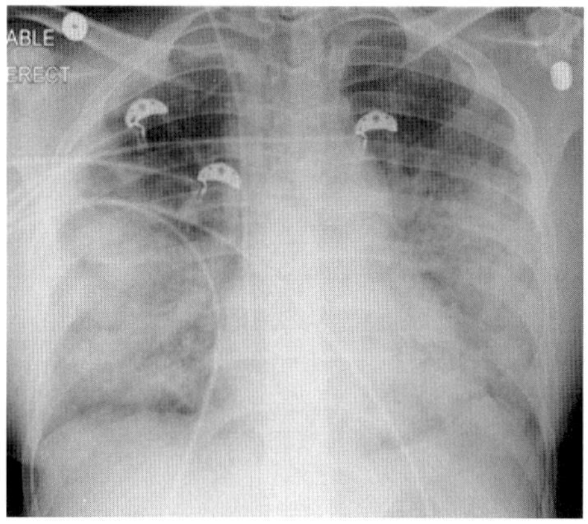

Figure 3

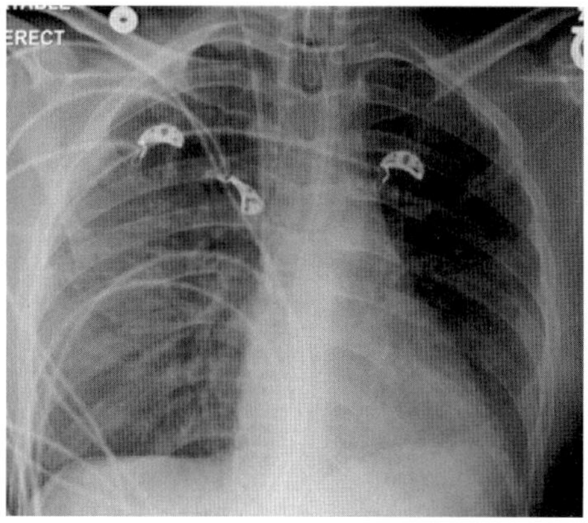

Figure 4

receiving four liters of intravenous volume resuscitation with 0.9% saline. Norepinephrine infusion was required and vancomycin and piperacillin/tazobactam was initiated. The patient's central venous catheter, suspected to be the source of the bacteremia, was promptly removed and a new central venous catheter placed. On hospital day 2, the patient experienced worsened dyspnea and hypoxemia that necessitated noninvasive positive pressure ventilation (NIPPV). Repeat chest imaging revealed more remarkable opacities (Figure 2). On hospital day 3, hypoxemia and radiographic abnormalities became more significant (Figure 3). The patient was intubated and invasive mechanical ventilation begun for apparent sepsis-associated acute respiratory distress syndrome (ARDS). Bronchoscopy performed at this time yielded no pathogens. Low tidal volume ventilation (6 cc/kg of ideal body weight, followed by a reduction to 4 cc/kg of ideal body weight) with high positive end expiratory pressure was initiated employing assist/control pressure/control ventilation. Despite this approach, the patient remained profoundly hypoxemic (PaO_2/FiO_2 ratio, 63 mm Hg). Intravenous vitamin C (50 mg/kg every 6 hours) was initiated on hospital day 4. Chest imaging via AP chest X-ray film on hospital day 5 revealed significantly improved bilateral opacities (Figure 4). PaO_2/FiO_2 ratio improved significantly to 190 mm Hg. On hospital day 7, the patient was successfully extubated.

Six weeks following initial hospitalization, the patient re-presented to the emergency department once again with headaches, fevers, and myalgia. The patient was hypotensive on admission (62/37 mm Hg). Fluid resuscitation was undertaken. Hypotension persisted and she was admitted to medical ICU where she was ultimately intubated for respiratory failure. Figure 5 shows the patient's initial chest X-ray. Despite invasive mechanical ventilation, oxygenation deteriorated and the criteria for ARDS were again met. Neuromuscular paralysis (cisatracurium) was required on ventilator day 3 due to elevated peak airway pressures and ventilator dyssynchrony. Despite this, oxygenation remained severely depressed (PaO_2/FiO_2 = 100). On ventilator day 4, intravenous vitamin C (50 mg/kg every 6 hours) was initiated (Figure 6). Within two days (ventilator day 6), chest imaging dramatically improved (Figure 7) as did oxygenation (PaO_2/FiO_2 ratio = 316 mm Hg). On ventilator day 10, the patient was weaned and was successfully extubated.

3. Discussion

We report here the application of high dose intravenous vitamin C employed as an interventional drug treatment

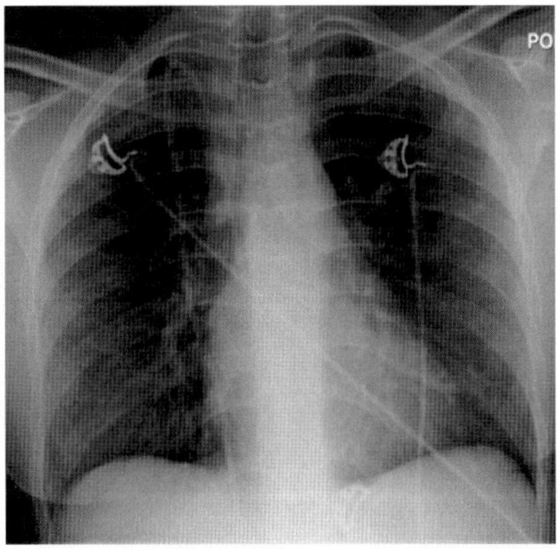

Figure 5

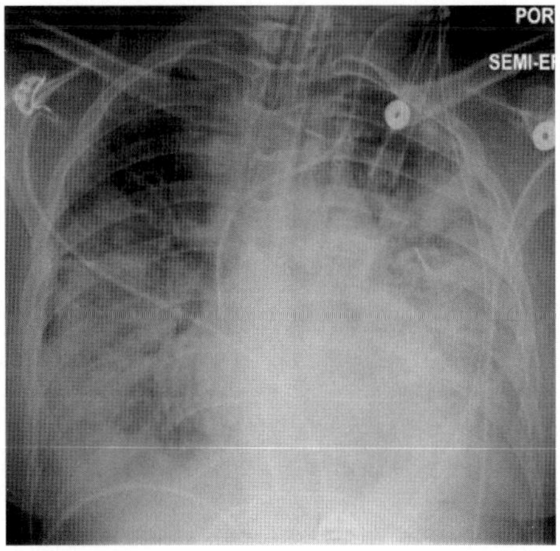

Figure 6

for ARDS. Very few studies in critically ill patients with ARDS have reported the use of intravenous vitamin C. The use of vitamin C to treat lung injury is still investigational. Nathens et al. infused ascorbic acid at 1 gram every 8 hours combined with oral vitamin E for 28 days in 594 surgically critically ill patients and found a significantly lower incidence of acute lung injury and multiple organ failure [1]. Tanaka et al. infused ascorbic acid continuously at 66 mg/kg/hour for the first 24 hours in patients with greater than 50% surface area burns and showed significantly reduced burn capillary permeability [2]. A single report (published as abstract only) of a clinical study of large intravenous doses of ascorbic acid, and other antioxidants (tocopherol, N-acetyl-cysteine, and selenium), in patients with established ARDS showed reduction in mortality of 50% [3]. Clinical protocols currently in use for hospitalized septic patients fail to normalize ascorbic acid levels. Vitamin C dosages utilized in the treatment of the patient we describe in this case report arose from our previous human studies, infusing high dose intravenous vitamin C into critically ill patients with severe sepsis [4], and in our preclinical studies [5–7]. Our work thus far shows vitamin C to exert potent "pleotropic effects" when used as described in this report. We showed that septic patients receiving high

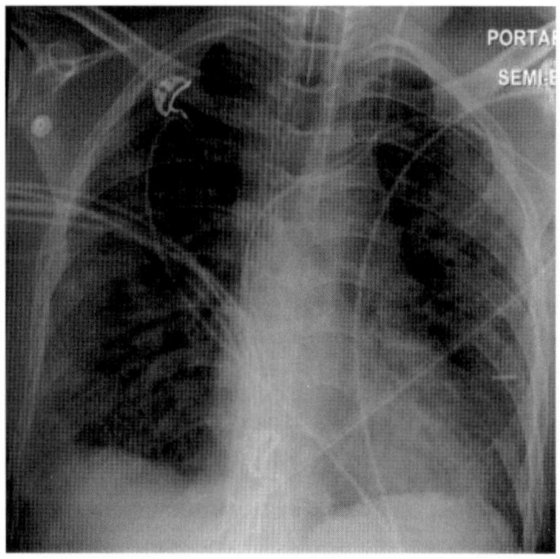

Figure 7

dose intravenous vitamin C exhibit significant reduction in multiple organ injury and reduced inflammatory biomarker levels [4]. Our preclinical work in septic lung-injured animals shows that vitamin C downregulates proinflammatory genes that are driven by transcription factor NF-κB. Furthermore, vitamin C significantly increases alveolar fluid clearance in septic lung-injured animals [7]. Finally, infused vitamin C's capability to downregulate liberated reactive oxygen and nitrogen species appears to be critical for attenuating lung injury [8].

Competing Interests

The authors declare that there is no conflict of interests regarding the publication of this paper.

Acknowledgments

This case report was presented at the annual international meeting of The American Thoracic Society in May of 2016. The preclinical work that led up to the use of vitamin C as an interventional agent in humans was supported by the Aubrey Sage McFarlane acute lung injury fund, the VCU Johnson Center for Critical Care and Pulmonary Research, and NIH/UM1 HL116885-02, Vitamin C Infusion for Treatment in Sepsis Induced Acute Lung Injury (CITRIS-ALI).

References

[1] A. B. Nathens, M. J. Neff, G. J. Jurkovich et al., "Randomized, prospective trial of antioxidant supplementation in critically III surgical patients," *Annals of Surgery*, vol. 236, no. 6, pp. 814–822, 2002.

[2] H. Tanaka, T. Matsuda, Y. Miyagantani, T. Yukioka, H. Matsuda, and S. Shimazaki, "Reduction of resuscitation fluid volumes in severely burned patients using ascorbic acid administration: a randomized, prospective study," *Archives of Surgery*, vol. 135, no. 3, pp. 326–331, 2000.

[3] M. A. J. Sawyer, J. J. Mike, and K. Chavin, "Antioxidant therapy and survival in ARDS," *Critical Care Medicine*, vol. 17, article S153, 1989.

[4] A. A. Fowler III, A. A. Syed, S. Knowlson et al., "Phase I safety trial of intravenous ascorbic acid in patients with severe sepsis," *Journal of Translational Medicine*, vol. 12, article 32, 2014.

[5] B. J. Fisher, I. M. Seropian, D. Kraskauskas et al., "Ascorbic acid attenuates lipopolysaccharide-induced acute lung injury," *Critical Care Medicine*, vol. 39, no. 6, pp. 1454–1460, 2011.

[6] B. J. Fisher, D. Kraskauskas, E. J. Martin et al., "Attenuation of sepsis-induced organ injury in mice by vitamin C," *Journal of Parenteral and Enteral Nutrition*, vol. 38, no. 7, pp. 825–839, 2014.

[7] B. J. Fisher, D. Kraskauskas, E. J. Martin et al., "Mechanisms of attenuation of abdominal sepsis induced acute lung injury by ascorbic acid," *American Journal of Physiology—Lung Cellular and Molecular Physiology*, vol. 303, no. 1, pp. L20–L32, 2012.

[8] M. M. Berger and H. M. Oudemans-van Straaten, "Vitamin C supplementation in the critically ill patient," *Current Opinion in Clinical Nutrition and Metabolic Care*, vol. 18, no. 2, pp. 193–201, 2015.

Cyclic Nonrespiratory Pulse Pressure Oscillations Caused by Atrioventricular Dissociation

László Rudas, Péter Hankovszky, András Lovas, Éva Zöllei, and Zsolt Molnár

Department of Anesthesiology and Intensive Care, Faculty of Medicine, University of Szeged, Szeged, Hungary

Correspondence should be addressed to László Rudas; rudasl@hotmail.com

Academic Editor: Kenneth S. Waxman

Dynamic preload assessment tests, especially pulse pressure variation (PPV) and stroke volume variation (SVV), are increasingly acknowledged in mechanically ventilated patients as being predictors of fluid responsiveness. However, the limitations of this method are often neglected or overlooked. One of the prerequisites for PPV and SVV evaluation, in addition to intermittent positive pressure ventilation, is a "regular heart rhythm," which may be an ambiguous term. We present a case where, despite a regular (paced) rhythm, atrioventricular dissociation was present and resulted in marked PPV elevation, which subsequently disappeared once sinus rhythm returned. Our case indicates that PPV and SVV should be interpreted with caution when atrioventricular dissociation is present.

1. Introduction

Traditional, "static" hemodynamic parameters, such as central venous and pulmonary artery occlusion pressures, have limited capacity for predicting cardiac output changes in response to volume administration. In contrast, the so-called dynamic parameters describe the dynamic interactions of hemodynamic variables in response to a defined perturbation, and the net response indicates the probable circulatory response to fluid therapy [1]. Based on the magnitude of the positive pressure ventilation-induced pulse pressure variation (PPV) or stroke volume variation (SVV), "volume responsiveness" can be defined, which predicts a substantial elevation in cardiac output in response to a fluid bolus [2]. One of the prerequisites of PPV/SVV evaluation is a "regular heart rhythm." However, this definition does not describe a universally accepted term. We hereby present a case where atrioventricular block necessitated ventricular pacing, and, in spite of the seemingly regular rhythm, the atrioventricular dissociation resulted in "nonrespiratory" PPV augmentation.

2. Case Report

A 70-year-old male with a long history of coronary artery disease was brought to our cardiac catheterization laboratory during the night where an acute inferior myocardial infarction was diagnosed. A critical stenosis on the proximal segment of the right coronary artery was successfully stented. However, third-degree atrioventricular (AV) block developed during the procedure necessitating in brief cardiopulmonary resuscitation and the insertion of a temporary ventricular pacemaker (VVI pacing mode, set frequency 80/min). He had to be anaesthetized, intubated, and mechanically ventilated during the catheter intervention, after which he was transferred to our intensive care unit (ICU).

On admission, he was hemodynamically unstable with marked arterial pressure fluctuation noted on the first ECG and arterial pressure curve recordings (Figure 1). Initially, his hypotension was treated with norepinephrine 0.5 μg/kg/min, which had to be increased up to 1.2 μg/kg/min to maintain an acceptable mean arterial pressure. Arterial blood gases showed severe metabolic acidosis with pH of 7.26, lactate of 4.5 mmol/l, HCO_3 of 13.4 mmol/l, and a base deficit of 13.6 mmol/l. Therefore, invasive hemodynamic monitoring was commenced with transpulmonary thermodilution and pulse contour analysis (PiCCO, PULSION, Germany). The first measurements revealed a low cardiac index (CI) of 2.2 l/min/m^2. Based on the corresponding hemodynamic indices (SVI: 26 ml/m^2, dP/dt_{max}: 1545, and

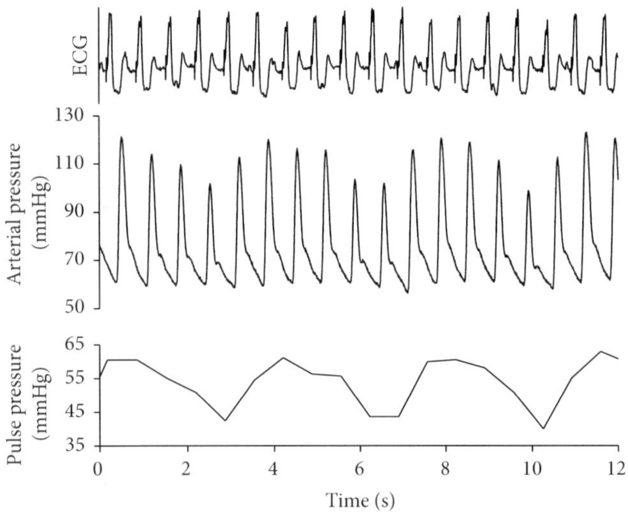

FIGURE 1: ECG, arterial pressure, and pulse pressure during pacemaker rhythm. The recording was taken shortly after the patient's arrival to the ICU. Pacemaker spikes can be seen before every heartbeat, and the arterial pressure and pulse pressure indicate substantial fluctuations. The recordings were analyzed offline, and a pulse pressure diagram was also added.

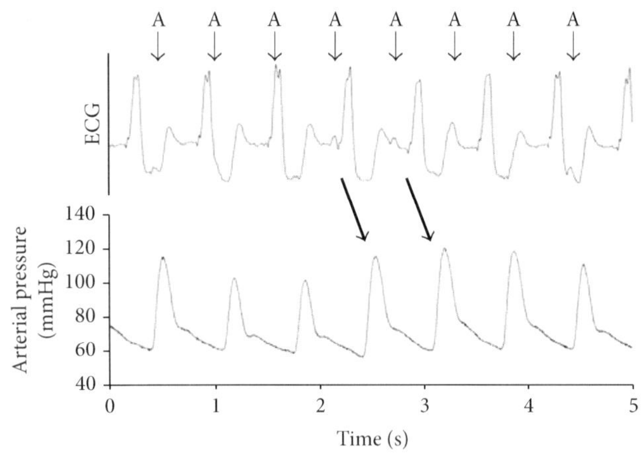

FIGURE 2: Relationship of sinus and paced cardiac activity and its effect on arterial pressure. The ECG strip shows a paced ventricular "regular" rhythm, where atrioventricular dissociation is still present. The small arrows indicate atrial activity ("A"). The coincidence of normal AV sequence results in substantial arterial pressure augmentation (indicated by the thick arrows). For more details, read the text.

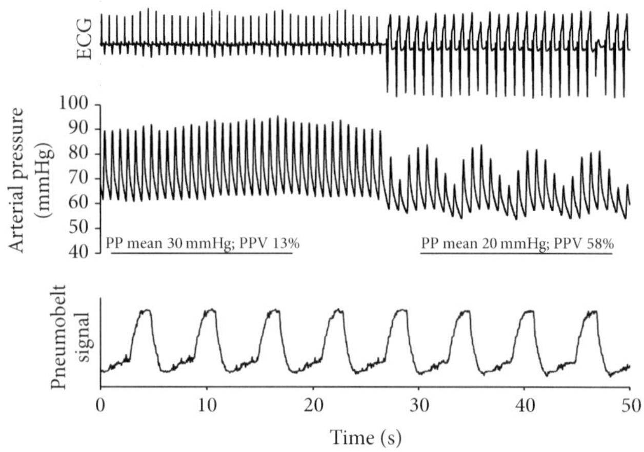

FIGURE 3: Change of pulse pressure variation (PPV) during sinus and pacemaker rhythm. ECG, arterial pressure, and noncalibrated pneumobelt signals were recorded during the dynamic preload test. While the initial segment of the arterial pressure panel during sinus rhythm indicates minimal changes in pulse pressure (PP) resulting in borderline PPV, the switch to ventricular pacemaker rhythm is accompanied by enormous pressure fluctuations and a severalfold increase in PPV. The straight lines indicate the 3 breathing cycles detected by the pneumobelt during the first and second part of recording. Based on the pneumobelt signal, the arterial pressure swings occurring during the pacemaker rhythm seem to be unrelated to the ventilation.

SVRI: 2230 dyn∗s∗cm^{-5}), dobutamine dose, 3.0 μg/kg/min, was added to the therapy. His spontaneous and paced rhythm alternated.

A more detailed evaluation of the ECG and blood pressure recordings revealed an obvious interference between the paced ventricular and spontaneous atrial (sinus) activities (Figure 2). When this interference resulted in a normal AV sequence, there was a substantial increase in the area under the arterial pressure curve, indicating an augmented stroke volume.

By the second day, his heart rate seemed regular, and intermittent restoration of the normal AV conduction was noted in addition to the paced rhythm. At this time, the patient was mechanically ventilated in pressure control mode with 10/min breathing frequency with no spontaneous breathing efforts as he was kept under deep sedation. Therefore, this scenario (regular rhythm, controlled mechanical ventilation) seemed ideal to assess fluid responsiveness using PPV. Furthermore, the alternative sinus and VVI-paced periods allowed comparison of the hemodynamic responses during these two different rhythms (Figure 3). For the brief period of the test, the tidal volume was increased to 9 ml/kg. In order to be able to record changes in cardiac and respiratory mechanics on the same recording, we applied a device called the pneumobelt, a silicone tube hooked around the abdomen, which measures pressure changes in response to mechanical ventilation. A switch from sinus rhythm to VVI pacemaker rhythm resulted in general hemodynamic deterioration. In addition to the drop in mean pulse pressure from an already low value of 30 mmHg to an even lower value of 20 mmHg, this change was accompanied by a large increase in PPV, from 13% to 58% (Figure 3). The 13% PPV during sinus rhythm was just around the cut-off range for volume responsiveness. However, the >4-fold increase in PPV when the VVI pacemaker took over by definition would normally suggest volume responsiveness. However, we decided not to give fluid, taking into consideration the full clinical picture, and we carried on treating him for cardiogenic shock.

The patient's subsequent course was uneventful. The sinus rhythm stabilized so that he could be successfully weaned

TABLE 1: Prerequisites for dynamic preload assessment using ventilation-induced hemodynamic alterations.

(i) Tidal volume > 8 ml/kg
(ii) Heart rate/respiratory rate ratio > 3.6
(iii) Closed chest
(iv) No abdominal hypertension
(v) No spontaneous respiratory efforts
(vi) No right ventricular failure
(vii) Regular rhythm

from the ventilator within 24 hours. The catecholamine support was also terminated by the third day of observation and eventually the pacemaker could be removed. Echocardiography revealed satisfactory global left ventricular function (EF 54%), with inferobasal akinesis. No significant mitral insufficiency was seen. He was discharged to the cardiology ward for further treatment.

3. Discussion

Dynamic preload assessment with PPV or SVV in mechanically ventilated patients is increasingly acknowledged in our daily routine but is still underused in clinical practice [3]. Despite the fact that these are considered to be the most sensitive and specific indicators of fluid responsiveness, there are several prerequisites for appropriate assessment and there are several circumstances that can limit the interpretation of the results (Table 1) [4–8]. Unfortunately, not all of these components are obvious or known by many anesthesiologists and intensivists [7]. "Regular rhythm" may seem like a simple requirement, but, surprisingly, the definition is ambiguous in various papers. Certain authors specify sinus rhythm [4, 7, 8] and others simply define regular rhythm as "lack of irregularity" [9] (at least for the duration of a single respiratory cycle [10]) and others talk about the absence of arrhythmia [5, 6]. These terms are confusing. Normal sinus rhythm, especially in healthy young subjects, can be quite irregular, and on the other hand certain forms of arrhythmias are actually regular.

In this current case, the patient had regular (paced) rhythm but the atrioventricular dissociation resulted in a "nonrespiratory" PPV augmentation. This response, however, is not "false" in the sense that it is related to true preload disturbances caused not by changes in the circulating blood volume but rather by the spontaneous atrial activity. Cyclic synchrony and dyssynchrony of the atrial "booster pump" resulted in varying ventricular filling ranging from optimal to very abnormal. The latter was the case when the atria and the ventricles contracted simultaneously, resulting in abnormally high atrial pressure waves, which actually impeded venous return.

One of the main clues in our case was the simultaneous assessment of the ECG trace and arterial pressure curves, which put in context the noninvasively measured breathing pattern detected by the pneumobelt. This revealed an asynchrony between the breathing cycle and the observed major changes in PPV. This information provided by the pneumobelt was only applied because we wanted real-time comprehensive documentation. However, this could easily be replaced by the observation of the ventilator monitor.

It is important to note that these observations do not necessarily mean that pacemaker rhythm always excludes the possibility of PPV assessment. In patients, for example, with complete AV block and VVI pacing in the setting of permanent atrial fibrillation or atrial standstill, a dynamic preload test still could be an informative procedure. We have learnt from cardiac resynchronization studies that modulation of AV delay has a tremendous impact on the pulse amplitude [11]. Cyclic changes in AV delay, as seen in our case, contaminate the PPV pattern.

4. Conclusion

Definition of a "regular rhythm," a prerequisite for dynamic preload tests in mechanically ventilated patients, is ambiguous. Our case shows that mechanistic implication of PPV as an indicator of fluid responsiveness when the heart rate is considered regular could have led to incorrect conclusions. However, this was overcome by thorough simultaneous observation of the ECG, arterial pressure curves, and the breathing cycle. We also feel that clarification of the current exclusion criteria may be warranted.

References

[1] M. R. Pinsky, "Functional Hemodynamic Monitoring," *Critical Care Clinics*, vol. 31, no. 1, pp. 89–111, 2015.

[2] F. Michard, S. Boussat, D. Chemla et al., "Relation between respiratory changes in arterial pulse pressure and fluid responsiveness in septic patients with acute circulatory failure," *American Journal of Respiratory and Critical Care Medicine*, vol. 162, no. 1, pp. 134–138, 2000.

[3] M. Cecconi, C. Hofer, J.-L. Teboul et al., "Fluid challenges in intensive care: the FENICE study: a global inception cohort study," *Intensive Care Medicine*, vol. 41, no. 9, pp. 1529–1537, 2015.

[4] S. Maguire, J. Rinehart, S. Vakharia, and M. Cannesson, "Respiratory variation in pulse pressure and plethysmographic waveforms: Intraoperative applicability in a North American academic center," *Anesthesia & Analgesia*, vol. 112, no. 1, pp. 94–96, 2011.

[5] M. Biais, A. Ouattara, G. Janvier, and F. Sztark, "Case scenario: Respiratory variations in arterial pressure for guiding fluid management in mechanically ventilated patients," *Anesthesiology*, vol. 116, no. 6, pp. 1354–1361, 2012.

[6] Y. Mahjoub, V. Lejeune, L. Muller et al., "Evaluation of pulse pressure variation validity criteria in critically ill patients: a prospective observational multicentre point-prevalence study," *British Journal of Anaesthesia*, vol. 112, no. 4, pp. 681–685, 2014.

[7] M.-O. Fischer, F. Dechanet, D. du Cheyron, J.-L. Gérard, J.-L. Hanouz, and J.-L. Fellahi, "Evaluation of the knowledge base of French intensivists and anaesthesiologists as concerns the interpretation of respiratory arterial pulse pressure variation,"

Anaesthesia Critical Care and Pain Medicine, vol. 34, no. 1, pp. 29–34, 2015.

[8] B. Delannoy, F. Wallet, D. Maucort-Boulch et al., "Applicability of Pulse Pressure Variation during Unstable Hemodynamic Events in the Intensive Care Unit: A Five-Day Prospective Multicenter Study," *Critical Care Research and Practice*, vol. 2016, Article ID 7162190, 5 pages, 2016.

[9] S. Preau, F. Dewavrin, V. Demaeght et al., "The use of static and dynamic haemodynamic parameters before volume expansion: A prospective observational study in six French intensive care units," *Anaesthesia Critical Care and Pain Medicine*, vol. 35, no. 2, pp. 93–102, 2016.

[10] F. Michard, "Volume Management Using Dynamic Parameters," *The good, the bad, and the ugly Chest*, vol. 128, no. 4, pp. 1902–1904, 2005.

[11] Z. I. Whinnett, J. E. R. Davies, K. Willson et al., "Haemodynamic effects of changes in atrioventricular and interventricular delay in cardiac resynchronisation therapy show a consistent pattern: Analysis of shape, magnitude and relative importance of atrioventricular and interventricular delay," *Heart*, vol. 92, no. 11, pp. 1628–1634, 2006.

Miliary Tuberculosis Presenting with ARDS and Shock: A Case Report and Challenges in Current Management and Diagnosis

Keevan Singh,[1] Saara Hyatali,[2] Stanley Giddings,[3] Kevin Singh,[2] and Neil Bhagwandass[2]

[1]*Anaesthesia and Intensive Care Department, San Fernando General Hospital and Department of Clinical Surgical Sciences, University of the West Indies, San Fernando, Trinidad, Trinidad and Tobago*
[2]*Internal Medicine Department, San Fernando General Hospital, San Fernando, Trinidad and Tobago*
[3]*Infectious Disease Unit, San Fernando General Hospital and Department of Clinical Medical Sciences, University of the West Indies, San Fernando, Trinidad, Trinidad and Tobago*

Correspondence should be addressed to Keevan Singh; keevansingh@gmail.com

Academic Editor: Chiara Lazzeri

Miliary tuberculosis, complicated by ARDS and septic shock, is a rare and lethal presentation of this disease. Here we present a case of such a patient, following which we discuss the management of tuberculosis in the ICU and some of the challenges that may be faced. A young HIV negative female presented to us with an acute history of worsening shortness of breath on a background of weight loss, nonproductive cough, and fever. CXR and CT scan showed bilateral miliary type opacities and the patient was admitted to the hospital. Within forty-eight hours of admission she became hypoxemic and was intubated and transferred to the ICU. There she experienced worsening organ dysfunction and developed circulatory shock. Despite escalating doses of noradrenaline, she continued to decline and died before specific anti-TB treatment could be started. Timely diagnosis and treatment initiation are the keys to improving outcomes in critically ill TB patients. However there are many challenges in doing so, especially in a general ICU located in a country with a low TB incidence.

1. Introduction

Globally, there has been a decline in the incidence as well as number of tuberculosis (TB) deaths [1]. However the disease continues to have a significant burden with more than ten million cases and one million deaths recorded in 2015 [1]. The Southeast Asian Region bears a large part of this disease burden, with significantly lower disease rates recorded in many western countries [1, 2].

Trinidad and Tobago lying in the Southern Caribbean has an incidence of approximately 17 cases per 100 000 persons [3]. With this relatively low incidence rate, tuberculosis is seldom seriously considered among the primary diagnoses, especially in the setting of ARDS and shock where other diagnoses are more likely.

Although outcome data shows an 83% success rate for TB treatment, presentation to an ICU setting with multiorgan failure can carry an extremely poor prognosis [1, 4, 5]. Delayed diagnosis and treatment initiation due to lack of recognition in low incidence countries are some of the chief contributors to this mortality [4, 6].

The following case illustrates this in the rapid decline of a young HIV negative female with miliary TB who presented to us with acute respiratory failure. The patient's condition progressed quickly to fatal circulatory shock despite supportive ICU care. Following the case, we also discuss the prognosis and current ICU management and challenges in identifying and managing a critically ill TB patient.

2. Case Report

A 16-year-old female was admitted to hospital with a one-week history of gradually worsening shortness of breath. For more than two months, she described having a nonproductive cough, nocturnal fever, significant weight loss, joint pains, and fatigue.

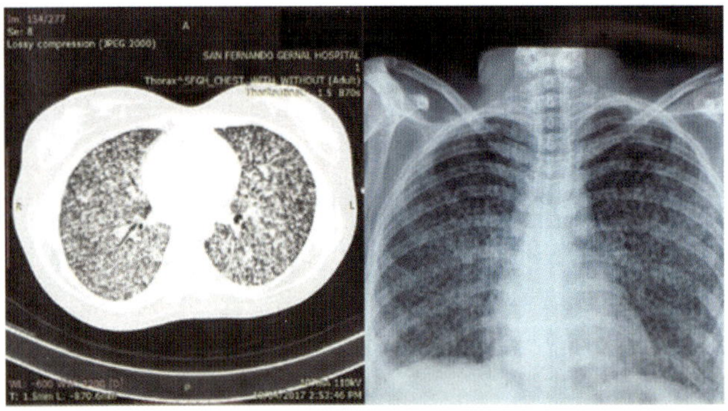

Figure 1: CT scan and CXR of patient showing bilateral miliary opacification.

The patient had previously sought treatment from her local primary care physician for a cough and fever approximately two months prior to this presentation. At this time, a HIV test was done which was negative. No further follow-up was done until her subsequent deterioration and presentation at our hospital.

On presentation the patient was tachypnoeic and tachycardic, with a respiratory rate of 40 bpm, a heart rate of 148 bpm, and a temperature of 37.8°C. Her oxygen saturation was 100% on facemask oxygen at 6 L/min with a blood pressure of 123/85 mmHg. Crepitations were heard throughout both lung fields. The remainder of the physical exam was normal with the patient noted to be alert and oriented.

An urgent CXR was requested which showed multiple miliary opacities scattered throughout both lung fields (Figure 1). Laboratory results at this time were significant for microcytic anemia, leukocytosis (Hb, 7.6 g/dL, MCV, 76 fL, and WBC, 15.4×10^9/L) and a normal platelet count (332×10^9/L). Serum creatinine and electrolytes were grossly normal. A CT scan of the chest confirmed miliary opacities, with no mediastinal or hilar lymphadenopathy (Figure 1).

Differential diagnoses at this time included pneumocystis pneumonia, viral/fungal pneumonia, miliary tuberculosis, and metastatic disease. Patient was reviewed by the Infectious Disease Unit and transferred to an isolation room on the medical ward.

An HIV rapid test was performed, which was subsequently reported as negative [Determine™ and UNI-GOLD™]. Due to the lack of any historical evidence suggesting frequent infections or an immunocompromised state, no immunological tests were requested. An interferon-gamma release assay [QuantiFERON™] was also requested and the patient was empirically started on levofloxacin, fluconazole, and acyclovir.

On day 2 of admission the patient deteriorated (SPO2 70% on Nonrebreather Mask set at 15 L/min), was transferred to the ICU, intubated, and placed on mechanical ventilation. Her P/F ratio at that time was 130 indicating moderate ARDS. After initial stabilization, worsening oxygenation (P/F ratio 113) prompted administration of bolus and infusion of cisatracurium. The patient was ventilated using a lung protective approach with a tidal volume of 330 ml (6 ml/kg), a PEEP of 10 cmH2O, RR of 20, and flow rate of 35 L/min. Sputum, via endotracheal tube suction catheter, was taken for testing at the regional public health lab. On a FiO2 setting ranging from 70 to 100%, the patient's oxygen saturation remained between 85% and 90%.

On further questioning of the patient's parents, it was revealed that she was in contact with a relative who had a nonproductive cough of unknown but prolonged duration. There was no testing or TB confirmation done in the family.

On admission day 3, patient was noted to be hypotensive with MAP's < 60 mmHg and persistently pyretic. Multiple polygeline fluid boluses were given and a noradrenaline infusion was started. As her condition continued to deteriorate, the noradrenaline dose increased to a max of 50 ug/min. Despite this the patient's hypotension persisted and she progressed to a fatal cardiac arrest early on the fourth day.

Shortly after her demise, Nucleic Acid Amplification [Xpert™ MTB/RIF] results from her sputum became available and it was positive for *Mycobacterium tuberculosis* with no rifampin resistance being detected. No smear microscopy or culture was performed in this case. Previously requested QuantiFERON test was marred by postprocessing issues and a retest was suggested.

On the evening before her death, a decision had been made to empirically start antituberculosis therapy; however due to its infrequent presentation in our regional hospital, no drugs were kept in stock and they had to be sourced from our local TB treatment center. Unfortunately, the patient's death preempted this.

3. Discussion

3.1. Prognosis. Miliary TB is described as a form of disseminated TB that results from lymphatic and hematologic spread from a TB focus and is invariably fatal if left untreated [8]. Recent data from countries with a low to moderate incidence of TB shows a 14% mortality in treated patients with miliary TB [9]. However, mortality increases once ARDS and septic shock and multiorgan failure develop.

In a cohort of 469 ARDS patients, from a high incidence setting, only 3.6% of the cases were due to *Mycobacterium tuberculosis* (MTB) [10]. Similarly the incidence of MTB as the primary cause of septic shock was less than one percent in a large septic shock cohort from low-moderate incidence countries [4]. Although the incidence of both ARDS and septic shock secondary to MTB is quite low in the general cohort of ICU patients, patients with TB needing ICU admission can have a > 90% rate of developing ARDS [5].

Kethireddy et al. showed that in patients with MTB septic shock the mortality rate was 79% (versus 49% in those with non-MTB septic shock) and only one patient who received anti-TB therapy after 24 hours survived [4]. In patients with ARDS secondary to MTB, recent data has shown a similar mortality rate to nontuberculous ARDS; however older studies have indicated mortality rates of 60–88% for MTB ARDS [10–12].

Overall, quoted ICU mortality can range from 26 to 66% for patients admitted with TB [5, 6, 13]. Mortality predictors

Histoplasmosis
Sarcoidosis
Hypersensitivity Pneumonia
Tumor Metastases (thyroid, renal cell)
Bronchogenic carcinoma
Pyogenic spread/septic embolization

Box 1: Causes of miliary type opacifications. Modified from [7].

included delayed treatment initiation by >1 month, baseline organ dysfunction, and number of organ failures [6, 10].

3.2. Diagnosis. In low incidence countries, miliary TB presenting as ARDS or septic shock can be easily missed, especially given the scarcity of these presentations in HIV negative patients even in endemic regions [4, 10]. However, given the high mortality rate associated with delayed treatment, it is important that the diagnosis be confirmed early so that treatment can be started promptly.

In addition to historical features, which can be variable, miliary type opacifications may be found in more than 80% of patients with miliary TB [9, 14]. As such, finding miliary opacifications should prompt rapid and further diagnostic testing so as to facilitate early treatment initiation. Other causes of miliary opacification are listed in Box 1.

Diagnosis of TB can be time consuming and challenging. This is especially true in the ICU patient where a delayed diagnosis can prove fatal and an appropriate specimen can be difficult to obtain. Standard diagnostic testing involves AFB smear microscopy followed by liquid and solid mycobacterial culture [15]. Mycobacterial culture can take up to a month to be available, while molecular techniques, as was done in this case, can give a result in hours and is recommended by consensus guidelines [15, 16]. In the critically ill patient where a high degree of clinical suspicion exists for disseminated or pulmonary TB, consideration should be given to obtain a sputum sample urgently for molecular testing and drug sensitivity.

3.3. ICU Management. High quality, supportive ICU care is essential in managing the TB patient with organ dysfunction. In patients with miliary TB presenting with ARDS and respiratory failure, particular attention should be paid to low tidal volume ventilation, conservative fluid administration, early use of neuromuscular blocking agents, and prone positioning in severe cases [16]. Of note the increased risk of pneumothorax in pulmonary TB would prompt the clinician to be vigilant in cases where high PEEP is used [17]. It is possible that the lower mortality rates seen in the recent work by Muthu et al. represent the effect of some of these changes [10].

In patients presenting with tuberculous septic shock, as in our case, standard management for bacterial shock should be followed. The core management principles involve early antibiotic use, fluid administration, and vasopressors to correct persisting hypotension—as described in the early goal directed protocol by Rivers et al. [18]. Although current evidence does not support a rigid application of this early goal directed protocol, the core principles in the management of septic shock remain the same [19].

Initiating anti-TB therapy can be challenging in the ICU patient. Issues include poor oral absorption, lack of parenteral formulations for some agents, and the presence of renal and hepatic dysfunction which is commonly seen in the critically ill patient. Standard therapy for TB involves a combination of three or more agents and usually contains isoniazid and rifampicin both of which are hepatotoxic [20]. Early consultation with an infectious disease specialist can help guide effective therapy. Additional options include the use of Therapeutic Drug Monitoring when oral dosing is used in critically ill patients, especially when delayed gastric emptying is an issue, and use of parenteral fluoroquinolones and aminoglycosides when liver dysfunction is a concern [20].

3.4. Challenges in the ICU. Despite efforts to contain and minimize the spread of contagious diseases in the ICU, several challenges remain in isolating and nursing such patients. Tuberculosis, though of low incidence, is no exception.

The main mode of transmission of TB is via droplet nuclei, dispersal of which is very common in the ICU setting during endotracheal intubation, suctioning, bronchoscopy, sputum induction, and administration of aerosolized medication [21]. According to the CDC, at least an N95 level of airway protection should be used for any healthcare worker entering a room with an infectious TB patient and especially during any of these procedures [21]. Consideration may be made for higher levels of respiratory protection during bronchoscopy as there is a higher risk of transmission. N95 masks are usually available in most healthcare settings; however there is often a lack of PAPRs (powered air-purifying respirators) if further protection is needed.

Most ICUs are designed with a fixed number of negative pressure isolation rooms. The number of these rooms is dependent on the function and case mix of the ICU [22]. In ICUs that deal with a low number of highly infectious cases, isolation room numbers may be quite small, whereas negative pressure rooms situated outside of the ICU are inadequate to deal with a critically ill patient. Such rooms are the standard of care for housing hospitalized patients with active pulmonary TB [21].

In many low incidence countries TB is treated in specialized centers. As a result, many smaller hospitals and ICUs may not have easy access to rapid confirmatory testing. Also, oral and parenteral TB drugs may not be available in a general ICU in these settings. All of these contribute to delays which may prove fatal in the critically ill patient.

4. Conclusion

ARDS and septic shock are rare presentations of miliary TB even in countries with a high TB incidence. Our case describes a patient who presented with both shock and respiratory failure and her subsequent fatal course. In addition to organ support, these patients need early definitive anti-TB treatment. Miliary shadowing observed on imaging a critically ill patient with organ failure may warrant molecular methods in testing for TB, so as to facilitate prompt treatment. Availability of parenteral anti-TB drugs and droplet transmission and availability of negative pressure isolation rooms are further challenges that can be faced, especially in smaller ICUs.

Authors' Contributions

Keevan Singh is a major contributor in reviewing the literature and writing all parts of the manuscript. Saara Hyatali is a major contributor in reviewing the literature and writing parts of the discussion. Stanley Giddings is a contributor to the diagnosis and management section. Kevin Singh contributed to the case description and clinical course. Neil Bhagwandass contributed to the case description and clinical course. All authors approved the final manuscript.

References

[1] World Health Organization, "Global tuberculosis report," 2016, http://www.who.int/tb/publications/global_report/en/.

[2] Centre for Disease Control and Prevention, "Trends in Tuberculosis - United States," 2014, https://www.cdc.gov/tb/publications/factsheets/data.htm.

[3] World Health Organization, "Tuberculosis country profiles," 2015, http://www.who.int/tb/country/data/profiles/en/.

[4] S. Kethireddy, R. B. Light, Y. Mirzanejad et al., "Mycobacterium tuberculosis septic shock," *CHEST*, vol. 144, no. 2, pp. 474–482, 2013.

[5] D. R. Silva, D. M. Menegotto, L. F. Schulz, M. B. Gazzana, and P. T. R. Dalcin, "Mortality among patients with tuberculosis requiring intensive care: a retrospective cohort study," *BMC Infectious Diseases*, vol. 10, article no. 54, 2010.

[6] J.-R. Zahar, E. Azoulay, E. Klement et al., "Delayed treatment contributes to mortality in ICU patients with severe active pulmonary tuberculosis and acute respiratory failure," *Intensive Care Medicine*, vol. 27, no. 3, pp. 513–520, 2001.

[7] J. Bernando, "Clinical manifestations, diagnosis, and treatment of miliary tuberculosis," in *UpToDate*, C. Reyn, Ed., UpToDate Inc, Waltham, Mass, USA, 2017.

[8] S. K. Sharma, A. Mohan, A. Sharma, and D. K. Mitra, "Miliary tuberculosis: new insights into an old disease," *The Lancet Infectious Diseases*, vol. 5, no. 7, pp. 415–430, 2005.

[9] A. Mert, F. Arslan, T. Kuyucu et al., "Miliary tuberculosis: Epidemiologicaland clinical analysis of large-case series from moderate to low tuberculosis endemic Country," *Medicine*, vol. 96, no. 5, p. e5875, 2017.

[10] V. Muthu, S. Dhooria, A. N. Aggarwal, D. Behera, I. S. Sehgal, and R. Agarwal, "Acute Respiratory Distress Syndrome Due To Tuberculosis in a Respiratory ICU Over a 16-Year Period," *Critical Care Medicine*, vol. 45, no. 10, pp. e1087–e1090, 2017.

[11] C. Penner, D. Roberts, D. Kunimoto, J. Manfreda, and R. Long, "Tuberculosis as a primary cause of respiratory failure requiring mechanical ventilation," *American Journal of Respiratory and Critical Care Medicine*, vol. 151, no. 3 I, pp. 867–872, 1995.

[12] A. R. Piqueras, L. Marruecos, A. Artigas, and C. Rodriguez, "Miliary tuberculosis and adult respiratory distress syndrome," *Intensive Care Medicine*, vol. 13, no. 3, pp. 175–182, 1987.

[13] R. Erbes, K. Oettel, M. Raffenberg, H. Mauch, M. Schmidt-Ioanas, and H. Lode, "Characteristics and outcome of patients with active pulmonary tuberculosis requiring intensive care," *European Respiratory Journal*, vol. 27, no. 6, pp. 1223–1228, 2006.

[14] A. Mert, M. Bilir, F. Tabak et al., "Miliary tuberculosis: Clinical manifestations, diagnosis and outcome in 38 adults," *Respirology*, vol. 6, no. 3, pp. 217–224, 2001.

[15] D. M. Lewinsohn, M. K. Leonard, P. A. Lobue et al., "Official American thoracic society/Infectious diseases society of America/Centers for disease control and prevention clinical practice guidelines: diagnosis of tuberculosis in adults and children," *Clinical Infectious Diseases*, vol. 64, no. 2, pp. 111–115, 2017.

[16] T. Bein, S. Grasso, O. Moerer et al., "The standard of care of patients with ARDS: ventilatory settings and rescue therapies for refractory hypoxemia," *Intensive Care Medicine*, vol. 42, no. 5, pp. 699–711, 2016.

[17] R. J. Wilder, E. G. Beacham, and M. M. Ravitch, "Spontaneous pneumothorax complicating cavitary tuberculosis," *The Journal of Thoracic and Cardiovascular Surgery*, vol. 43, pp. 561–573, 1962.

[18] E. Rivers, B. Nguyen, S. Havstad et al., "Early goal-directed therapy in the treatment of severe sepsis and septic shock," *The New England Journal of Medicine*, vol. 345, no. 19, pp. 1368–1377, 2001.

[19] The ARISE Investigators and the ANZICS Clinical Trials Group, "Goal-directed resuscitation for patients with early septic shock," *The New England Journal of Medicine*, vol. 371, no. 16, pp. 1496–1506, 2014.

[20] G. Hagan and N. Nathani, "Clinical review: tuberculosis on the intensive care unit," *Critical Care*, vol. 17, no. 5, article 240, 2013.

[21] P. A. Jensen, L. A. Lambert, M. F. Iademarco, and R. Ridzon, "Guidelines for preventing the transmission of Mycobacterium tuberculosis in health-care settings, 2005.," *MMWR. Recommendations and reports : Morbidity and mortality weekly report. Recommendations and reports / Centers for Disease Control*, vol. 54, no. 17, pp. 1–141, 2005.

[22] A. Valentin and P. Ferdinande, "Recommendations on basic requirements for intensive care units: structural and organizational aspects," *Intensive Care Medicine*, vol. 37, no. 10, pp. 1575–1587, 2011.

48

Fulminant Cerebral Fat Embolism: Case Description and Review of the Literature

Giorgio Berlot,[1] Rossana Bussani,[2] Vennus Shafiei,[2] and Nadia Zarrillo[3]

[1] *University of Trieste, Dept. of Anesthesia and Intensive Care, Cattinara Hospital, Strada di Fiume 447, 34149 Trieste, Italy*
[2] *University of Trieste, Dept. of Pathology, Cattinara Hospital, Strada di Fiume 447, 34149 Trieste, Italy*
[3] *Caserta Hospital, Dept. of Anesthesia and Intensive Care, Via Ferdinando Palasciano, 81100 Caserta, Italy*

Correspondence should be addressed to Giorgio Berlot; berlot@inwind.it

Academic Editor: Gil Klinger

The release of fat and bone marrow fragments is a common occurrence following traumatic and nontraumatic events. In most cases, they go symptomless or cause only minor disturbances, but occasionally they can determine a multiorgan dysfunction whose severity ranges from mild to fatal. The authors describe the case of a patient who became deeply comatose and ultimately died after a traffic accident in which he suffered the exposed right femoral and tibial fracture in the absence of other injuries. He underwent the external fixation of the fractured bones 2 hours after the admission under general anesthesia. Three hours later, he failed to awake at the suspension of the anesthetic agents and became anisocoric; a CT scan demonstrated a diffuse cerebral edema with the herniation of the cerebellar tonsils; these abnormalities were unresponsive to the treatment and the brain death was one day later. The causes, the mechanisms, the symptoms, the prevention, and the treatment of the syndrome are reviewed and discussed.

1. Introduction

A number of traumatic as well nontraumatic circumstances can determine the passage of bone components such as fat and hemopoietic tissue into the bloodstream [1–3]. Independently from the triggering event, the ensuing fat and bone marrow emboli (FE and BME, respectively) can reach the systemic circulation crossing the lung capillaries, through intrapulmonary physiologic shunts or via a patent foramen ovale (PFO) [4].

In most cases, FE and BME cause no or only minor clinical consequences and only few patients develop systemic complications, a condition usually known as Fat Embolism Syndrome (FES). However, despite its widespread use, this denomination ignores the relevant role played by the BME especially in younger subjects. Whatever acronym is used, two different and not mutually exclusive mechanisms have been hypothesized in its pathogenesis: the first consists in the obstruction of the microvascular network by one or both components (mechanical hypothesis) whereas the other advocates the irritative effects exerted by the free fatty acids released by the interaction between the FE and the lung lipases on the endothelium and the subsequent activation of the inflammatory and coagulative cascades (biochemical hypothesis) [4].

The subsequent dysfunction(s) and related symptoms can occur alone or in combination and are primarily related to the end organ(s) involved. The most common clinical presentations include a noncardiogenic pulmonary edema, disturbances of the central nervous system (CNS) of variable severity, and coagulative alterations. Remarkably, despite the high number of predisposing circumstances, the occurrence of a full-blown FES is reported only occasionally [5, 6]. In the absence of a specific treatment, the early fixation of long-bone fractures and the avoidance of the intramedullary reaming represents the only measures that are able to prevent the syndrome and/or to reduce the related complications [6, 7].

Here we describe the case of a trauma patient who developed a fulminant cerebral FES approximately two hours after the trauma when he underwent urgent orthopaedic surgery under general anesthesia.

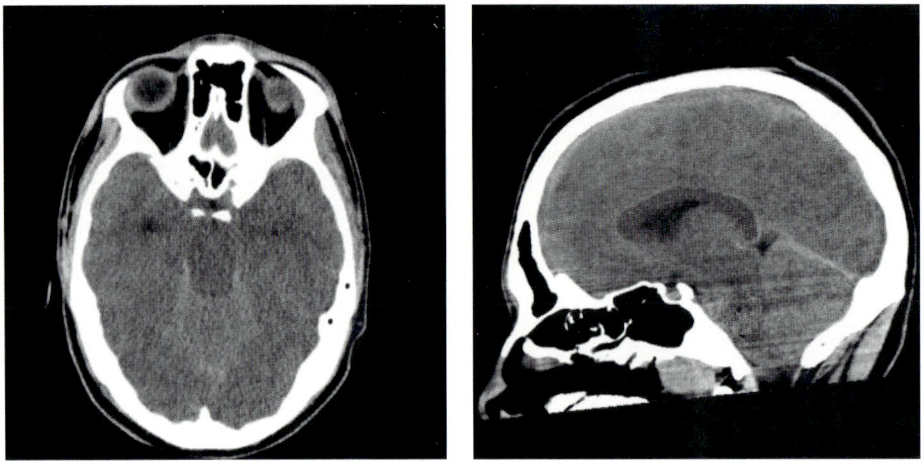

FIGURE 1: a (left): brain CT scan showing a diffuse edema with the disappearance of the gray/white matter limitation; b (right): herniation of the cerebellar tonsils.

2. Case Description

A 17-year-old man was involved in a road accident in which he suffered the open fractures of the right femur and tibia. At the arrival to the Emergency Dept (ED), he was alert and hemodynamically stable and the Glasgow Coma Scale (GCS) was 15; the initial alignment of the fractured ends was performed in the ED with a gentle traction performed under sedation with iv. ketamine; a total body CT did not demonstrate other injuries. Approximately two hours after the admission the patient was taken to the surgical theatre for the external fixation of the fractured bones; at entering the operating room, the GCS was 8, the arterial pressure was 115/80 mm Hg, the heart rate was 115 bpm, and the arterial oxygen saturation (SPO_2) was 85 at room air; the procedure was performed under general iv anesthesia with propofol and remifentanyl; the standard monitoring included the ECG, the noninvasive arterial pressure, the SPO_2, and the end-tidal CO_2 ($ETCO_2$); during the intervention, the SPO_2 rose to 100% at a FIO_2=40% and all the other variables remained stable throughout the procedure after the 3-hour-long intervention in which the complete alignment of the bony ends was achieved; the patient was transferred to the Intensive Care Unit (ICU) still intubated and mechanically ventilated; the iv anaesthetics were gradually tapered until the complete suspension. Two hours later, the $SpaO_2$ and the $ETCO_2$ slightly decreased and anisocoria was observed; and an urgent CT scan of the head demonstrated a diffuse cerebral edema and the herniation of the cerebellar tonsils (Figures 1(a) and 1(b), respectively). At this time, the pupils became bilaterally mydriatic and the EEG was almost isoelectric; due to the severity of the conditions, a MR scan was considered unnecessary. On the basis of the clinical and radiologic findings repeated boluses of iv. mannitol and steroids were given in the following hours aiming to reduce the intracranial pressure. An echocardiogram demonstrated a severe right ventricular depression with an ejection fraction of 20%. On the following day, the patient was declared brain dead according to the current Italian law.

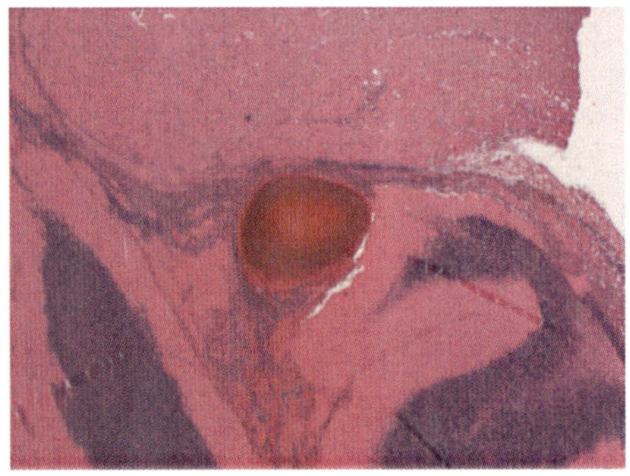

FIGURE 2: Large vascular thrombus in the cerebellum (H & E, $*$ 2.5).

At the autopsy, the cerebral microvascular network appeared diffusely plugged with BME (Figures 2–4) and ischemia-related microcalcifications were scattered throughout the brain (Figure 5); other organs were less extensively involved; no PFO was demonstrated.

3. Discussion

In trauma patients, the diagnosis of FES can be challenging because the symptoms (a) are not specific, ranging from mild dyspnoea to severe disturbances of the central nervous system (CNS) and possibly death; (b) appear after variable intervals of time after the injury; and, finally, (c) can overlap with those caused by the initiating event. Then, it is likely that this clinical entity goes largely undiagnosed either in adult or in pediatric patients [11–13] as reflected also by the wide variations of its incidence and time of onset reported in different studies, ranging from $\leq 1\%$ to 35% and from ≤ 6 to > 48 hours, respectively [2, 14].

Once triggered, the outcome of patients with FES is related to different circumstances, including the amount of BME and FE released, their final location, and the severity of the end organ dysfunction. The fulminant clinical course

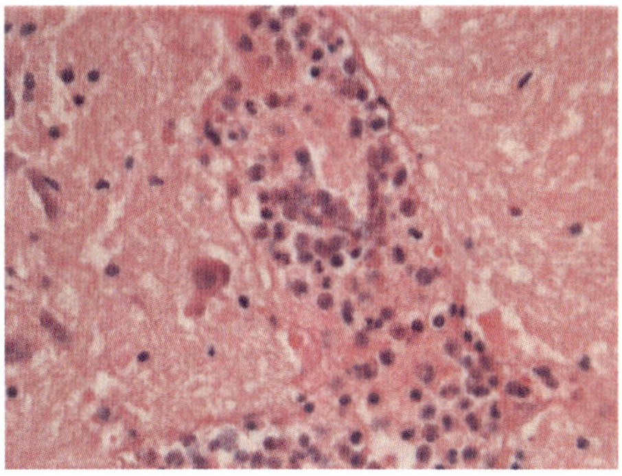

FIGURE 3: A cerebral vein completely obliterated by normally non-circulating bone marrow components (promyelocytes and myelocytes) (H & E, *40).

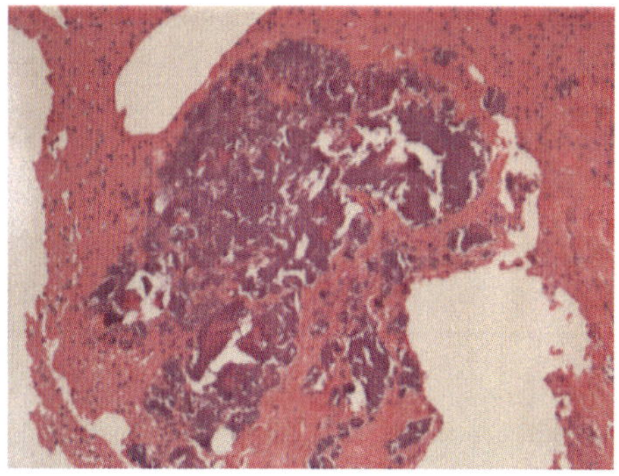

FIGURE 5: Coarse calcification in the cerebral parenchyma (H & E, * 10).

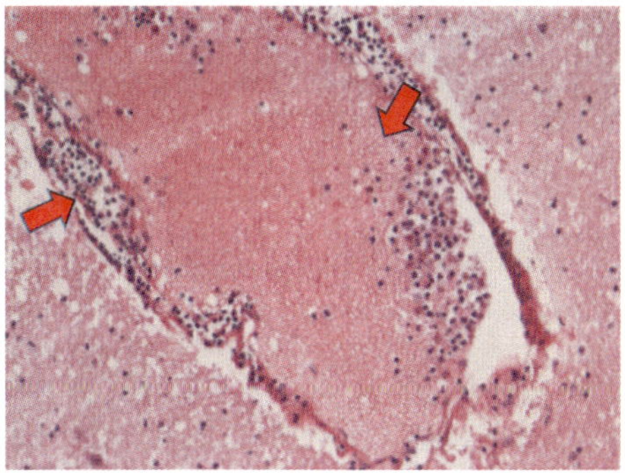

FIGURE 4: Venular occlusion by erythrocytes, promyelocytes, and myelocytes (arrows) (H & E, * 20).

and the poor outcome of our patient despite the immediate external fixation, which is considered the gold standard for patients at risk, deserve some remarks. [15, 16].

First, the double long-bone fracture likely determined a massive release of FE and BME. Actually, both their amount and the velocity of bloodstream invasion have been associated with the outcome: Kamenar et al. [16] observed up to 100 fat globules /mm^2 of brain area in an autoptical study performed in a patient with a femoral shaft fracture and Cui et al. [17] demonstrated that the velocity of infusion of BM-derived mesenchymal stem-cells as well as their dose was positively associated with the appearance of cerebral ischemic lesions in a rodent model of cell-based therapy for stroke. More recently, also Jarmer et al. [18] observed a correlation between the severity of the fractures, the amount of pulmonary FE, and the outcome. As occurred in our patient, FE and BME can get the systemic circulation via pathways other than a PFO, including the lung microvascular network and the intrapulmonary physiologic shunts.

Second, it is likely that the embolic spread towards the brain initiated immediately after the trauma and continued during both the initial stabilization and the intervention due to the manipulations of the fractured bone ends; the progressive ischemic and cytotoxic damage to the lung and the brain caused by the FE and [4] likely account for the deterioration of the SPO_2 and of the neurologic conditions observed at the arrival in the surgical theatre. Actually, it appears that both the severity and the timing of the initial CNS symptoms are related to the outcome: in a recent review, Kellogg et al. [19] reported that no or only minor mental status changes, focal deficits, or seizures at the admission were associated with a good outcome in 90,6% of patients, but this rate dropped to 57,6% in the presence of coma or abnormal posturing; other investigators demonstrated that the duration of the free interval is associated with the outcome, being worse in patients whose symptoms were present already in an earlier phase (1-8 hours) as compared with those whose neurological deterioration appeared later on [14, 19]. As far as the imaging is concerned, the CT scan is considered not sensible enough especially in the initial phases of the disease and a MR scan is warranted in order to detect the scattered (so-called "starfield pattern") or confluent areas of cytotoxic edema caused by the plugging of the cerebral vascular network [19]. This imaging was not obtained in our patient due to the absence of any therapeutic option other than the administration of mannitol and steroids able to reverse or limit the already established severe neurologic damage.

Third, both the SPO_2 and the $ETCO_2$ did not change during the surgical procedure, possibly due to the better cardiopulmonary functional reserves of a young subject, and started to deteriorate only after the ICU admission. Actually, the lack of specific signs and symptoms directly ascribable to BME of FE makes the diagnosis elusive and a number of scoring systems have been developed to overcome these difficulties (Table 1) [4, 8, 9, 20]; however, all of them require, among other signs, a deterioration of gas exchanges in association with acute changes in CNS function; yet, we could not observe alterations of these due to the general anesthesia and mechanical ventilation.

Fourth, the presence of BME is far less common that that of FE: actually, Dettmer et al. [10] studied a group of 982 patients (age 75,7±11,9 years) who died following trauma and orthopaedic procedures and observed that (a) a BE or a FE was present in only 34 (3,4%) cases; (b) a BME was present in only 3% of them; and (c) they were mutually exclusive, the BE being primarily associated with the resuscitative manoeuvres and the FE with orthopaedic procedures and/or bone disease; this finding leads the authors to hypothesize

TABLE 1: Scoring systems used for the diagnosis of FES. CNS: central nervous system; ESR: erythrocyte sedimentation rate.

Author	Features
A.R. Gurd et al. [8] (FES= 1 major + 4 minor + fat microglobulinemia)	**Major criteria** Respiratory insufficiency, CNS involvement, petechial rash **Minor Criteria** Pyrexia, tachycardia, jaundice, oliguria/anuria, thrombocytopenia, elevated ESR, fat microglobulinemia
B.G. Shonfeld et al. [9] (FES ≥ 5 points)	Diffuse petechiae (5 points) Alveolar infiltrates (4 points) Hypoxemia (paO_2 < 70 mm Hg) CNS involvement (1 point) Fever ≥ 38°C Heart rate > 120 beats/min Respiratory rate > 30 min
B.G. Lindeque et al. [10] (FES = femur fracture ± tibial fracture + 1 feature)	PaO_2 < 60 mm Hg $PaCO_2$ > 55 mmHg or pH < 7,3 Respiratory rate > 35/ min Dyspnea, anxiety, use of accessory respiratory muscles

that whereas BME had been released from the ribs broken during the CPR the FE could have been derived from the subcutaneous tissue. In our patient, the remarkable amount of blood cells precursors obstructing the brain small vessels must be ascribed to their abundance in the bone marrow of a young subject as compared to that present in elderly patients observed by other investigators [10, 11] in whom the hemopoietic tissue is largely replaced by fat [21].

4. Conclusions

The occurrence of a trauma-associated full-blown FES represents a potentially catastrophic clinical condition whose diagnosis requires a high index of suspicion. Its severity largely depends on the extension of trauma and on the amount of BE and BME consequently released. The only risk-reducing measure is the early fixation avoiding the medullary reaming and the treatment is only supportive.

References

[1] K. Newbigin, C. A. Souza, C. Torres et al., "Fat embolism syndrome: State-of-the-art review focused on pulmonary imaging findings," *Respiratory Medicine*, 2015.

[2] P. D. Stein, A. Y. Yaekoub, F. Matta, and M. Kleerekoper, "Fat embolism syndrome," *The American Journal of the Medical Sciences*, vol. 336, no. 6, pp. 472–477, 2008.

[3] R. Gangaraju, V. V. B. Reddy, and M. B. Marques, "Fat embolism syndrome secondary to bone marrow necrosis in patients with hemoglobinopathies," *Southern Medical Journal*, vol. 109, no. 9, pp. 549–553, 2016.

[4] S. Akhtar, "Fat Embolism," *Anesthesiology Clinics*, vol. 27, no. 3, pp. 533–550, 2009.

[5] E. E. Husebye, T. Lyberg, and O. Røise, "Bone marrow fat in the circulation: clinical entities and pathophysiological mechanisms," *Injury*, vol. 37, no. 4, p. -S18, 2006.

[6] T. J. Blokhuis, H. Pape, and J. Frölke, "Timing of definitive fixation of major long bone fractures: Can fat embolism syndrome be prevented?" *Injury*, vol. 48, Supplement 1, pp. S3–S6, 2017.

[7] N. Shaikh, "Emergency management of fat embolism syndrome," *Journal of Emergencies, Trauma, and Shock*, vol. 2, no. 1, pp. 29–33, 2009.

[8] B. Lindeque, H. Schoeman, G. Dommisse, M. Boeyens, and A. Vlok, "Fat embolism and the fat embolism syndrome. A double-blind therapeutic study," *The Journal of Bone & Joint Surgery*, vol. 69, no. 1, pp. 128–131, 1987.

[9] S. A. Schonfeld, Y. Ploysongsang, R. DiLisio et al., "Fat embolism prophylaxis with corticosteroids. A prospective study in high-risk patients," *Annals of Internal Medicine*, vol. 99, no. 4, pp. 438–443, 1983.

[10] M. S. Dettmer, N. Willi, T. Thiesler, P. Ochsner, and G. Cathomas, "The impact of pulmonary bone component embolism: An autopsy study," *Journal of Clinical Pathology*, vol. 67, no. 4, pp. 370–374, 2014.

[11] E. A. Eriksson, D. C. Pellegrini, W. E. Vanderkolk, C. T. Minshall, S. M. Fakhry, and S. D. Cohle, "Incidence of pulmonary fat embolism at autopsy: An undiagnosed epidemic," *Journal of Trauma - Injury Infection and Critical Care*, vol. 71, no. 2, pp. 312–315, 2011.

[12] E. A. Eriksson, "Fat embolism in pediatric patients: an autopsy evaluation of incidence and etiology," *Journal of Critical Care*, vol. 30, no. 1, pp. 221-e1, 2015.

[13] D. A. Godoy, M. Di Napoli, and A. A. Rabinstein, "Cerebral Fat Embolism: Recognition, Complications, and Prognosis," *Neurocritical Care*, pp. 1–8, 2017.

[14] T. J. Blokhuis, H. Pape, and J. Frölke, "Timing of definitive fixation of major long bone fractures: Can fat embolism syndrome be prevented?" *Injury*, vol. 48, pp. S3–S6, 2017.

[15] T. White, B. A. Petrisor, and M. Bhandari, "Prevention of fat embolism syndrome," *Injury*, vol. 37, no. 4, pp. S59–S67, 2006.

[16] E. Kamenar and P. C. Burger, "Cerebral fat embolism: A neuropathological study of a microembolic state," *Stroke*, vol. 11, no. 5, pp. 477–484, 1980.

[17] L. Cui, A. Bakreen, F. Nitzche et al., "The cerebral embolism evoked by intra-arterial delivery of allogeneic bone marrow mesechimal stem cell in rats is related to cell dose and infusion velocity," *Stem Cell Research & Therapy*, vol. 6, pp. 11–20, 2015.

[18] J. Jarmer, G. Ampanozi, M. J. Thali, and S. A. Bolliger, "Role of Survival Time and Injury Severity in Fatal Pulmonary Fat Embolism," *The American Journal of Forensic Medicine and Pathology*, vol. 38, no. 1, pp. 74–77, 2017.

[19] R. G. Kellogg, R. B. V. Fontes, and D. K. Lopes, "Massive cerebral involvement in fat embolism syndrome and intracranial pressure management," *Journal of Neurosurgery*, vol. 119, no. 5, pp. 1263–1270, 2013.

[20] A. R. Gurd and R. I. Wilson, "The fat embolism syndrome," *The Journal of Bone & Joint Surgery*, vol. 56B, no. 3, pp. 408–416, 1974.

[21] S. R. Tuljapurkar, T. R. McGuire, S. K. Brusnahan et al., "Changes in human bone marrow fat content associated with changes in hematopoietic stem cell numbers and cytokine levels with aging," *Journal of Anatomy*, vol. 219, no. 5, pp. 574–581, 2011.

49

Severe Progressive Diffuse Alveolar Hemorrhage in a Patient with Systemic Lupus Erythematosus

Munenori Kusunoki, Takeshi Umegaki, Tomohiro Shoji, Kota Nishimoto, Natsuki Anada, Akiko Ando, Takeo Uba, Kanako Oku, Saya Hakata, Satoshi Hagihira, and Takahiko Kamibayashi

Department of Anesthesiology, Kansai Medical University Hospital, Osaka, Japan

Correspondence should be addressed to Takeshi Umegaki; umegakit@hirakata.kmu.ac.jp

Academic Editor: Kenneth S. Waxman

Diffuse alveolar hemorrhage (DAH) refers to the effusion of blood into the alveoli due to damaged pulmonary microvasculature. The ensuing alveolar collapse can lead to severe hypoxemia with poor prognosis. In these cases, it is crucial to provide respiratory care for hypoxemia in addition to treating the underlying disease. Here, we describe our experience with a case involving a 46-year-old woman with severe DAH-induced hypoxemia accompanying systemic lupus erythematosus (SLE). Mechanical ventilation was managed using airway pressure release ventilation (APRV) after intubation. Through APRV-based respiratory care and treatment of the underlying disease, hemoptysis was eliminated and oxygenation improved. The patient did not experience significant barotrauma and was successfully weaned from mechanical ventilation after 25 days in the intensive care unit. This case demonstrates that APRV-based control for respiratory management can inhibit the effusion of blood into the alveoli and achieve mechanical hemostasis, as well as mitigate alveolar collapse. APRV may be a useful method for respiratory care in patients with severe DAH-induced hypoxemia.

1. Introduction

Diffuse alveolar hemorrhage (DAH) is a clinicopathological syndrome characterized by intra-alveolar bleeding from damaged pulmonary microvasculature, which can arise due to factors such as pulmonary capillaritis or humoral immune responses [1–3]. This condition can lead to hemoptysis or alveolar collapse resulting in hypoxemia [1–3]. In some cases, DAH can result in acute respiratory failure and death.

DAH is a particularly important potentially fatal complication in patients with systemic lupus erythematosus (SLE) [4], and physicians face difficulties in managing both the underlying disease and respiratory dysfunction in these patients.

This case report describes severe DAH in a 46-year-old woman with SLE who developed severe hypoxemia. Mechanical ventilation was performed using airway pressure release ventilation (APRV). The patient was successfully treated with the combined use of APRV, immunosuppressive therapy, and high-dose corticosteroid therapy.

2. Case Presentation

A 46-year-old Japanese woman with known SLE was admitted to our hospital due to sudden weight loss and respiratory distress. Her vitals on arrival were a temperature of 37.1°C, heart rate of 96 bpm, blood pressure of 148/82 mmHg, respiratory rate of 18 per minute, and oxygen saturation of 95% in room air. The patient was given 50 mg of oral prednisolone immediately after admission.

Approximately 3 weeks after the start of treatment, the dosage of prednisolone was reduced to 45 mg/day. However, the patient suddenly developed hemoptysis and respiratory distress. A chest X-ray (Figure 1) revealed infiltrative shadows in both lung fields, with greater density in the right lung. A computed tomography (CT) scan showed pulmonary

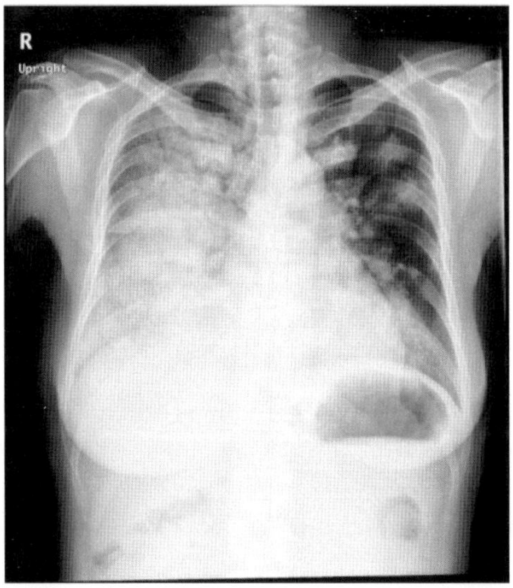

FIGURE 1: Chest radiograph upon the start of high-dose corticosteroid therapy. Infiltrative shadows are clearly observed in both lung fields.

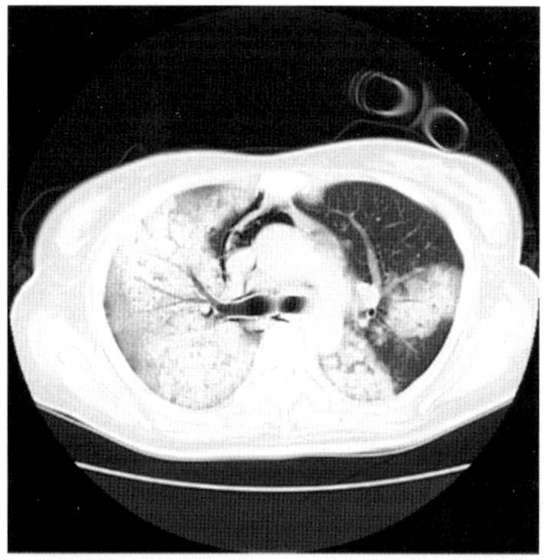

FIGURE 2: CT scan upon the start of high-dose corticosteroid therapy. The scan shows bilateral pulmonary infiltrates along the peripheral bronchovascular bundles and ground-glass opacities with a panlobular distribution.

infiltrates along the peripheral bronchovascular bundles and ground-glass opacities (Figure 2). We diagnosed the patient with DAH-induced hypoxemia accompanying SLE and initiated high-dose corticosteroid therapy (methylprednisolone 500 mg/day). However, respiratory distress worsened, and we began immunosuppressive therapy (cyclophosphamide 750 mg/day) 3 days after the start of high-dose corticosteroid therapy. The patient was also transferred to the intensive care unit (ICU) and placed on mechanical ventilation. Although the patient produced copious quantities of bloody secretions after intubation, the secretions were reduced when APRV was set to the highest airway pressure (35 cmH_2O). We administered oxygen through an oxygen mask (flow rate: 6 L/min) while in the ICU. Under these conditions, the arterial oxygen partial pressure (PaO_2) was 55.1 mmHg, and the ratio of arterial oxygen partial pressure to fractional inspired oxygen (P/F ratio) was 125.2. APRV resulted in substantial improvements to respiratory function, with a fraction of inspired oxygen (FiO_2) of 0.60 and a PaO_2 of 117.6 mmHg.

High-dose corticosteroid therapy was administered using 500 mg/day of methylprednisolone for 3 days, 250 mg/day of methylprednisolone for 3 days, and 125 mg/day of methylprednisolone for 3 days, after which the patient was given 50 mg/day of intravenous prednisolone every day while in the ICU. During approximately 3 consecutive weeks of APRV and steroid therapy, the patient demonstrated gradual improvements in respiratory function, and a CT scan after extubation showed that the pulmonary infiltrates and ground-glass opacities had disappeared (Figure 3). Mechanical ventilation was discontinued 25 days after admission to the ICU. The patient was moved to the general ward and continued on oral steroid therapy (methylprednisolone 16 mg/day) until discharge. The patient's respiratory and hemodynamic parameters from admission to ICU discharge are summarized in Table 1. The patient was successfully discharged from hospital 102 days after admission.

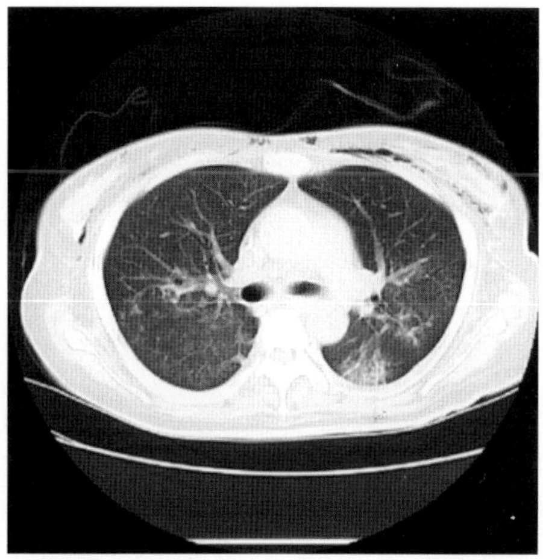

FIGURE 3: CT scan after extubation. The pulmonary infiltrates and ground-glass opacities had disappeared.

3. Discussion

The requirement for mechanical ventilation in SLE patients with DAH has been reported to be associated with higher mortality [5, 6]. The case described here provides valuable findings that the use of APRV and high-dose corticosteroid therapy can contribute to the alleviation of respiratory distress in an SLE patient with severe DAH. To the best of our knowledge, this is the first report to describe a case of severe DAH where respiratory dysfunction was successfully resolved with this unique approach.

DAH is associated with primary vasculitis (due to conditions such as microscopic polyarteritis, Wegener's granulomatosis, and Churg-Strauss syndrome) and secondary

Table 1: Respiratory and hemodynamic parameters from hospital admission to ICU discharge.

Variables	Oxygen therapy	FiO_2 (%)	P_{high} (cmH_2O)	SpO_2 (%)	PaO_2 (mmHg)
ICU admission prior to intubation	Mask 6 L/min	0.44	-	≤90	55.1
Two hours after intubation	APRV	0.60	35	100	117.6
ICU Day 7	APRV	0.30	35	100	97.6
ICU Day 14	APRV	0.30	30	100	102.2
ICU Day 21	CPAP	0.30	15	100	100.5
One hour after extubation	HFNC 40 L/min	0.40	-	100	122.9

APRV, airway pressure release ventilation; CPAP, continuous positive airway pressure; FiO2, fraction of inspiratory oxygen; HFNC, high-flow nasal cannula; ICU, intensive care unit; PaO_2, partial pressure of arterial oxygen; P_{high}, peak inspiratory pressure; SpO_2, oxygen saturation of peripheral artery.

vasculitis accompanying connective tissue diseases (such as SLE and malignant rheumatoid arthritis) [7]. DAH frequently presents as diffuse bleeding into the alveoli as a result of microvascular injury, and cases like the one described here may result in fatal consequences if treatment is unsuccessful [8, 9].

The development of barotrauma has been reported to have little effect on ventilator parameters such as peak pressure, positive end-expiratory pressure, and tidal volume [10]. However, patients with acute respiratory distress syndrome are at increased risk of barotrauma arising from high airway pressure if consistently exposed to peak pressures of 35 cmH_2O or more during mechanical ventilation [11]. Therefore, the risk of barotrauma must be considered when performing respiratory management with high peak pressures in these patients.

As there are currently no established evidence-based treatment protocols for DAH, cases are generally treated with high-dose corticosteroid therapy or immunosuppressive therapy (e.g., cyclophosphamide), which target pulmonary capillaritis and vasculitis [12]. However, positive pressure mechanical ventilation can be useful for recruitment maneuvers and hemostasis for collapsed alveoli, such as in the successful treatment of DAH using high-frequency oscillation ventilation [13]. In our patient, the combination of high-dose corticosteroid therapy, immunosuppressive therapy, and APRV was used to improve DAH and acute respiratory distress. APRV is characterized by relatively long high-pressure phases with intermittent short pressure release phases. The short durations for pressure release prevent alveolar collapse and ventilator-associated lung injury and allow for the steady expansion of the alveoli and improvement of oxygenation [14]. The maintenance of positive pressure using APRV in our patient may have contributed to the prevention of intra-alveolar bleeding, improvement of alveolar collapse, and alleviation of respiratory distress.

4. Conclusions

This case report describes the successful use of APRV-based respiratory management to inhibit the effusion of blood into the alveoli and achieve mechanical hemostasis, as well as mitigating alveolar collapse. APRV may be a useful method for respiratory care in SLE patients with severe DAH-induced hypoxemia when used in combination with high-dose corticosteroid therapy and immunosuppressive therapy to control the exacerbation of SLE.

References

[1] O. C. Ioachimescu and J. K. Stoller, "Diffuse alveolar hemorrhage: Diagnosing it and finding the cause," *Cleveland Clinic Journal of Medicine*, vol. 75, no. 4, pp. 258–280, 2008.

[2] A. R. Lara and M. I. Schwarz, "Diffuse alveolar hemorrhage," *CHEST*, vol. 137, no. 5, pp. 1164–1171, 2010.

[3] S. L. Primack, R. R. Miller, and N. L. Muller, "Diffuse pulmonary hemorrhage: clinical, pathologic, and imaging features," *American Journal of Roentgenology*, vol. 164, no. 2, pp. 295–300, 1995.

[4] M. U. Martínez-Martínez and C. Abud-Mendoza, "Diffuse alveolar hemorrhage in patients with systemic lupus erythematosus: Clinical manifestations, treatment, and prognosis," *Reumatología Clínica*, vol. 10, no. 4, pp. 248–253, 2014.

[5] M. U. Martínez-Martínez and C. Abud-Mendoza, "Predictors of mortality in diffuse alveolar haemorrhage associated with systemic lupus erythematosus," *Lupus*, vol. 20, no. 6, pp. 568–574, 2011.

[6] S.-K. Kwok, S.-J. Moon, J. H. Ju et al., "Diffuse alveolar hemorrhage in systemic lupus erythematosus: Risk factors and clinical outcome: Results from affiliated hospitals of Catholic University of Korea," *Lupus*, vol. 20, no. 1, pp. 102–107, 2011.

[7] R. J. Green, S. J. Ruoss, S. A. Kraft, G. J. Berry, and T. A. Raffin, "Pulmonary capillaritis and alveolar hemorrhage: Update on diagnosis and management," *CHEST*, vol. 110, no. 5, pp. 1305–1316, 1996.

[8] D. Lauque, J. Cadranel, R. Lazor et al., "Microscopic Polyangiitis with Alveolar Hemorrhage A Study of 29 Cases and Review of the Literature," *Medicine*, vol. 79, no. 4, pp. 222–233, 2000.

[9] M. R. Zamora, M. L. Warner, R. Tuder, and M. I. Schwarz, "Diffuse alveolar hemorrhage and systemic lupus erythematosus: clinical presentation, histology, survival, and outcome," *Medicine*, vol. 76, no. 3, pp. 192–202, 1997.

[10] A. Anzueto, F. Frutos-Vivar, A. Esteban et al., "Incidence, risk factors and outcome of barotrauma in mechanically ventilated patients," *Intensive Care Medicine*, vol. 30, no. 4, pp. 612–619, 2004.

[11] T. Umegaki, S. Sakamoto, K. Nishi et al., "Impact of steroid medication before hospital admission on barotrauma in mechanically ventilated patients with acute respiratory distress syndrome in intensive care units," *Journal of Anesthesia & Clinical Research*, vol. 28, no. 5, pp. 681–686, 2014.

[12] M. Shen, X. Zeng, X. Tian et al., "Diffuse alveolar hemorrhage in systemic lupus erythematosus: A retrospective study in China," *Lupus*, vol. 19, no. 11, pp. 1326–1330, 2010.

[13] A. Markland, G. Hansen, A. Banks, R. Chibbar, and D. Adamko, "A Pediatric Case of Diffuse Alveolar Hemorrhage Secondary to Poststreptococcal Glomerulonephritis," *Case Reports in Critical Care*, vol. 2017, pp. 1–5, 2017.

[14] M. B. P. Amato, C. S. V. Barbas, D. M. Medeiros et al., "Beneficial effects of the 'open lung approach' with low distending pressures in acute respiratory distress syndrome: A prospective randomized study on mechanical ventilation," *American Journal of Respiratory and Critical Care Medicine*, vol. 152, no. 6 I, pp. 1835–1846, 1995.

50

Fatal Septic Shock in a Patient with Hemophagocytic Lymphohistiocytosis Associated with an Infectious Mononucleosis

Giorgio Berlot,[1] Ariella Tomasini,[1] Lorenzo Zandonà,[2] Eugenio Leonardo,[2] Rossana Bussani,[2] and Nadia Zarrillo[3]

[1] *University of Trieste, Department of Anesthesia and Intensive Care, Cattinara Hospital, 447, 34149, Trieste, Italy*
[2] *University of Trieste, Department of Pathology, Cattinara Hospital, 447, 34149, Trieste, Italy*
[3] *Caserta Hospital, Department of Anesthesia and Intensive Care, Italy*

Correspondence should be addressed to Giorgio Berlot; berlot@inwind.it

Academic Editor: Zsolt Molnár

The authors describe the case of a young woman who developed a clinical pictures resembling a septic shock-related multiple organ dysfunction syndrome a couple of months after having been diagnosed suffering from a hemophagocytic lymphohistiocytosis associated with an infectious mononucleosis. Despite the aggressive treatment, which included antibiotics, vasopressors, IV immunoglobulins, and the use of an extracorporeal device aimed to remove mediators released both during sepsis and the cytokine storm determined by the hemophagocytic lymphohistiocytosis, the patient died. At the autopsy, an extremely uncommon aggressive lymphoma of Epstein-Barr virus-positive T-lymphocytes with systemic involvement was discovered.

1. Introduction.

Although most patients with infectious mononucleosis (IM) recover without major clinical sequelae, a number of harmful complications can occur, including hepatitis, splenic rupture, and hematological abnormalities [1]; among the latter, the hemophagocytic lymphohistiocytosis (HLH) is particularly harmful because it is characterized by the massive production and release of inflammatory mediators caused by the uncontrolled activation of T-lymphocytes, NK-cells, and macrophages; the ensuing clinical picture resembles septic shock and can determine a multiple organ dysfunction syndrome (MODS) [2–4]. The HLH is increasingly recognized in patients admitted to the Intensive Care Units (ICU) due to different conditions including hematologic and solid tumors, autoimmune diseases, and bacterial and viral infections. [4–6]; as far IM-associated HLH is concerned, its occurrence has been ascribed to the persistence of the Epstein-Barr virus (EBV) in the tissues and the outcome is particularly poor [3].

Independently of the underlying triggering cause(s) the differential diagnosis of secondary HLH is difficult and relies mainly on a high index of suspicion and a number of hematological and biochemical criteria basically derived from those used in the pediatric form which is mostly caused by genetic abnormalities [7], making their use less useful in the acquired form (Table 1).

Here we describe the case of a patient who developed à rapidly evolving MODS a couple of months after the occurrence of an IM complicated by HLH.

2. Case Description

A 24-year-old woman was admitted to the Department of Infectious Disease with fever (T = 38,3°C) which was attributed to a relapse of a IM-HLH occurring about two months prior to the current hospitalization. At that time, the diagnosis of IM was confirmed by the presence of EBV DNA in the bloodstream and the diagnosis of HLH was suspected on the basis of the clinical findings such as persisting fever, the enlargement of the liver and the spleen as well as of blood abnormalities including pancytopenia, abnormally elevated values of ferritin (> 15.000 mcg/ml),

TABLE 1: Diagnostic criteria of HLH.

Molecular diagnosis consistent with HLH.
Or 5 of the following criteria
(1) Fever
(2) Splenomegaly
(3) Cytopenia affecting ≥ 2 lineages
(a) Hemoglobin < 9g / dl
(b) Platelets < 90.000 / ml
(c) Neutrophils < 1000 /ml
(4) Hypertrigliceridemia and/or hypofibrinogemia
(a) Triglycerides > 265 mg/dl
(b) Fibrinogen < 150 mg/dl
(5) Hemophagocytosis in bone marrow, spleen or nodes
(6) Low/absent NK cell activity
(7) Ferritin ≥ 500 mcg/ml
(8) sCD25 (sIL2R) ≥ 2400U/ml

triglycerides (789 mg/dl), and liver enzymes (AST 175 U/L, AST 120 U/L); a bone marrow biopsy confirmed the presence of hemophagocytosis and viral RNA in many cells by means of in situ hybridization (EBER) [7]; a genetic screening excluded the presence of gene mutations associated with HLH. During that hospitalization, she received steroids, etoposide, rituximab, cyclosporine, granulocyte-stimulating factor, and intravenous immunoglobulins (IvIg) and was ultimately discharged 38 days after the initial admission without viral DNA detectable in the bloodstream. During her stay at home, which lasted 3 weeks, the patient received prednisone, cyclosporine, trimethoprim-sulphametoxazole and acyclovir through a peripherally inserted central venous catheter (PICC). Thirty-six hours after the current admission during which rituximab was added to the ongoing treatment she was transferred to the ICU due to the deterioration of the consciousness, arterial hypotension, and fever. At the ICU admission, the patient presented high fever (40,5°C), disseminated intravascular coagulation, arterial hypotension, and acute kidney injury requiring renal replacement therapy (RRT): a methicillin-resistant *Staph. aureus* (MRSA) was isolated from the blood cultures and a septic shock-related MODS possibly in association with a cytokine storm caused by the HLH were hypothesized; the patient was intubated and mechanically ventilated and treated with IV vasopressors at incremental doses, IV vancomycin, meropenem, and caspofungin; the PICC was removed and replaced with a central venous catheter; as the patient remained unresponsive to the treatment, a Coupled Plasma Filtration and Adsorption treatment (CPFA, LYNDA®, Bellco, Mirandola, Italy) that aimed at removing the inflammatory mediators was added to the RTT along with the IV administration of IgM and IgA-enriched IvIg (Pentaglobin®, Biotest; Dreieich, Germany). Despite this increasingly aggressive approach, the MODS further worsened and the patient died 18 hours after the ICU admission.

At the autopsy, the liver and the spleen appeared enlarged, weighting 3110 g and 1230 g, respectively. Microscopically, the spleen showed lymphocyte depletion and the scattered necrosis of Malpighi's follicles (Figure 1(a)) combined with subversion of the general architecture due to a proliferation of T-lymphocytes (CD3+) with predominant expression of CD8 (Figure 1(b)). The lymphocyte population B (CD20+, PAX-5+) was virtually absent, while there was a significant increase in monocyte-macrophage component sometimes associated with hemophagocytosis. The EBER highlighted several lymphocytes with integrated EBV RNA in the nucleus (Figure 1(c)). The liver showed several perivascular infiltrates of polymorphic lymphocytes likewise those found in the spleen and many monocyte-macrophage cells (CD14+, CD64+). In the bone marrow there were multiple lymphocyte with polymorphic or abnormal nucleuses (Figure 2(a)) that appeared to be almost exclusively CD8+ T-lymphocytes (Figure 2(b)). Most of these cells were EBER positive (Figure 2(c)); B-lymphocytes (CD20+, PAX-5+) were almost absent while there was an expansion of the monocyte-macrophage series (CD14 +, CD64 +). The three hematopoietic lines appeared contracted but with preserved maturation. Mediastinal lymph nodes showed a diffuse proliferation of medium/large sized lymphoid elements, sometimes with single or multiple polymorphic nuclei (Figure 3(a)). The lymphocyte population was composed by CD3+ CD8+ T-lymphocytes with a limited presence of lymphocytes CD3+ CD4+ and absence of B cells (CD20 +, PAX-5 +).

3. Discussion

Different pathologic conditions, including macrophage activation syndrome (MAS), adult onset Still's disease (AOSD), catastrophic antiphospholipid syndrome (cAPS), and septic shock share a similar clinical presentation characterized by fever, arterial hypotension, and multisystem involvement due to the action of a number of inflammatory mediators [8]. This overlap of symptoms makes the diagnosis elusive and the appropriate approach can be delayed in the absence of other information. This difficulty is substantial because the treatments differ widely among the various clinical entities: as an example, in the AOSD, MAS, and CAPS, the administration of immunosuppressant agents is warranted [6, 9] but is strongly contraindicated in septic shock whose treatment is based on the prompt administration of large-spectrum antibiotics [10], which in many ICUs is combined with the administration of eIg and the use of blood purification techniques. This uncertainty can be particularly represented in hematological patients, in whom the onset of MODS can represent the final common pathway of different conditions, including immunosuppression-related sepsis, the cytokine release syndrome induced by novel cancer immunotherapies, and HLH [8, 11, 12]. Moreover, the proposed diagnostic criteria could not help in a critically ill patient, as none of them is sensible and sensitive enough and/or they are time-consuming: as an example, a recent study demonstrated the even extremely elevated blood ferritin levels were not predictive of LHL in adult patients [6]. Indeed, the described patient lied in the grey area in which an inappropriate approach means the difference between life and death. To overcome the risks associated with a wrong diagnosis and

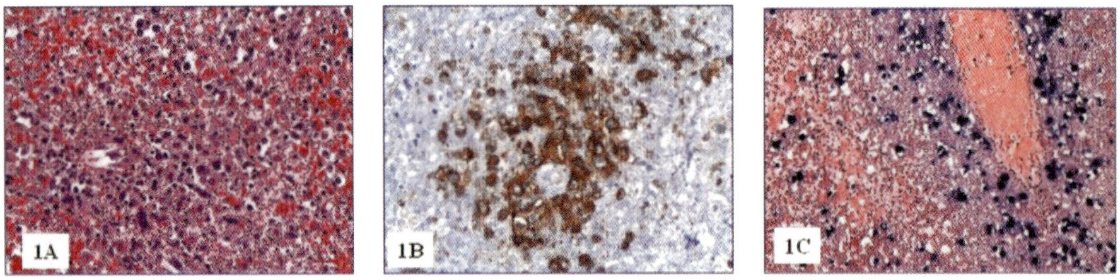

(a) (b) (c)

Figure 1: (a) Spleen tissue (H&E 200x); (b) CD8 positive spleen lymphocytes (200x); (c) spleen EBV positive cells (EBER, 200x).

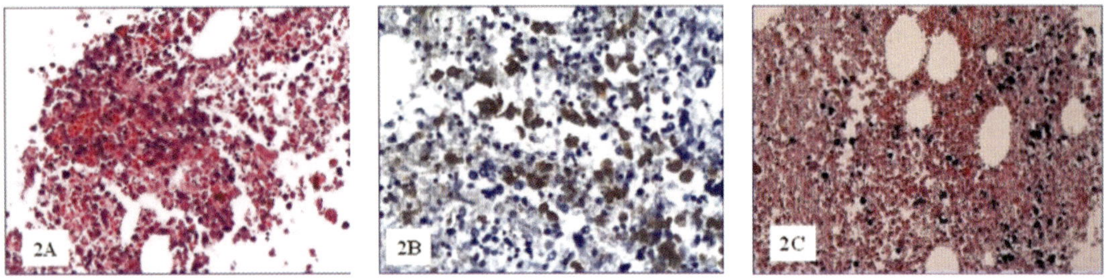

(a) (b) (c)

Figure 2: (a) Bone marrow pleomorphic lymphocytes (H&E 200x); (b) CD8 positive bone marrow lymphocytes (200x); (c) bone marrow EBV positive lymphocytes (EBER, 200x).

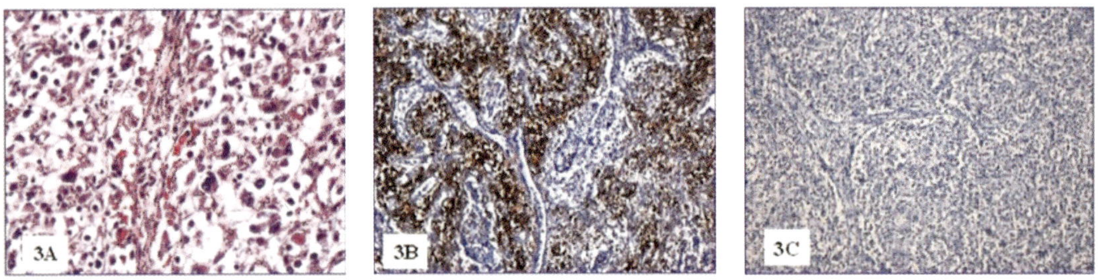

(a) (b) (c)

Figure 3: (a) Mediastinal lymph node (H&E 200x); (b) CD8 positive lymph node lymphocytes (200x); (c) PAX-5 negative lymph node lymphocytes (200x).

treatment we hypothesized that a septic shock was superimposed to a relapsed HLH and added to the already running therapies the CPFA aiming to remove the inflammatory mediators involved in both circumstances. Unfortunately, also this approach failed to modify the fulminant clinical course and the patient ultimately died. Moreover, it has been hypothesized an increased virulence and/or a reduced sensitivity to vancomycin in MRSA causing infections in patients with solid or hematologic malignancies [13].

The autoptical findings demonstrated that the septic shock occurred concomitantly with an aggressive lymphoma with multiorgan involvement; actually, it is likely that long-term treatment with immunosuppressant agents, albeit indicated for the treatment of the HLH, may have determined the evolution of the underlying chronic active EBV infection towards the aggressive T-cell lymphoma with systemic involvement. This is an extremely uncommon finding, as the tropism of EBV for B-lymphocyte has been associated with B-cells cancers, including Burkitt, Hodgkin, and diffuse large cell lymphomas [14, 15]; conversely EBV-positive T-cell lymphoma is exceedingly uncommon in western populations and has been attributed either to a possible antiapoptotic action exerted by the viral DNA hosted in the infected T-cells and/or to signals transmitted by some viral proteins such as Latent Membrane Protein 1 causing the continuous stimulation of members of the TNF receptors [2, 16]. Actually, it appears that in patients with EBV-related infections the chronic persistence of an elevated viral load represents a risk factor for HLH as well for other severe hematologic complications, including disseminated intravascular coagulation and lymphoma [2, 14]. In the described patient, however, viral DNA was absent at the discharge from the previous admission and this finding contrasts with the massive presence of EBV in all tissues demonstrated at the autopsy. It is likely that the immunosuppressant agents given to treat the HLH and to prevent its relapse acted as a double-edged sword: from one side they abated the hemophagocytosis, which was present only marginally at the post mortem examination of the bone marrow but from the other one triggered the reactivation of the EBV and the rapidly developing lymphoma.

4. Conclusions

The occurrence of EBV infection-associated HLH and the prevention of its relapse consists in the prolonged administration of immunosuppressant agents possibly associated with bone-marrow transplantation. Similar to other conditions associated with the decrease of the immune capabilities, this treatment exposes the patients to infectious complications, including viral reactivation and overwhelming bacterial infections. The occurrence of aggressive hematologic cancers is uncommon but must be kept into consideration in patients with HLH admitted with conditions resembling septic shock.

Authors' Contributions

All authors contributed equally to the preparation of the manuscript

References

[1] K. Luzuriaga and J. L. Sullivan, "Infectious mononucleosis," *The New England Journal of Medicine*, vol. 362, no. 21, pp. 1993–2000, 2010.

[2] K. Tawfik, Y. Liron, A. R. Ayman, R. Schneider, D. Wolf, and L. Ronen, "A heart breaking case of rapidly developing severe hemophagocytic syndrome secondary to chronic active EBV infection; a case report and review of the literature," *Journal of Clinical Virology*, vol. 67, pp. 14–16, 2015.

[3] S. Buyse, L. Teixeira, L. Galicier et al., "Critical care management of patients with hemophagocytic lymphohistiocytosis," *Intensive Care Medicine*, vol. 36, no. 10, pp. 1695–1702, 2010.

[4] G. E. Janka and K. Lehmberg, "Hemophagocytic syndromes—an update," *Blood Reviews*, vol. 28, no. 4, pp. 135–142, 2014.

[5] F. Gauvin, B. Toledano, J. Champagne, and J. Lacroix, "Reactive hemophagocytic syndrome presenting as a component of multiple organ dysfunction syndrome," *Critical Care Medicine*, vol. 28, no. 9, pp. 3341–3345, 2000.

[6] A. M. Schram and N. Berliner, "How I treat hemophagocytic lymphohistiocytosis in the adult patient," *Blood*, vol. 125, no. 19, pp. 2908–2914, 2015.

[7] N. Neparidze and J. Lacy, "Malignancies associated with Epstein-Barr virus: Pathobiology, clinical features and evolving treatments," *Clinical Advances in Hematology & Oncology*, vol. 6, pp. 358–371, 2014.

[8] C. Rosário, G. Zandman-Goddard, E. G. Meyron-Holtz, D. P. D'Cruz, and Y. Shoenfeld, "The hyperferritinemic syndrome: macrophage activation syndrome, Still's disease, septic shock and catastrophic antiphospholipid syndrome," *BMC Medicine*, vol. 11, article 185, 2013.

[9] M. B. Jordan, "Emergence of targeted therapy for hemophagocytic lymphohistiocytosis," *The Hematologist*, vol. 15, no. 2, 2018.

[10] A. Rhodes, L. E. Evans, W. Alhazzani et al., "Surviving sepsis campaign: international guidelines for management of sepsis and septic shock: 2016," *Intensive Care Medicine*, vol. 43, pp. 304–377, 2017.

[11] A. Shimabukuro-Vornhagen, P. Gödel, M. Subklewe et al., "Cytokine release syndrome," *Journal for ImmunoTherapy of Cancer*, vol. 6, article 56, 2018.

[12] E. Azoulay, F. Pène, M. Darmon et al., "Managing critically Ill hematology patients: time to think differently," *Blood Reviews*, vol. 29, no. 6, pp. 359–367, 2015.

[13] O. Blennow and P. Ljungman, "The challenge of antibiotic resistance in haematology patients," *British Journal of Haematology*, vol. 172, no. 4, pp. 497–511, 2016.

[14] S. A. Rezk and L. M. Weiss, "Epstein-Barr virus-associated lymphoproliferative disorders," *Human Pathology*, vol. 38, no. 9, pp. 1293–1304, 2007.

[15] K. Lehmberg and S. Ehl, "Diagnostic evaluation of patients with suspected haemophagocytic lymphohistiocytosis," *British Journal of Haematology*, vol. 160, no. 3, pp. 275–287, 2013.

[16] S. Park and Y. H. Ko, "Epstein-Barr virus-associated T/natural killer-cell lymphoproliferative disorders," *The Journal of Dermatology*, vol. 41, no. 1, pp. 29–39, 2014.

51

Cytokine Reduction in the Setting of an ARDS-Associated Inflammatory Response with Multiple Organ Failure

Karl Träger,[1] Christian Schütz,[1] Günther Fischer,[1] Janpeter Schröder,[1] Christian Skrabal,[2] Andreas Liebold,[2] and Helmut Reinelt[1]

[1]*Department of Cardiac Anesthesia, University Hospital Ulm, 89070 Ulm, Germany*
[2]*Clinic for Cardiothoracic and Vascular Surgery, University Hospital Ulm, 89070 Ulm, Germany*

Correspondence should be addressed to Karl Träger; karl.traeger@uni-ulm.de

Academic Editor: Zsolt Molnar

A 45-year-old male was admitted to our hospital with a small bowel obstruction due to torsion and was immediately scheduled for surgical intervention. At anesthesia induction, the patient aspirated and subsequently developed a severe SIRS with ARDS and multiple organ failure requiring the use of ECMO, CRRT, antibiotics, and low dose steroids. Due to a rapid deterioration in clinical status and a concurrent surge in inflammatory biomarkers, an extracorporeal cytokine adsorber (CytoSorb) was added to the CRRT blood circuit. The combined treatment resulted in a rapid and significant reduction in the levels of circulating inflammatory mediators. This decrease was paralleled by marked clinical stabilization of the patient including a significant improvement in hemodynamic stability and a reduced need for norepinephrine and improved respiratory function as measured by PaO_2/FIO_2, ventilator parameters, lung mechanics, and indirect measures of capillary leak syndrome. The patient could be discharged to a respiratory weaning unit where successful respiratory weaning could be achieved later on. We attribute the clinical improvement to the rapid control of the hyperinflammatory response and the reduction of inflammatory mediators using a combination of CytoSorb and these other therapies. CytoSorb treatment was safe and well tolerated, with no device-related adverse effects observed.

1. Introduction

Pulmonary aspiration of gastric or oropharyngeal fluid is a serious complication of general anesthesia that can lead to the development of acute respiratory distress syndrome (ARDS) in up to 30% of patients, the need for extracorporeal membrane oxygenation (ECMO), and the high risk of mortality [1]. Patients often develop a severe systemic inflammatory response syndrome (SIRS) that can lead to hemodynamic instability and multiple organ dysfunction syndrome (MODS), further complicating treatment [2]. A recently introduced extracorporeal cytokine hemoadsorption device called CytoSorb (CytoSorbents Corporation, USA) has gained interest in the field of critical care and cardiac surgery as a strategy to help control severe SIRS. Unlike metabolic approaches to anti-inflammation, CytoSorb is designed to directly capture and reduce mid-molecular weight inflammatory mediators (~10–60 kDa) in blood including both pro- and anti-inflammatory cytokines, chemokines, and bacterial exotoxins [3–5]. It works with standard hemodialysis or CRRT machines to purify blood extracorporeally. The technology is based on highly porous, biocompatible nonpolar polymer beads that are capable of capturing these inflammatory mediators from whole blood through size exclusion and nonspecific surface adsorption throughout the entire bead. The device is concentration dependent, reducing substances at high concentration efficiently, while having significantly less activity on substances at low concentration. This presumably is partially responsible for the observed reduction, but not complete elimination (which would be undesirable), of cytokines and other inflammatory mediators in patients treated with CytoSorb.

We herein report on a patient with an extreme SIRS response, cytokine storm, ARDS, and severe hemodynamic impairment following pulmonary aspiration during anesthesia induction, who was successfully treated with a combination of hemoadsorption with CytoSorb, ECMO, CRRT, antibiotics, and low dose steroids.

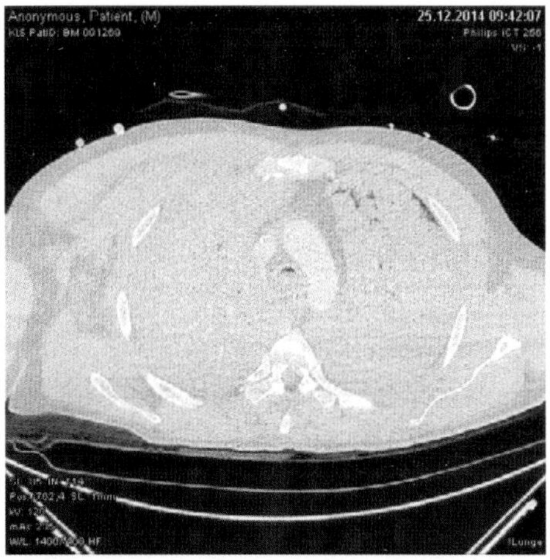

FIGURE 1: Lung computer tomography confirmed severe bilateral pulmonary consolidation with only minor residual ventilated lung areas.

2. Case Presentation

A 45-year-old male patient was admitted to our hospital with a small bowel obstruction due to torsion and was immediately scheduled for surgical intervention. Prior medical history included an anterior rectal resection requiring an enterostomy due to anastomotic insufficiency. At anesthesia induction, the patient aspirated and immediately underwent bronchoscopy which confirmed pulmonary aspiration. Laparotomy was performed and decompression of the small bowel was achieved. However, during the ongoing operation (4 hours in total), the patient developed progressive and severe respiratory failure (paO_2 48 mmHg, FIO_2 1,0, paO_2/FIO_2 ratio 48, and $paCO_2$ 75 mmHg, pH 7.09) despite mechanical ventilatory support. Therefore, the patient was switched to venovenous ECMO (VV-ECMO). However, four hours later, insufficient VV-ECMO flow and the rapid development of right ventricular failure necessitated a switch to central venoarterial ECMO (VA-ECMO). Sufficient ECMO flow was restored with an improvement in gas exchange (paO_2 83 mmHg, $paCO_2$ 38 mmHg, pH 7.39). Twelve hours after the start of VA-ECMO, lung computer tomography confirmed severe bilateral pulmonary consolidation (see Figure 1).

However, the patient's condition continued to worsen with clinical and functional signs of severe exudative ARDS with alveolar edema (paO_2 49 mmHg, $paCO_2$ 43 mmHg, and lung compliance <15 mL/cm H_2O), systemic vasoplegia (norepinephrine dose 0.31 μg/kg/min), and marked capillary leak syndrome (fluid balance + 4,080 mL after 12 hours in the ICU). In addition, the patient exhibited leukocytopenia (0.2 Giga/L), requiring the application of the granulocyte colony-stimulating factor analog filgrastim (Neupogen, Amgen) and acute kidney injury (AKIN Stage 3) necessitating continuous renal replacement therapy (CRRT-CVVHD, multiFiltrate, Fresenius Medical Care) [6]. At this time, the patient exhibited a massive increase in inflammatory biomarkers (IL-6 20,000 pg/mL, IL-8 24,656 pg/mL, and PCT > 100 μg/L). Microbiological findings of intraoperative abdominal swabs revealed *Klebsiella*, *E. coli*, and Enterococci, while material from the respiratory tract indicated growth of *E. coli* and *Candida*. Combined treatment with meropenem (primed continuous infusion), linezolid, and anidulafungin was initiated. Further treatment included bronchoscopy, continued VA-ECMO combined with protective ventilation, kinetic positioning using a Rotorest (KCI) bed, and application of the sepsis bundle including administration of low dose hydrocortisone.

Despite these interventions, the patient remained in septic shock and was in critical status with regard to vasoplegia, hemodynamics, and capillary leakage. On post-op Day 1, an extracorporeal cytokine hemoadsorption cartridge (CytoSorb, CytoSorbents Corp., USA) was added in series to the CRRT system (Fresenius multiFiltrate) in a predialyzer position. During CytoSorb treatment, antibiotics were administered routinely as follows: meropenem 500 mg bolus followed by infusion of 1.45 mg/kg/h, anidulafungin prolonged infusion at 200 mg per day, and linezolid prolonged infusion 600 mg twice a day. A total of three treatments with a combination of CytoSorb and CRRT were consecutively performed for a total of 85 hours (20 hours + 35 hours + 29 hours) at a blood flow rate of 100–140 mL/min. Regional anticoagulation was achieved using a citrate-based protocol. Of note, the first treatment was interrupted for 4.5 hours due to a thoracic CT scan and surgical revision in order to reposition the arterial ECMO cannula to improve blood flow. When treatment was paused, the blood circuit was flushed with saline and was then later safely restarted. Following the addition of CytoSorb, a pronounced decrease in the concentrations of IL-6 and IL-8 was observed which continued to decrease further in the following days (see Figure 2). As shown in Figure 2, when the patient was on CRRT and VA-ECMO alone on Day 0, prior to CytoSorb usage, there was no change in the plasma levels of either IL-6 and IL-8. This cytokine reduction was associated temporally with a stabilization of clinical parameters. The patient stabilized hemodynamically under continued CytoSorb, VA-ECMO, and CRRT treatment, and the need for norepinephrine was significantly reduced (Figure 3). In addition, respiratory function improved during the treatment course, with a disappearance of any signs of alveolar exudation as confirmed by daily bronchoscopy. In parallel, the severity of capillary leakage as demonstrated by daily fluid needs and daily fluid balance became less apparent (Figure 4).

At postoperative Day 12, therapy was started with methylprednisolone following the Meduri protocol, in order to inhibit fibroproliferation in the lung and risk of fibrosis during ARDS [7]. Gradual additional improvements in lung recruitment and alveolar ventilation were observed. A percutaneous tracheostomy was performed on Day 13. By postoperative Day 18, the patient's respiratory function, along with gas exchange and lung mechanics, on mechanical ventilation had sufficiently improved such that VA-ECMO was discontinued. CRRT had to be continued for a period of 20 days and could then be stopped after sufficient recovery of renal function.

On Day 27, the patient was transferred to a respiratory weaning unit where the patient was subsequently successfully

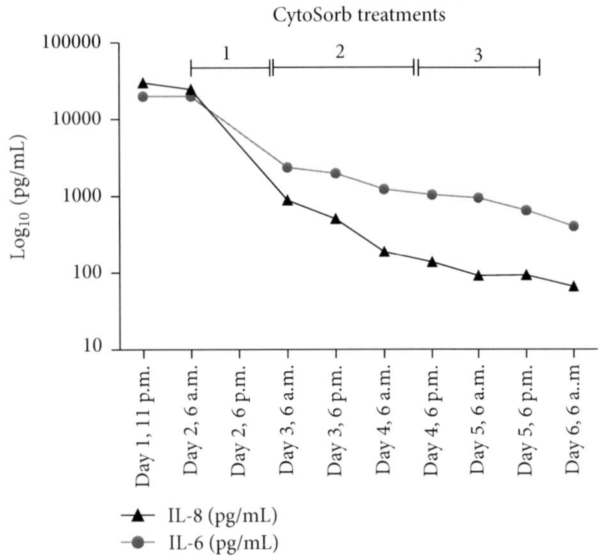

FIGURE 2: Course of IL-6 and IL-8 throughout the three treatments with the CytoSorb hemoadsorption device. Note that the y-axis is depicted in log 10 scale.

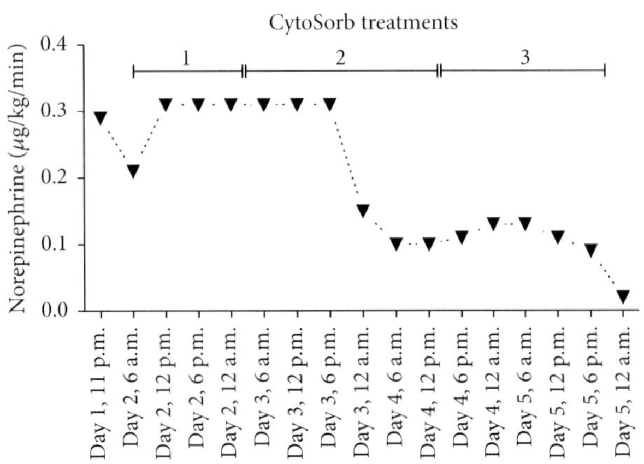

FIGURE 3: Need for norepinephrine throughout the treatment period.

weaned off mechanical ventilation, with a discontinuation of CRRT and the recovery of renal function.

Informed consent to use clinical data for scientific purposes was obtained from the patient's legal caregiver.

3. Discussion

This case report highlights the stabilization and successful treatment of a complicated pulmonary aspiration postsurgical patient with septic shock and polymicrobial infection, severe exudative ARDS, renal failure, and a severe SIRS response with pronounced hypercytokinemia. Treatment encompassed a combination of cytokine reduction and inflammation reduction with CytoSorb, extracorporeal oxygenation and support with VA-ECMO, renal support with CRRT, low dose hydrocortisone treatment per sepsis bundle guidelines, and infection source control with broad

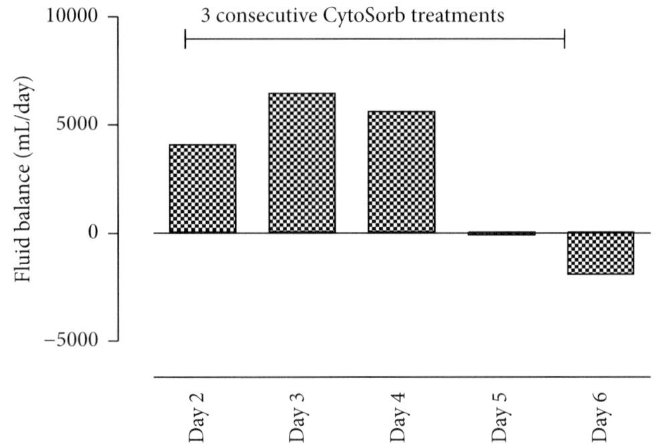

FIGURE 4: Fluid balance during the three consecutive CytoSorb treatments.

spectrum antibiotics. Underlying the multiple organ failure was a severe SIRS/sepsis response, despite initial leukopenia, with extremely high levels of IL-6 (20,000 pg/mL) and IL-8 (24,656 pg/mL), exudative alveolar edema, systemic vasoplegia, and marked capillary leak syndrome. The use of a CytoSorb cytokine adsorber with this multipronged therapeutic approach resulted in a profound decrease in plasma concentrations of both IL-6 and IL-8, both classic inflammatory mediators. This reduction was paralleled by a significant clinical stabilization of the patient during the course of the combined treatment. Importantly, the treatment bundle was able to reverse the systemic vasoplegia and hemodynamic collapse, which is unlikely to be fully explained by the limited circulatory support of central VA-ECMO. In addition, the combined treatment reversed the highly exudative phase of ARDS, as demonstrated by bronchoscopy, and appeared to decrease capillary leak syndrome and alveolar fluid accumulation, as evidenced by improved respiratory function, a significantly reduced need for fluid resuscitation, and achievement of a negative fluid balance shortly after therapy initiation. Although a causal relationship cannot be proven, we presume that controlling the excessive inflammatory response helped to stabilize the patient. These observations are in line with a number of recently published case reports using CytoSorb in septic patients, correlating the positive effects of cytokine adsorption on inflammation, hemodynamics, and organ recovery [3, 4].

More randomized controlled studies using CytoSorb in critically ill patients will help to establish the true benefit of the therapy. Certainly, this case report that uses multiple interventions to treat this complex patient prevents us from ascribing the patient's positive outcome to any one treatment modality. In addition, cytokine levels could have gradually decreased on their own due to the use of antibiotics (e.g., improved source control reduces stimulation of the immune response), as was observed in the largest community acquired pneumonia and sepsis study (GenIMS) [2], or low dose hydrocortisone (administered here according to sepsis bundle guidelines) which has been previously associated with reduced concentrations of IL-6 and diminished *de novo* production of several interleukins [8]. We would note, however, that none of these approaches are mutually exclusive. In fact, they may all be synergistic with each other and may be needed to achieve the elusive improvements in mortality that no single sepsis treatment has yet been able to demonstrate or maintain.

In conclusion, we believe that control over the patient's initial hyperinflammatory response was a key element in helping clinically stabilize the patient, allowing for organ recovery and ultimately survival. In this very challenging clinical case, we used all of the tools available to us to do so, including CytoSorb cytokine adsorption, CVVH, VA-ECMO, antibiotics, and steroids. CytoSorb is the newest therapy in our toolkit and was safe and well tolerated with no device-related adverse events and easy to implement as part of the CVVH circuit. Based upon our positive clinical experience with CytoSorb as an adjunctive therapy to standard of care therapy for critical illnesses to date, we look forward to future systematic clinical trials that will clarify its contribution and potential in the treatment of severe sepsis and septic shock.

References

[1] O. Bartusch, M. Finkl, and U. Jaschinski, "Aspiration syndrome: epidemiology, pathophysiology, and therapy," *Anaesthesist*, vol. 57, no. 5, pp. 519–532, 2008.

[2] J. A. Kellum, L. Kong, M. P. Fink et al., "Understanding the inflammatory cytokine response in pneumonia and sepsis: results of the Genetic and Inflammatory Markers of Sepsis (GenIMS) study," *Archives of Internal Medicine*, vol. 167, no. 15, pp. 1655–1663, 2007.

[3] S. R. Mitzner, M. Gloger, J. Henschel, and S. Koball, "Improvement of hemodynamic and inflammatory parameters by combined hemoadsorption and hemodiafiltration in septic shock: a case report," *Blood Purification*, vol. 35, no. 4, pp. 314–315, 2013.

[4] F. Bruenger, L. Kizner, J. Weile, M. Morshuis, and J. F. Gummert, "First successful combination of ECMO with cytokine removal therapy in cardiogenic septic shock: a case report," *The International Journal of Artificial Organs*, vol. 38, no. 2, pp. 113–116, 2015.

[5] F. Born, M. Pichlmair, S. Peterß, N. Khaladj, and C. Hagl, "Systemic inflammatory response syndrome in der herzchirurgie: neue therapiemöglichkeiten durch den einsatz eines cytokin-adsorbers während EKZ?" *Kardiotechnik*, no. 2, pp. 41–46, 2014.

[6] R. L. Mehta, J. A. Kellum, S. V. Shah et al., "Acute Kidney Injury Network: report of an initiative to improve outcomes in acute kidney injury," *Critical Care*, vol. 11, no. 2, article R31, 2007.

[7] G. U. Meduri, E. A. Tolley, G. P. Chrousos, and F. Stentz, "Prolonged methylprednisolone treatment suppresses systemic inflammation in patients with unresolving acute respiratory distress syndrome: evidence for inadequate endogenous glucocorticoid secretion and inflammation-induced immune cell resistance to glucocorticoids," *American Journal of Respiratory and Critical Care Medicine*, vol. 165, no. 7, pp. 983–991, 2002.

[8] M. Oppert, R. Schindler, C. Husung et al., "Low-dose hydrocortisone improves shock reversal and reduces cytokine levels in early hyperdynamic septic shock," *Critical Care Medicine*, vol. 33, no. 11, pp. 2457–2464, 2005.

Permissions

All chapters in this book were first published in CRCC, by Hindawi Publishing Corporation; hereby published with permission under the Creative Commons Attribution License or equivalent. Every chapter published in this book has been scrutinized by our experts. Their significance has been extensively debated. The topics covered herein carry significant findings which will fuel the growth of the discipline. They may even be implemented as practical applications or may be referred to as a beginning point for another development.

The contributors of this book come from diverse backgrounds, making this book a truly international effort. This book will bring forth new frontiers with its revolutionizing research information and detailed analysis of the nascent developments around the world.

We would like to thank all the contributing authors for lending their expertise to make the book truly unique. They have played a crucial role in the development of this book. Without their invaluable contributions this book wouldn't have been possible. They have made vital efforts to compile up to date information on the varied aspects of this subject to make this book a valuable addition to the collection of many professionals and students.

This book was conceptualized with the vision of imparting up-to-date information and advanced data in this field. To ensure the same, a matchless editorial board was set up. Every individual on the board went through rigorous rounds of assessment to prove their worth. After which they invested a large part of their time researching and compiling the most relevant data for our readers.

The editorial board has been involved in producing this book since its inception. They have spent rigorous hours researching and exploring the diverse topics which have resulted in the successful publishing of this book. They have passed on their knowledge of decades through this book. To expedite this challenging task, the publisher supported the team at every step. A small team of assistant editors was also appointed to further simplify the editing procedure and attain best results for the readers.

Apart from the editorial board, the designing team has also invested a significant amount of their time in understanding the subject and creating the most relevant covers. They scrutinized every image to scout for the most suitable representation of the subject and create an appropriate cover for the book.

The publishing team has been an ardent support to the editorial, designing and production team. Their endless efforts to recruit the best for this project, has resulted in the accomplishment of this book. They are a veteran in the field of academics and their pool of knowledge is as vast as their experience in printing. Their expertise and guidance has proved useful at every step. Their uncompromising quality standards have made this book an exceptional effort. Their encouragement from time to time has been an inspiration for everyone.

The publisher and the editorial board hope that this book will prove to be a valuable piece of knowledge for researchers, students, practitioners and scholars across the globe.

List of Contributors

Mohsin Ijaz and Dmitry Lvovsky
Division of Pulmonary and Critical Care Medicine, Department of Medicine, Bronx Lebanon Hospital Center, 1650 Selwyn Avenue, Suit No. 12 F, Bronx, NY 10457, USA

Hassan Tariq
Department of Medicine, Bronx Lebanon Hospital Center, 1650 Selwyn Avenue, Suit No. 10 C, Bronx, NY 10457, USA

Masooma Niazi
Department of Pathology, Bronx LebanonHospital Center, 1650 Selwyn Avenue, SuitNo. 10 C, Bronx, NY 10457, USA

Jerrold L. Perrott
Departments of Pharmacy and Critical Care, Royal Columbian Hospital, New Westminster, BC, Canada
Faculty of Pharmaceutical Sciences, University of British Columbia, Vancouver, BC, Canada

Michelle T. Co
Department of Pharmacy, Ridge Meadows Hospital, Maple Ridge, BC, Canada

Steven C. Reynolds
Department of Critical Care, Royal Columbian Hospital, New Westminster, BC, Canada
Department of Medicine, University of British Columbia, Vancouver, BC, Canada

Derek J. R. Gunning
Departments of Cardiac Surgery and Critical Care, Royal Columbian Hospital, New Westminster, BC, Canada

Mohsin Ijaz
Division of Critical Care Medicine, Montefiore Medical Center, Albert Einstein College of Medicine, Bronx, NY 10467, USA

Arsalan Rafiq
Division of Cardiology, Mount Sinai St. Luke'sHospital, New York, NY 10025, USA

Sindhaghatta Venkatram and Gilda Diaz-Fuentes
Division of Pulmonary and Critical Care Medicine, Bronx-Lebanon Hospital Center, Bronx, NY 10457, USA

Sam Ghali, Keith Lewis, Viviane Kazan, Neezam Altorok, Jamil Taji, Mohammad Taleb, Kiranmayee Lanka and Ragheb Assaly
The University of Toledo Medical Center, Toledo, OH 43614, USA

Muhammad S. Khan
Department of Medicine, University of Oklahoma Health Sciences Center,Williams Pavilion 1130, Oklahoma City, OK 73190, USA

Muhammad K. Ishaq and Kellie R. Jones
Department of Pulmonary and Critical Care Medicine, University of Oklahoma Health Sciences Center,Williams Pavilion 1130, Oklahoma City, OK 73190, USA

Eduardo Martinez, Sindhaghatta Venkatram and Gilda Diaz-Fuentes
Division of Pulmonary and Critical Care Medicine, Bronx Lebanon Hospital Center, Bronx, NY 10457, USA
Albert Einstein College of Medicine, Bronx, NY 10461, USA

Raza Alvi
Albert Einstein College of Medicine, Bronx, NY 10461, USA
Department of Internal Medicine, Bronx Lebanon Hospital Center, Bronx, NY 10457, USA

Saptarshi Biswas, Catherine Price and Sunil Abrol
Brookdale University Hospital and Medical Center, 1 Brookdale Plaza, Brooklyn, NY 11212, USA

F. A. Zeiler, J. Silvaggio, A. M. Kaufmann and M.West
Section of Neurosurgery, University of Manitoba, GB-1 820 Sherbrook Street, Winnipeg, MB, Canada R3A 1R9

L. M. Gillman
Section of Critical Care, Department of Medicine, University of Manitoba, RoomGC425, 820 Sherbrook Street, Winnipeg, MB, Canada R3T 2N2

Filipa Pereira and Paula Sá
Serviço de Anestesiologia, Centro Hospitalar do Porto, Largo Professor Abel Salazar, 4099-001 Porto, Portugal

Teresa Cardoso
Unidade de Cuidados Intensivos Polivalente, Centro Hospitalar do Porto, Largo Professor Abel Salazar, 4099-001 Porto, Portugal

Michael Gale and Thierry Mallet
Division of Cardiology, Department of Medicine,Woodhull Medical Center, 760 Broadway, Suite 3B320, Brooklyn, NY 11206, USA

Brooks Mirrer and Ronny Cohen
Division of Cardiology, Department of Medicine,Woodhull Medical Center, 760 Broadway, Suite 3B320, Brooklyn, NY 11206, USA
NYU School of Medicine, 550 First Avenue, New York, NY 10016, USA

Pablo Loarte
Department of Medicine, Yale-New Haven Hospital, 20 York Street, CB2041, New Haven, CT 06510, USA

Louis Salciccioli
Division of Cardiology, Department of Medicine, SUNY DownstateMedical Center, 450 Clarkson Avenue, Brooklyn, NY 11203, USA

Alison Petrie
Saint George's University School of Medicine, 3500 Sunrise Highway, Great River, NY 11739, USA

Michael Barrie
Department of Emergency Medicine, The Ohio State University Wexner Medical Center, Columbus, OH 43210, USA

Lucas McKnight
Department of Internal Medicine and Department of Pediatrics, The Ohio State University Wexner Medical Center, Columbus, OH 43210, USA

Pallavi Solanki
Division of Cardiovascular Medicine, Department of Internal Medicine and The Dorothy M. Davis Heart and Lung Research Institute, The Ohio State University Wexner Medical Center, Columbus, OH 43210, USA

Mark D. Salter
TheUniversity of Sydney, NSW2006, Australia
Emergency Medicine Department, Nepean Hospital, Penrith, NSW 2751, Australia

Yu-Jin Lee
Department of Human Biology, Stanford University, Stanford, CA 94305, USA

D. Scott Smith
Department of Infectious Disease and Geographic Medicine, Kaiser Permanente, Redwood City, CA 94063, USA

Vivek A. Rao and Alexander C. Flint
Department of Neuroscience, Kaiser Permanente, Redwood City, CA 94063, USA

Robert D. Siegel
Department of Microbiology and Immunology, Stanford University, Stanford, CA 94305, USA

Jon Kosek
Department of Pathology, Veterans Affairs Palo Alto Health Care System, Palo Alto, CA 94304, USA

Carol A. Glaser
Center for Infectious Diseases, California Department of Public Health, Richmond, CA 94804, USA

R. Cornejo, D. Ugalde, O. Llanos, P. Bisbal, L. De la Barrera, C. Romero, R. Neira and Roberto González
Unidad de Pacientes Críticos, Departamento de Medicina, Hospital Clínico, Universidad de Chile, Chile

J. Gajardo
Unidad de Pacientes Cr´ıticos, Complejo Asistencial Hospital Barros Luco Trudeau, Chile

Saptarshi Biswas, Sujana Dontukurthy, Mathew G. Rosenzweig, Ravi Kothuru and Sunil Abrol
Department of General Surgery, Brookdale University Hospital Medical Center, Brooklyn, NY 11212, USA

Daniel L. Roberts
Division of Hospital Internal Medicine, Department of Medicine, Mayo Clinic, Phoenix, AZ 85054, USA

David A. Galbreath
Kansas City Family Medical Clinic, Kansas City, MO 64114, USA

Bhavesh M. Patel
Department of Critical Care Medicine, Mayo Clinic, Phoenix, AZ 85054, USA

Timothy J. Ingall
Department of Neurology, Mayo Clinic, Phoenix, AZ 85054, USA

Amer Khatib
Division of Gastroenterology, Faculty of Medicine, University of Jordan, Amman 11942, Jordan

Daniel J. Johnson
Department of Surgery, Mayo Clinic, Phoenix, AZ 85054, USA

Kenneth R. Hoffman and Sean W. Chan
Intensive Care Unit, Canberra Hospital, Yamba Drive, Canberra, ACT 2605, Australia

Andrew R. Hughes
Neurology Department, Canberra Hospital, Yamba Drive, Canberra, ACT 2605, Australia

Stephen J. Halcrow
Neurosurgical Unit, Canberra Hospital, Yamba Drive, Canberra, ACT 2605, Australia

Aditya Shah and Sorabh Kothari
University of Illinois at Chicago, Chicago, IL, USA
Advocate Christ Medical Center, Oak Lawn, IL, USA

Samir Patel and Jennifer Denk
Advocate Christ Medical Center, Oak Lawn, IL, USA

J. Scott Baird
Department of Pediatrics, Division of Critical Care Medicine, Columbia University, New York, NY, USA

N. Houari, S. Touzani, A. El Bouazzaoui, B. Boukatta and N. Kanjaa
Anesthesiology and Intensive Care Unit A4, Hassan II University Hospital, Fez, Morocco

H. Salhi and H. El Ouahabi
Endocrinology Department, Hassan II University Hospital, Fez, Morocco

M.-Y. Alaoui Lamrani and M. Maâroufi
Imaging and Interventional Radiology Department, Hassan II University Hospital, Fez, Morocco

K. Ibnmajdoub and K. Maazaz
Visceral Surgery Department, Hassan II University Hospital, Fez, Morocco

Asma Abu-Abed Abdin
Jordan University for Science and Technology, Irbid 22110, Jordan

Muhammad Hamza
Department of Medicine, Dow Medical College, Baba-E-Urdu Road, Karachi 74200, Pakistan

Muhammad S. Khan and Awab Ahmed
Section of Pulmonary and Critical Care Medicine, University of Oklahoma Health Sciences Center, 920 Stanton L Young Boulevard, Oklahoma City, OK 73104, USA

Nupur Sinha, Sindhaghatta Venkatram and Gilda Diaz-Fuentes
Division of Pulmonary and Critical Care Medicine, Bronx Lebanon Hospital Center and Albert Einstein College of Medicine, Bronx, NY 10457, USA

Nao Umei and Shingo Ichiba
Department of Surgical Intensive Care Medicine, Nippon Medical School Hospital, Tokyo, Japan

Vivek Alaigh
Department of Medicine, University of CT Health Center, 263 Farmington Avenue, Farmington, CT 06030, USA

Debapriya Datta
Division of Pulmonary-Critical Care Medicine, University of CT Health Center, Farmington, CT 06030, USA

Giorgio Berlot, Adriano Rinaldi, Marco Moscheni, Massimo Ferluga and Perla Rossini
Anesthesia and Intensive CareDepartment, Cattinara Hospital, Azienda Sanitaria Universitaria Integrata di Trieste, University of Trieste, Strada di Fiume 447, 34149 Trieste, Italy

Bashar Alzghoul and Ayoub Innabi
Department of Internal Medicine, University of Arkansas for Medical Sciences, Little Rock, AR, USA

Aditya Chada, Ahmad R. Tarawneh, Krishna Kakkera and Khaled Khasawneh
Division of Pulmonary and Critical Care Medicine, University of Arkansas for Medical Sciences, Little Rock, AR, USA

Leonardo Cordeiro de Souza
Medical Science Post-Graduation Program, Universidade Federal Fluminense, Niterói, RJ, Brazil
Intensive Care Division, Hospital e Clínica São Gonc¸alo, São Gonçalo, RJ, Brazil

Josué Felipe Campos, Leandro Possidente Daher, Priscila Furtado da Silva, Alex Ventura, Pollyana Zamborlini do Prado, Daniele Brasil and Debora Mendonça
Intensive Care Division, Hospital e Clínica São Gonc¸alo, São Gonçalo, RJ, Brazil

Jocemir Ronaldo Lugon
Nephrology Division, Department of Medicine, Medical School, Universidade Federal Fluminense, Niterói, RJ, Brazil

Jacob R. Miller, Muhammad F. Masood, Keki R. Balsara and Akinobu Itoh
Division of Cardiothoracic Surgery,Washington University, St. Louis, MO, USA

Warren Isakow and Patrick Aguilar
Division of Pulmonary Critical Care,Washington University, St. Louis, MO, USA

Kristen M. Sanfilippo
Division of Hematology,Washington University, St. Louis, MO, USA

Dovile Leonaviciute
Department of Anaesthesiology and Intensive Care Medicine, Aalborg University Hospital, Aalborg, Denmark

Bodil S. Rasmussen
Department of Anaesthesiology and Intensive Care Medicine, Aalborg University Hospital, Aalborg, Denmark
Department of Clinical Medicine, Aalborg University, Aalborg, Denmark

Bo Madsen and Niels H. Buus
Department of Nephrology, Aalborg University Hospital, Aalborg, Denmark

Anne Schmedes
Department of Biochemistry and Immunology, Lillebaelt Hospital, Vejle, Denmark

Megan E. Kunka, Elizabeth A. Cady and Melissa L. Thompson Bastin
University of Kentucky HealthCare, 800 Rose Street, H110, Lexington, KY 40536, USA

Heejung C. Woo
University of Kentucky, Lexington, KY 40506, USA

Shilpa Desai, Luke Torre, Jason Seet and Emma Osnain
Sir Charles Gairdner Hospital, Nedlands, WA, Australia

Matthew Anstey and Bradley Wibrow
Sir Charles Gairdner Hospital, Nedlands, WA, Australia
School of Medicine, University of Western Australia, Crawley, WA, Australia

Máximo H. Trujillo and Carlos Fragachán G.
Critical Care Department, ICU, Instituto M´edico La Floresta (IMLF), Caracas 1060, Venezuela
Critical Care Department, University Hospital of Caracas, Caracas 1050, Venezuela

Stephanie Cull and Gebran Khneizer
Department of Internal Medicine, Saint Louis University School of Medicine, St. Louis, MO, USA

Zafar Jamkhana
Department of Internal Medicine, Saint Louis University School of Medicine, St. Louis, MO, USA
Division of Pulmonary, Critical Care and Sleep Medicine, Saint Louis University School of Medicine, St. Louis, MO, USA

Abhishek Krishna
Division of Pulmonary, Critical Care and Sleep Medicine, Saint Louis University School of Medicine, St. Louis, MO, USA

Razi Muzaffar and Sameer Gadani
Radiology Department, Saint Louis University, St. Louis, MO, USA

FlorentMoriceau, Johanne Prothet, Mathieu Page, Charles-Eric Ber and Jullien Crozon
Département d'Anesthésie-Réanimation, Hôpital Edouard Herriot, 5 place d'Arsonval, 69003 Lyon, France

Thomas Rimmelé
Département d'Anesthésie-Réanimation, Hôpital Edouard Herriot, 5 place d'Arsonval, 69003 Lyon, France
Université Claude Bernard Lyon 1, 43 Boulevard du 11 Novembre 1918, 69100 Villeurbanne, France

Benjamin J. Blaise
Département de Néonatologie et de Réanimation Néonatale, Hôpital Femme Mére Enfant, 32 Avenue Doyen Jean Lépine, 69500 Bron, France

Benoit Ben Said
Département d'Allergologie et d'Immunologie Clinique, Centre Hospitalier de Lyon-Sud, 165 Chemin du Grand Revoyet, 69310 Pierre-Bénite, France

Claudine A. Blum, Daniel Schneeberger, Matthias Lang, Marc Philippe Michot and Beat Müller
Medical University Clinic, Kantonsspital Aarau, Aarau, Switzerland

Janko Rakic
Medical University Clinic, Kantonsspital Aarau, Aarau, Switzerland
Department of Pneumology, Medical Clinic, Kantonsspital Baden, Baden, Switzerland

O'Dene Lewis Samina Afreen, Supo Folaranmi Marie Fidelia-Lambert Vishal Poddar and Alicia Thomas
Howard University Hospital, 2041 Georgia Ave. NW, Washington, DC 20060, USA

R. Singh, E. Arain, A. Buth, J. Kado, A. Soubani and N. Imran
Detroit Medical Center/Wayne State University, Detroit, MI, USA

Muhammad S. Khan and Ahmed Awab
Section of Pulmonary and Critical Care Medicine, University of Oklahoma Health Sciences Center, No.WP1310, 920 Stanton L Young Boulevard, Oklahoma City, OK 73117, USA

Najmi Shahbaz, Muhammad Hamza and Henna Iqbal
Dow University of Health Sciences, Mission Road, Karachi 74200, Pakistan

Hassaan A. Zia
Department of Internal Medicine, University of Oklahoma Health Sciences Center, No.WP1310, 920 Stanton L Young Boulevard, Oklahoma City, OK 73117, USA

John R. Woytanowski and Nausheen Hakim
Department of Internal Medicine, Drexel University College of Medicine, Philadelphia, PA, USA

Caytlin Deering and Sara Schultz
Department of Infectious Disease and HIV Medicine, Drexel University College of Medicine, Philadelphia, PA, USA

Pragya Punj, Prem kumar Nattanmai and Christopher R. Newey
Department of Neurology, University of Missouri, 5 Hospital Drive, CE 540, Columbia, MO 65211, USA

Pravin George
Cleveland Clinic, Cerebrovascular Center, Neurological Institute, 9500 Euclid Avenue, Cleveland, OH 44195-5245, USA

Sara E. Parli and Melissa L. Thompson Bastin
Department of Pharmacy Services, University of Kentucky HealthCare, Lexington, KY 40536, USA
Department of Pharmacy Practice and Science, University of Kentucky College of Pharmacy, Lexington, KY 40536, USA

Daniel A. Lewis
Department of Pharmacy Services, South Pointe Hospital, Cleveland Clinic, Cleveland, OH 44195, USA

Kenichi Nitta, Hiroshi Imamura, Akihiro Yashio, Satoko Kashima and Katsunori Mochizuki
Department of Emergency and Critical Care Medicine, Shinshu University School of Medicine, Nagano, Japan

Samantha Mc Kenzie Stancu
"Carol Davila" University of Medicine and Pharmacy Bucharest, 37 Dionisie Lupu Street, District 1, 020021 Bucharest, Romania

Catalin Gabriel Cirstoveanu
"Carol Davila" University of Medicine and Pharmacy Bucharest, 37 Dionisie Lupu Street, District 1, 020021 Bucharest, Romania
"Marie S. Curie Children's Emergency Hospital" Bucharest, Neonatal Intensive Care Unit, 20 Constantin Brancoveanu Street, District 4, 041451 Bucharest, Romania

Ileana Barascu
"Marie S. Curie Children's Emergency Hospital" Bucharest, Neonatal Intensive Care Unit, 20 Constantin Brancoveanu Street, District 4, 041451 Bucharest, Romania

Alessandro Ghiani, Konstantinos Tsitouras and Claus Neurohr
Schillerhoehe Lung Clinic (Robert-Bosch Hospital), Department of Pneumology and Critical Care Medicine, Solitudestr. 18, 70839 Gerlingen, Germany

Matthias Hansen
Schillerhoehe Lung Clinic (Robert-Bosch Hospital), Department of Anesthesiology and Critical Care Medicine, Solitudestr. 18, 70839 Gerlingen, Germany

Amit Bharara, Catherine Grossman, Daniel Grinnan, Aamer Syed, Bernard Fisher, Christine DeWilde, Ramesh Natarajan and Alpha A. (Berry) Fowler
Division of Pulmonary Disease and Critical Care Medicine, Department of Internal Medicine,The VCU Johnson Center for Critical Care and Pulmonary Research, Virginia Commonwealth University School of Medicine, Richmond, VA, USA

László Rudas, Péter Hankovszky, András Lovas, Éva Zöllei and Zsolt Molnár
Department of Anesthesiology and Intensive Care, Faculty of Medicine, University of Szeged, Szeged, Hungary

Keevan Singh
Anaesthesia and Intensive Care Department, San Fernando General Hospital and Department of Clinical Surgical Sciences, University of the West Indies, San Fernando, Trinidad, Trinidad and Tobago

Saara Hyatali, Kevin Singh and Neil Bhagwandass
Internal Medicine Department, San Fernando General Hospital, San Fernando, Trinidad and Tobago

Stanley Giddings
Infectious Disease Unit, San Fernando General Hospital and Department of Clinical Medical Sciences, University of the West Indies, San Fernando, Trinidad, Trinidad and Tobago

Giorgio Berlot
University of Trieste, Dept. of Anesthesia and Intensive Care, Cattinara Hospital, Strada di Fiume 447, 34149 Trieste, Italy

Rossana Bussani and Vennus Shafiei
University of Trieste, Dept. of Pathology, Cattinara Hospital, Strada di Fiume 447, 34149 Trieste, Italy

Nadia Zarrillo
Caserta Hospital, Dept. of Anesthesia and Intensive Care, Via Ferdinando Palasciano, 81100 Caserta, Italy

Munenori Kusunoki, Takeshi Umegaki, Tomohiro Shoji,Kota Nishimoto, Natsuki Anada, Akiko Ando, Takeo Uba, Kanako Oku, Saya Hakata, Satoshi Hagihira and Takahiko Kamibayashi
Department of Anesthesiology, Kansai Medical University Hospital, Osaka, Japan

Giorgio Berlot and Ariella Tomasini
University of Trieste, Department of Anesthesia and Intensive Care, Cattinara Hospital, 447, 34149, Trieste, Italy

Lorenzo Zandonà Eugenio Leonardo and Rossana Bussani
University of Trieste, Department of Pathology, Cattinara Hospital, 447, 34149, Trieste, Italy

Nadia Zarrillo
Caserta Hospital, Department of Anesthesia and Intensive Care, Italy

Karl Träger, Christian Schütz, Günther Fischer, Janpeter Schröder and Helmut Reinelt
Department of Cardiac Anesthesia, University Hospital Ulm, 89070 Ulm, Germany

Christian Skrabal and Andreas Liebold
Clinic for Cardiothoracic and Vascular Surgery, University Hospital Ulm, 89070 Ulm, Germany

Index

R

S

T

U

V